Atlas of
Ear, Nose and Throat Pathology

Current Histopathology

Consultant Editor
Professor G. Austin Gresham, TD, ScD, MD, FRCPath.
Professor of Morbid Anatomy and Histology, University of Cambridge

Volume Sixteen

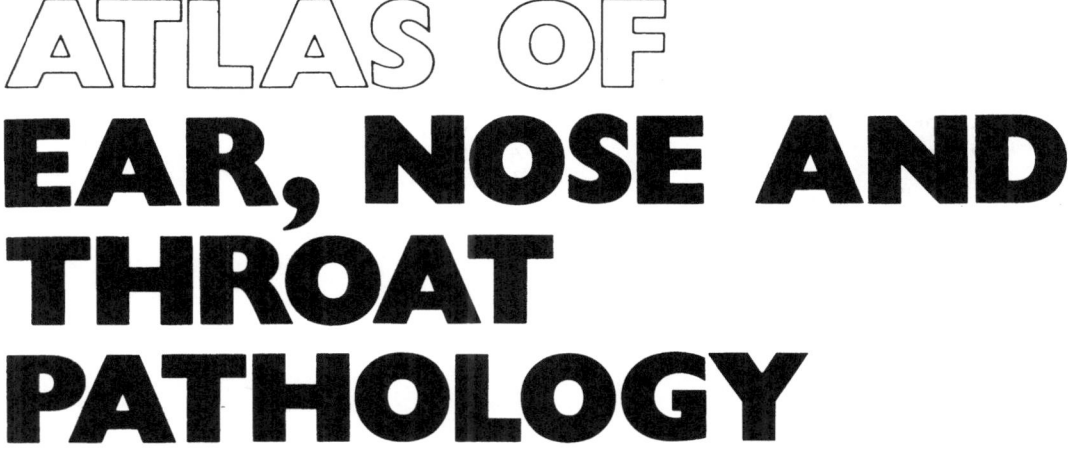

ATLAS OF EAR, NOSE AND THROAT PATHOLOGY

BY

L. MICHAELS
Professor of Pathology
Department of Histopathology
University College and Middlesex School of Medicine
Institute of Laryngology and Otology
330 Gray's Inn Road
London, WC1X 8EE
England

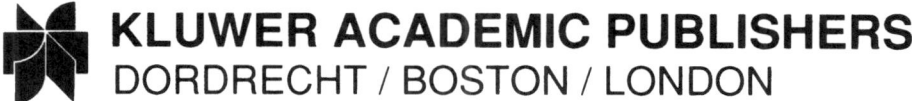
KLUWER ACADEMIC PUBLISHERS
DORDRECHT / BOSTON / LONDON

Distributors

for the United States and Canada: Kluwer Academic Publishers, PO Box 358, Accord Station, Hingham, MA 02018-0358, USA
for all other countries: Kluwer Academic Publishers Group, Distribution Center, PO Box 322, 3300 AH Dordrecht, The Netherlands

Published in the United Kingdom by Kluwer Academic Publishers, PO Box 55, Lancaster, UK.

Kluwer Academic Publishers BV incorporates the publishing programmes of D. Reidel, Martinus Nijhoff, Dr W. Junk and MTP Press.

Typeset and originated by Speedlith Photolitho Ltd., Longford Trading Estate, Thomas Street, Stretford, Manchester M32 0JT
Printed in Great Britain by Gibbons Barford, Willenhall, West Midlands, UK
Bound by Butler and Tanner Ltd., Frome and London

British Library Cataloguing in Publication Data

Michaels, L. (Leslie), *1925–*
   Atlas of ear, nose and throat pathology.
   1. Man. Ears, nose & throat. Diseases
   I. Title II. Series
   617.51
ISBN-13:978-94-010-6812-3   e-ISBN-13:978-94-009-0727-0
DOI: 10.1007/978-94-009-0727-0

Library of Congress Cataloging in Publication Data

Michaels, L. (Leslie)
   Atlas of ear, nose, and throat pathology / by L. Michaels.
      p. cm. — (Current histopathology ; v. 16)
   Includes bibliographic references.
   ISBN-13:978-94-010-6812-3
   ($140.00 U.S.)
   1. Ear—Histopathology—Atlases. 2. Nose—Histopathology—Atlases. 3. Throat—Histopathology—Atlases. I. Title. II. Series.
[DNLM: 1. Otorhinolaryngologic Diseases––pathology—atlases. 2. Otorhinolaryngologic Neoplasms—pathology—atlases. W1 CU788JBA v. 16 / WV 17 M621a]
RF47.5M5   1990
617.5'1075'0222—dc20
DNLM/DLC   90-4191
for Library of Congress   CIP

Contents

Current Histopathology Series

Consultant Editor's Note

At the present time books on morbid anatomy and histopathology can be divided into two broad groups: extensive textbooks often written primarily for students and monographs on research topic.

This takes no account of the fact that the vast majority of pathologists are involved in an essentially practical field of general diagnostic pathology providing an important service to their clinical colleagues. Many of these pathologists are expected to cover a broad range of disciplines and even those who remain solely within the field of histopathology usually have single and sole responsibility within the hospital for all this work. They may often have no chance for direct discussion on problem cases with colleagues in the same department. In the field of histopathology, no less than in other medical fields, there have been extensive and recent advances, not only in new histochemical techniques but also in the type of specimen provided by new surgical procedures.

There is a great need for the provision of appropriate information for this group. This need has been defined in the following terms:-

1. It should be aimed at the general clinical pathologist or histopathologist with existing practical training, but should also have value for the trainee pathologist.
2. It should concentrate on the practical aspects of histopathology taking account of the new techniques which should be within the compass of the worker in a unit with reasonable facilities.
3. New types of material, e.g. those derived from endoscopic biopsy should be covered fully.
4. There should be an adequate number of illustrations on each subject to demonstrate the variation in appearance that is encountered.
5. Colour illustrations should be used wherever they aid recognition.

The present concept stemmed from this definition but it was immediately realized that these aims could only be achieved within the compass of a series, of which this volume is one. Since histopathology is, by its very nature, systemized, the individual volumes deal with one system or where this appears more appropriate with a single organ.

Accounts of pathological processes in the nose and ear are not numerous. Nevertheless pathologists are meeting such problems more frequently. This atlas supplies an important addition to this series and will be of considerable value to diagnosticians dealing with biopsies from the ear, nose and throat. In this field, as in others, accurate diagnosis often determines appropriate therapy, as for example in Wegener's granulomatosis. This book will provide much needed assistance in this regard.

G. Austin Gresham
Cambridge

Introduction

Many pathologists have little acquaintance with ear, nose and throat pathology. Some receive few specimens from ENT tissues; others are deterred from deeper study of material that emanates from regions the normal anatomy of which is so forbidding in its complexity and holds no familiarity through autopsy investigation, for, apart from the larynx, there is usually no compelling indication for examination of the ear, nose or throat at postmortem. Yet, equally with biopsy specimens from other parts of the body, the pathologist's report is consequential for the efficient handling of ear, nose and throat illnesses and sometimes even for the patient's survival.

Otolaryngology has progressed in recent years as rapidly as any other form of surgery and many of its advances have similarly brought the need for a greater understanding of the histological alterations revealed in its biopsies. The middle ear is now frequently explored for chronic otitis media, cholesteatoma and otosclerosis and neoplasms of that region are less rare than was hitherto thought to be the case. Some nasal and nasopharyngeal inflammatory and neoplastic lesions are now more successfully treated; biopsy decisions play an important role in the type of therapy to be administered. Laryngeal endoscopy and its concomitant biopsy have become commonplace in the management of throat disorders. It is hoped that, by the publication of this Atlas, pathologists receiving only occasional specimens will be guided in their provision of a report helpful to the clinician and those who are involved with a larger ENT service may be provided with a guide to the deeper understanding of the subject.

The modern tendency in publication of histopathological microphotographs is to omit any statement of their magnification, since it will usually be clear to the reader what order of enlargement is involved. In this Atlas, however, to prevent the occasional source of confusion, a similar practice has been adopted to that used in the *Atlas of Skin Pathology* of this series, i.e. the power of the objective used has been indicated by 'A' for the scanning low-power ($\times 2.5 - \times 4.0$), 'B' for medium-power ($\times 10 - \times 25$), 'C' for high-power ($\times 40$) and 'D' for oil-immersion ($\times 1000$).

Many surgeons, physicians, pathologists and medical laboratory scientific officers have helped by the provision or processing of material which is used in this work and the author expresses his gratitude to them.

Removal of the Temporal Bone

Useful information is obtained by examination of the temporal bone, even 20 h after death and longer, particularly for studies of the bone or connective tissue structures. For examination of the membranous labyrinth, perilymphatic space perfusion with fixative soon after death is necessary (see below).

The skullcap and brain are first removed. In doing so, the dura should be treated carefully and left adherent to the temporal bone in order not to damage the endolymphatic sac. The seventh and eighth cranial nerves should be cut at the orifice of the internal auditory meatus so as to leave portions of the nerve trunks within the temporal bone specimen. A vibrating electric saw with triangular blade is used and three vertical and one horizontal cuts are made (Figures 1.1 and 1.2):

I   The first cut is set medial to the internal auditory meatus and extends vertically through the petrous temporal bone at right angles to the superior and posteromedial surfaces to a depth of approximately 2.5 cm.

II . The second cut is made parallel with the first and at least 2.5–3.0 cm posterolateral to it at the lateral end of the temporal bone. It also passes vertically to a depth of 2.5 cm. This cut leaves out most of the mastoid air cell system. A more extensive procedure by which these cells may be removed involves extending cut III laterally to the lateral surface of the squamous temporal bone anterior to the bony orifice of the external auditory meatus, after dissecting the pinna, scalp and cartilaginous canal away from the latter. Cut IV is also extended laterally posterior to the mastoid process and the two cuts are joined together below the bony ear canal (Figure 1.3). With care, this extended temporal bone resection does not result in an unsightly external disfigurement as long as cut I on each side is placed just medial to the internal auditory meatus and not further medially.

III. The third vertical cut is made connecting the forward ends of the two previous cuts, approximately parallel with the free (posterior) end of the petrous temporal bone at the anterior extent of the middle cranial fossa.

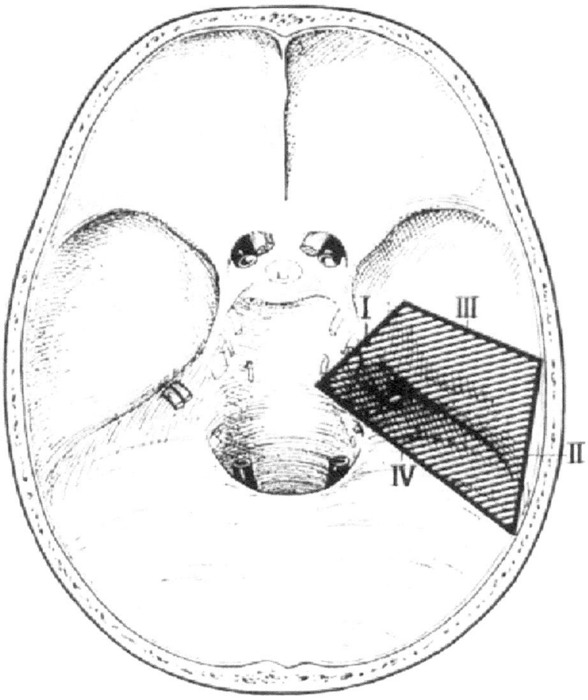

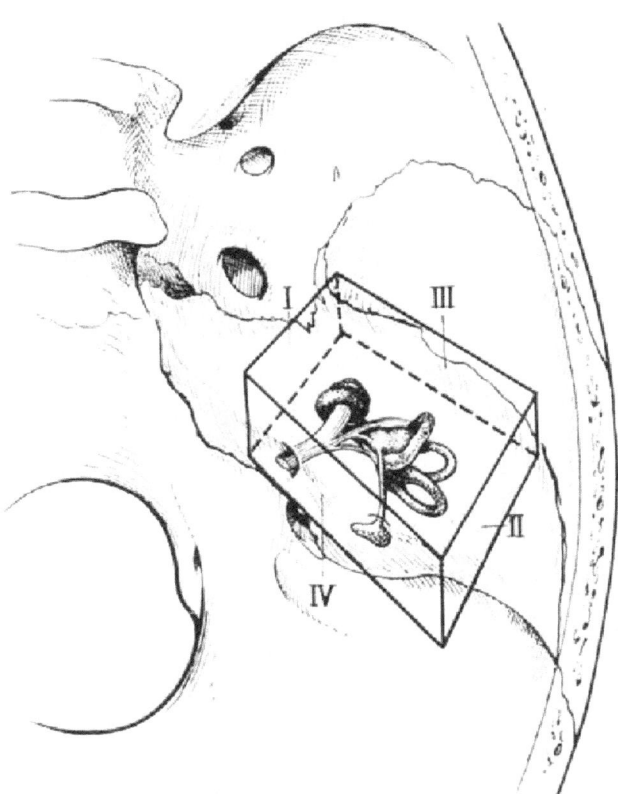

Figure 1.1 Base of skull showing position of four saw cuts (Roman numerals) which are required in removal of temporal bone. A more extensive procedure by which the mastoid process is removed is described in the text and shown in Figure 1.3. (From reference 2 with permission of the authors and publishers)

Figure 1.2 Wedge of temporal bone which is removed from the base of the skull for histological examination. The outlines of the membranous labyrinth drawn in Roman numerals refer to the saw cuts required to remove the temporal bone. A more extensive procedure by which the mastoid process may be removed is shown in Figure 1.3. (From reference 2 with permission)

IV. A horizontal cut is made beneath the petrous temporal bone at about 2.5 cm below the upper surface and parallel with it. The block can now be removed by gently 'rocking' and cutting the ligamentous structures on its inferior surface. So removed, it will include a portion of the external auditory canal, the tympanic membrane, the middle ear, the labyrinthine structures and the petrous portion of the seventh and eighth cranial nerves.

Serial Sectioning of the Temporal Bone

The standard method of histological examination of the temporal bone is by serial sectioning after celloidin embedding. Fixation is required for approximately 4 weeks. The bone should be roughly sawn to size before fixation. To decalcify, the whole temporal bone is placed in 10% formic acid for a period of 4–8 weeks, taking X-rays every week to check the progress of decalcification. On its completion, the final trimming of the specimen can be done by using a strong-bladed knife. Keeping the specimen down to a moderate size is important for proper diffusion of impregnating substances during the subsequent processing of the bone; the trimmed block should measure not more than 4.0 cm long × 2.5 cm wide × 5.5 cm high. Dehydration is carried out by placing it for 1 day in ascending grades of alcohol and alcohol—ether as follows: 30%, 50%, 95%, 100%, 100%, equal parts alcohol and ether. Impregnation in a celloidin base dissolved in a mixture of equal parts of alcohol and ether is then required. In my laboratory, low-viscosity nitrocellulose is used. For microtomy, a long heavy stellite-tipped knife, such as may be obtained from Deloro Stellite, a subsidiary of British Oxygen Company, is preferable. This knife should be sharpened to a final cutting edge bevel of about 28 degrees. Sections are cut at 20 μm thickness and between 50 and 100 sections can be obtained from one bone. It is necessary to stain only every tenth section, keeping the intermediate sections interleaved in vellum tissue, which may be stored indefinitely with the uncut blocks in 70% alcohol. Staining of sections may be carried out by the haematoxylin and eosin method (preferably using Ehrlich's haematoxylin) as well as by a wide variety of other routine histological stains.

The Microslicing Technique

The serial sectioning technique does not afford an opportunity for the pathologist to examine the gross changes within the temporal bone. A slicing method in which this can be carried out is in routine use in our laboratory for the examination of the temporal bones of all cases except fetuses before 20 weeks gestation[1]. In the sliced temporal bones so prepared, not only may gross and regular microscopic studies be carried out, but also special microscopic studies, including histochemistry and electron microscopy, as well as certain biochemical investigations on selected areas.

The temporal bone is removed at postmortem as described above. Fixation should take place for a minimum of 4 days. The bone is trimmed so that it is no larger than about 2.5 × 2.5 × 2.5 cm. It is then mounted with molten dental wax on a glass plate measuring 6 × 2.5 cm with a thickness of approximately 0.5 cm. The surface to be presented for slicing is arranged perpendicular to the glass plate. The latter, with the surface of the temporal bone that is to be cut to the front, is now mounted on the metal plinth attached with dental wax to the inner end of the lever of a special slicing machine (Figure 1.4) (Microslice 2 Precision Annular Saw, available from Malvern Instruments Ltd., Spring Lane South, Malvern, Worcestershire, WR14 12BR, England). This is a cutting machine with a circular steel blade which is bolted to the machine at 16 points to prevent lateral vibration. Cutting proceeds around a circular inner opening where the blade is tipped with diamond. The cutting edge is lubricated by a continuous jet of cold water. The lever with the specimen is advanced by the required length before each slice is made so that the thickness of the specimen can be regulated. Slices of 1, 2 or 3 mm thickness may be prepared. Slicing is carried out by gently lowering the weighted left-hand counterpoised end of the lever so that the specimen rotates up and is applied against the cutting edge. With this system, the specimen backs away from the blade when a particularly hard area is encountered, so avoiding excessive mechanical and thermal stresses. The slices adhere together and are removed from the machine after the whole temporal bone has been treated. Each slice is X-rayed. Selected areas of the whole or of a single slice may be subjected to celloidin or paraffin embedding for light microscopy, special histological or histochemical methods or even for electron microscopy if adequate fixation has been carried out.

Anatomy of Ear in Microsliced Temporal Bone
(Figures 1.5 and 1.6)

Transverse microslices, starting from the superior surface, allow the structures of the temporal bone to be easily examined by gross methods. The upper transverse slices contain the deeper osseous portion of the external auditory meatus terminating in the tympanic membrane. The handle of the malleus is attached to the latter. The joints between the malleus and the incus and between the incus and the stapes are identified. The footplate, the horizontal bar of the stapes, between the crura, is placed in the orifice of the vestibule (oval window). The Eustachian tube opens onto the anterior wall of the middle ear passing medially to communicate with the nasopharynx. At its commencement, it is surrounded by bone and more laterally by cartilage. The tensor tympani muscle lies in a canal above the Eustachian tube and is attached to the malleus in the middle ear cavity. The facial nerve enters the temporal bone through the internal auditory meatus where it lies above the eighth cranial nerve. The facial nerve makes a right-angle bend at the genu. At this point there are ganglion cells in the nerve, constituting the geniculate ganglion. The nerve then courses posteriorly and slightly downwards in the posterior wall of the middle ear. The stapedius muscle occupies a niche of the bony wall near the facial nerve and is attached to the posterior crus of the stapes. Mastoid air cells are very prominent in the posterior wall of the ear canal and are in communication with the main middle ear cavity. Air cells may spread to wide areas of the temporal bone. I have found them near the apex of the temporal bone in the vicinity of the jugular foramen in some 16% of adult temporal bones.

In the lower slices, the inner ear is well displayed. It consists of a bony labyrinth and a membranous one which lies within the former and contains the organs of hearing and balance. The bony labyrinth consists of a central part called the vestibule, a coiled tube, the bony cochlea and three bony semicircular canals, superior, lateral and posterior, which are in planes at right angles to each other. They open by only five openings into the vestibule, since one end of the superior and posterior canals join to form a common canal, the crus commune.

The bony cochlea consists of a bony tube coiled two and a half times around a bony pillar called the modiolus. The basal coil of the cochlea is the widest and the apical the narrowest. The cavity of the tube is incompletely divided into two chambers by a bony septum called the osseous spiral lamina, which is attached to the modiolus. The scala vestibuli opens and the scala tympani ends at the round window, an opening into the cochlea, which is separated from the middle ear by the secondary tympanic membrane. At the apex of the cochlea, the two scalae join at a point called the helicotrema.

The membranous labyrinth lies inside the bony labyrinth. It has three parts like the bony labyrinth:

1. Three membranous semicircular canals inside the corresponding bony canals.

2. Two sacs, the utricle and saccule, within the bony vestibule. The saccule is joined to the cochlear duct by a narrow canal called the canalis reuniens. The utricle receives the five openings of the membranous semicircular canals. A small duct is given off from both utricle and saccule and these join to form the endolymphatic duct, which passes through the aqueduct of the vestibule, a bony canal, to the posterior surfaces of the petrous temporal bone.

3. The cochlear duct (scala media) within the canal of the bony cochlea. This duct contains the structures constituting the organ of hearing.

The Surface Preparation Method

The surface preparation method has been applied mainly to the analysis of the hair cells of the organ of Corti and is best used in temporal bones in which the perilymphatic space has been perfused by fixative within 24 h after death; the autolysis which takes place in the hair cells beyond that time renders them unsuitable for this type of examination. Electron microscopy, particularly by the scanning method, is also frequently used to study specimens which have been perfused within 3 h after death.

Perilymphatic perfusion may be carried out directly on the cadaver in the autopsy room[2] or in the histopathology laboratory on a temporal bone which has been removed by the method described above. Using an ear speculum, the upper posterior part of the tympanic membrane is folded forwards. The incudostapedial joint is divided and the stapes is luxated from the oval window. It can be left in the middle ear hanging from the stapedial muscle tendon or removed for further study. The round window membrane is perforated with a small hook directed forwards (in the direction of the Eustachian tube). Fixative is injected with a fine unsharpened needle into the oval window and the perilymphatic space is perfused for about 15 min by repeated infusions of fixative (Figure 1.7).

Sampling the membranous labyrinth

The method of drilling away the bony labyrinth to sample the membranous labyrinth was described by Johnsson and Hawkins[3]. The method is difficult, requiring special training and a detailed knowledge of temporal bone anatomy. Because of its difficulty, damage to the membranous labyrinth is likely; a high degree of skill is required to carry out the procedure and each specimen requires many hours of work. A further disadvantage is that, in order to expose the membranous labyrinth in this way, it is necessary to destroy other parts of the middle and inner ear.

By contrast, the microsliced temporal bone prepared by the method described above may be used to sample the membranous labyrinth without drilling and with but very slight damage to inner ear structures. By this method the whole inner ear may be exposed within minutes. Vertical slicing may be utilized so as to sample the organ of Corti at measured lengths along its course.

A method of staining has been devised by Mr A. Frohlich in my department. After a short period of postfixation in dilute osmic acid solution, the sample is stained by an Alcian blue solution followed by phloxine—eosin counterstain. Hairs (stereocilia), hair cells, supporting cells, pillar cells and nerves are shown well by this method on ordinary light microscopy (Figures 1.8 and 1.9).

Normal Histology

External ear

The pinna consists of elastic cartilage with a covering of skin which follows all of the folds of the cartilage. The skin of the external meatus is continuous with that of the pinna and, like the latter, shows pronounced rete ridges in all areas except for the bony portion where the epidermis is usually flat. The skin over the pinna and cartilaginous portions shows the normal skin appendages of hair with sebaceous glands and hairs. Eccrine sweat glands are present on the pinna but absent in the external auditory canal. Apocrine (ceruminous) glands are present in the cartilaginous canal. The skin of the bony portion has no adnexal structures.

Tympanic membrane

The pars tensa represents all of the tympanic membrane except a loose upper portion, the pars flaccida. The pars tensa consists of an external layer of skin, a central collagenous zone composed of two layers of collagen and fibroblasts, and an internal mucosal layer (Figure 1.10).

The skin on the external surface is similar to that lining the bony portion of the external auditory meatus and shows strata corneum, granulosum and malpighii, the latter composed of four or five layers of 'prickle cells'. This epithelium possesses the property of 'migration', a means of cleansing the outer surface of the tympanic membrane from accumulation of keratin to ensure the preservation of the delicate mechanism of vibration in transmission of sound. Migration is demonstrated by placing an ink dot near the centre of the eardrum in the normal living subject. The dot moves towards the periphery on specific pathways based on embryological growth[4] and reaches the canal where the keratin is desquamated at the level of the junction of the bony and cartilaginous portions (Figures 1.11 and 1.12). A thin lamina of connective tissue with capillaries lies beneath the epithelium of the eardrum.

The connective tissue layer of the normal pars tensa shows a lateral layer of radially arranged collagenous fibres and a medial layer in which these fibres are arranged circularly.

The inner membranous surface – the mucosa of the middle ear – is a single layer of cuboidal epithelium which rests on a lamina propria of collagenous fibres and capillaries.

The pars flaccida shows an external covering of skin in which the epithelial cell layers are more numerous than in the pars tensa. The middle ear mucosa is similar in appearance to that lining the pars tensa. The intermediate, finely structured collagenous layers seen in the pars tensa are absent, however, and are replaced by a thicker zone of loose collagen and elastic fibres.

Epithelia of the middle ear

The epithelium of the Eustachian tube is of ciliated, pseudostratified columnar type. This may be continued into the anterior part of the middle ear cavity immediately adjacent to the Eustachian tube. Zones of ciliated pseudostratified epithelium may also be present elsewhere in the middle ear but usually the presence of such epithelium in the middle ear is considered to be a pathological response to the presence of inflammation. The normal middle ear covering is of simple (i.e. single-layered) squamous or simple cuboidal type. Stratified (i.e. multilayered) squamous epithelium is not a feature of the normal middle ear, but is found in cholesteatoma (see Chapter 2). Gland formation is also not a feature of the normal middle ear mucosa, but requires inflammatory change for its induction[5].

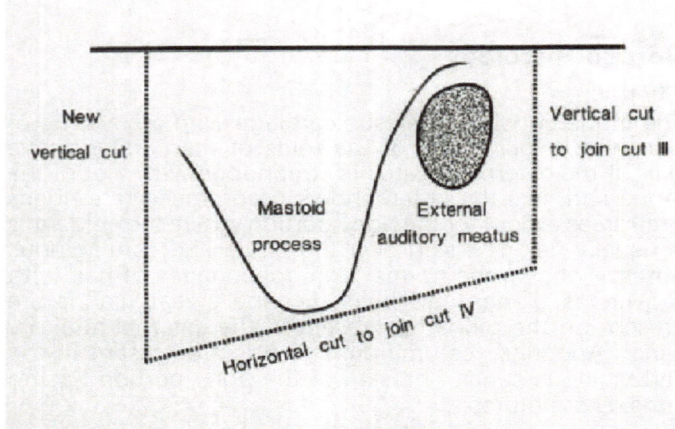

Figure 1.3 Diagram of the side view of the skull in the region of the external auditory meatus to indicate extended saw cuts which may be carried out to remove the mastoid process

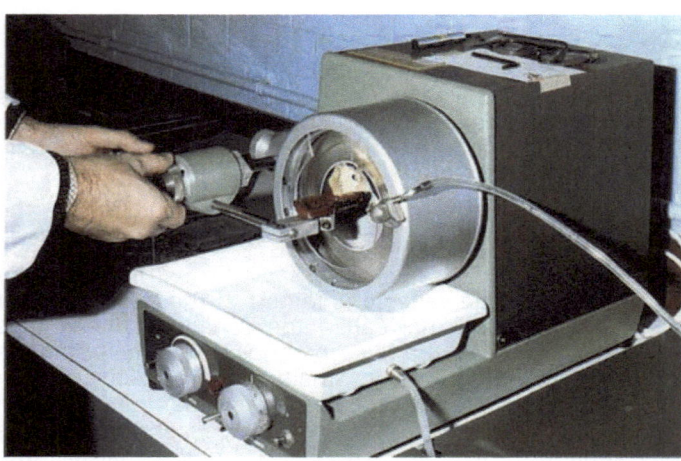

Figure 1.4 Microslice 2 Precision Annular Saw used to prepare slices of undecalcified temporal bone

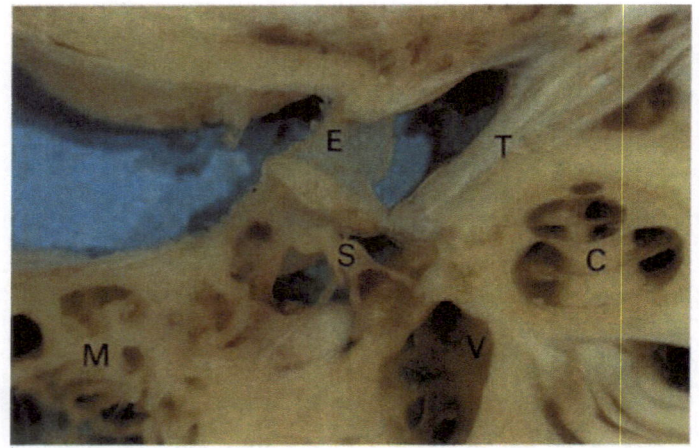

Figure 1.5 Microsliced normal temporal bone. C: cochlea; E: tympanic membrane; M: mastoid air cells; S: stapes; T: tensor tympani muscle; V: vestibule

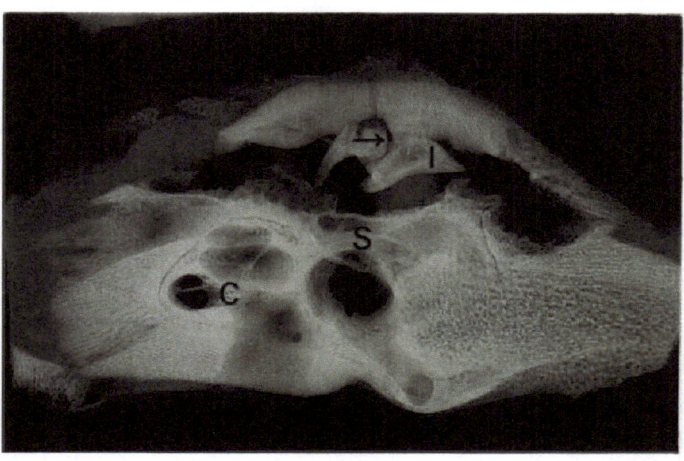

Figure 1.6 Radiograph of microslice of temporal bone at a level similar to that seen in Figure 1.5. Note the dense bone around the cochlea and vestibule.
Arrow: malleus; C: cochlea; I: incus; S: stapes; S. stapes; V: vestibule

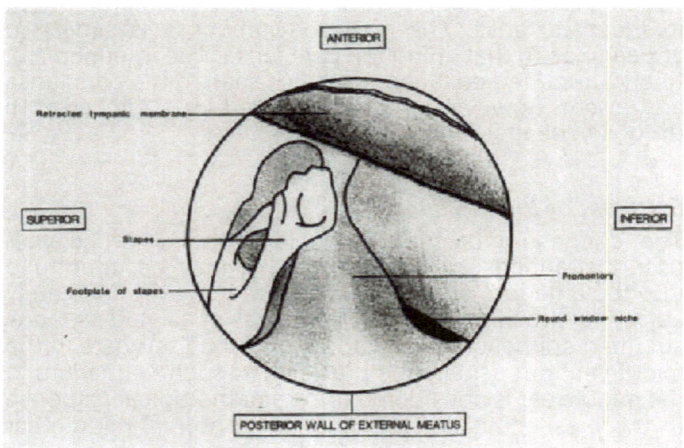

Figure 1.7 Diagram of appearances of normal middle ear observed during perilymphatic perfusion

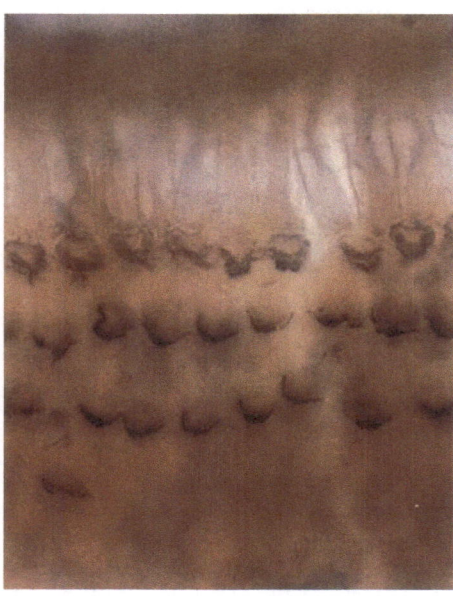

Figure 1.8 Outer hair cells of the basal coil of the cochlea in surface preparation. The stereocilia are short and arranged in a W formation in each hair cell. Frohlich staining method (D)

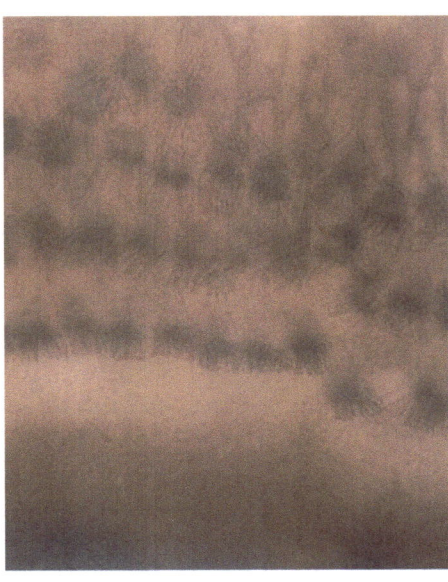

Figure 1.9 Outer hair cells of the middle coil of the cochlea. The stereocilia are long. Frohlich staining method (D)

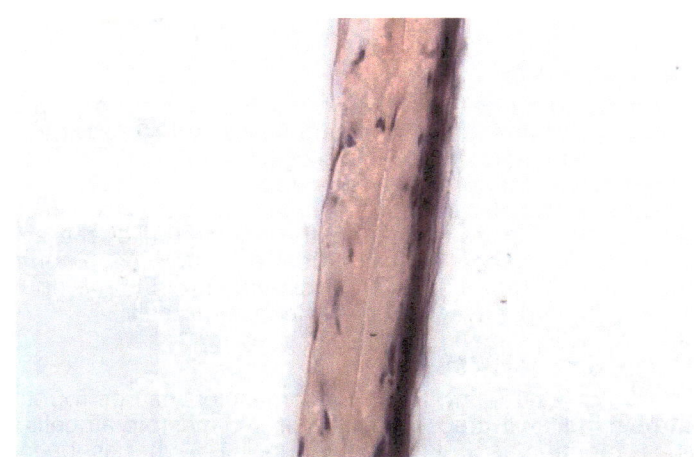

Figure 1.10 Transverse section of tympanic membrane showing outer layer of stratified squamous epithelium on left and inner layer of cubical epithelium on the right, between which are the outer radial and inner circular collagenous fibres. H & E (B)

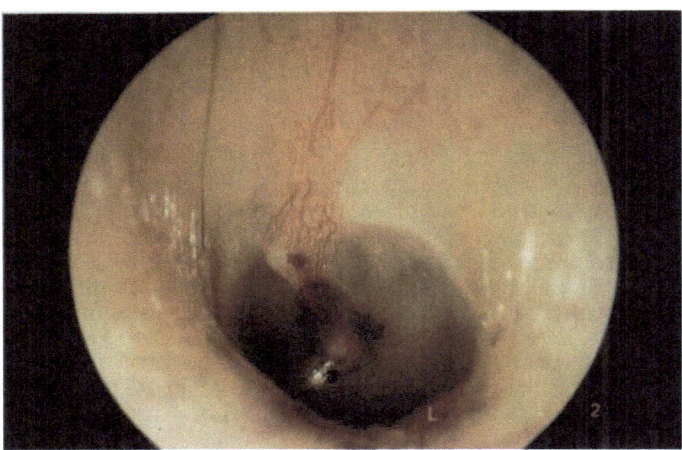

Figure 1.11 Normal tympanic membrane viewed otoscopically in the living subject. An ink dot has been near the lateral process of the malleus just before taking the photograph

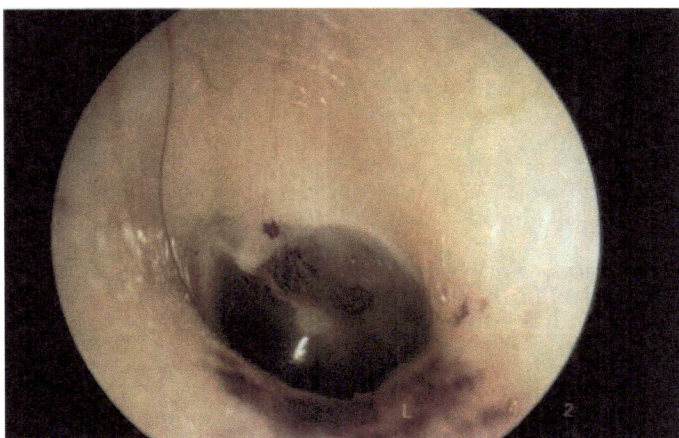

Figure 1.12 The same tympanic membrane as that seen in Figure 1.11, photographed 5 weeks later. The ink dot has travelled posteriorly across the eardrum and passed on to the edge of the external ear canal

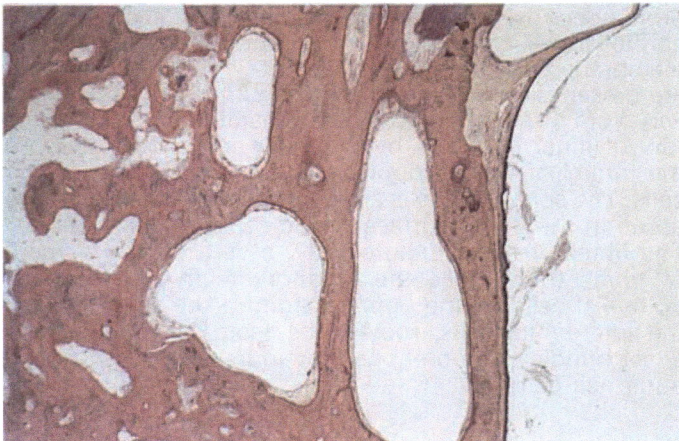

Figure 1.13 Mastoid air cells (centre), tympanic membrane (upper right) and squamous epithelium of the osseous portion of the ear canal (right). Note the extremely thin covering of the bone of the ear canal and its overlying epithelium. H & E (A)

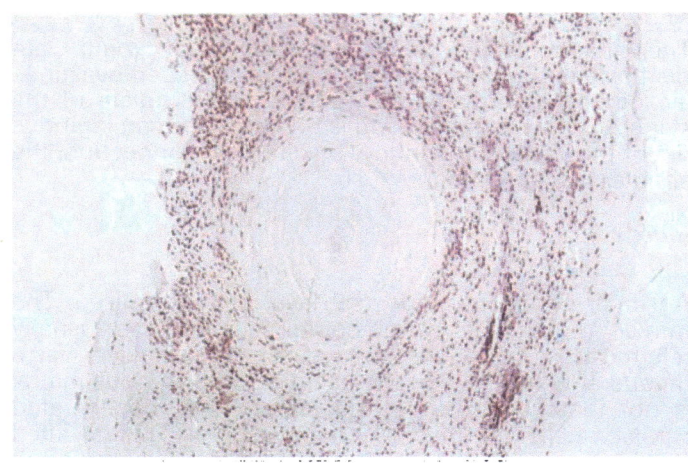

Figure 1.14 Middle ear corpuscle composed of many layers of concentric lamellae. H & E (A)

Mastoid air cells

The mastoid air cells, including the mastoid antrum, are a network of intercommunicating spaces which emanate from the tympanic cavity. The skeletal framework of each air cell is made up of a thin bony trabeculum of Haversian systems of lamellar bone. This is covered by a periosteal layer of fibrous tissue bearing the epithelium of the air cell. The epithelium is of cuboidal or simple squamous epithelium (Figure 1.13). Pseudostratified columnar epithelium is hardly ever found in the mastoid cells.

Middle ear corpuscles

Structures resembling Pacinian corpuscles may be found in the middle ear mucosa, usually in the mastoid air cells. Their function is unknown (Figure 1.14). It has been indicated that they are not true Pacinian corpuscles, since they lack the fine innervation of the latter structures and they are often bifurcated or even trifurcated[6].

Ossicles

Cartilage is retained as a thin horizontal lamina on the vestibular aspect of the footplate of the stapes and also covers the articular surfaces of the stapediovestibular joints (Figures 1.15 and 1.16). The vestibular surface of the stapes is lined by a single flattened thin squamous layer of cells characteristic of the perilymphatic space. A thin layer of bone is applied exteriorly to the cartilage of the footplate, so that the latter is bilaminar in constitution. The crura are formed of periosteal bone only. The head of the stapes is composed of endochondral bone capped by a cartilaginous layer at the incudostapedial joint (Figure 1.17).

The body and long process of the incus show an outer covering of periosteal bone and an inner core of endochondral bone both possessing well-formed Haversian systems. The short process of the incus has a tip of unossified cartilage, and cartilage also covers the articular surfaces of the incus at its two joints.

The structure of the head and upper part of the handle of the malleus is similar to that of the body and long process of the incus, with an outer shell of periosteal bone and an inner core of endochondral bone. Most of the malleus handle shows a layer of retained cartilage instead of periosteal bone. The inner core of the malleus handle is composed of endochondral bone like the rest of the malleus.

Middle ear joints

The incudomalleal and incudostapedial joints are diarthrodial (Figures 1.18 and 1.19). The stapediovestibular joint (the cartilaginous edge of the footplate of the stapes) is a synarthrosis, and is bound to the cartilaginous rim of the vestibular window by a fibrous connection, the annular ligament (Figure 1.16).

Inner ear

Otic capsule

An inner and outer periosteal layer are recognized. The former (lining the membranous labyrinth) is usually referred to as the endosteal layer. The middle layer has a unique structure in that the calcified cartilaginous matrix is not removed when the lacunae of the degenerated cartilage cells are lined by primitive bone. This calcified matrix accompanied by primitive bone persists into adult life as the 'globuli ossei' characteristic of the otic capsule (Figure 1.20). The bony tissue in the first months of life shows red bone marrow as in the development of long bones. This marrow is subsequently replaced by bone. The bone of the adult otic capsule is not lamellated, but still somewhat more differentiated than woven bone.

Thus, the otic capsule bone shows lack of removal and replacement of primitive cartilaginous and bony tissue. These persisting structures interweave to form a tissue which is of extremely hard consistency.

Cochlea

Modiolus (Figure 1.21): This is composed of spongy bone. It is penetrated by blood vessels and the nerve bundles of the cochlear branch of the eighth nerve. At the origin of the three cochlear coils, and forming nests within the thin core of the modiolus, lie the nerve cells of the spiral ganglion (Figure 1.22).

Spiral lamina: Emanating from the modiolus in a spiral manner is the spiral lamina, which separates the perilymph-containing space of the scala vestibuli from the similarly containing space, the scala tympani. The inner zone of the spiral lamina is the osseous spiral lamina, which contains thin trabeculae of bone and nerve fibres. The outer zone of this lamina is known as the basilar membrane (Figure 1.23). At the attachment of the latter to the cochlear wall, the periosteal connective tissue is thickened to form the spiral ligament. This appears in histological section as a crescentic structure with a protruding peak on its concave surface to which the basilar membrane is anchored. It is composed of collagenous fibres with a few fibroblasts. The fibres blend with the endosteum of the cochlear bony wall and the fibres of the basilar membrane.

Reissner's membrane: The cochlear canal is further subdivided by a thin membrane, Reissner's membrane, that extends from the spiral lamina to the outer wall of the bony cochlea, so producing an additional scala, the scala media or cochlear duct, which is inserted between the other two (Figure 1.23). Reissner's membrane consists of two thin layers of cells. The inner layer is ectodermal in origin; epithelial-appearing clusters may be often observed in this structure. The outer layer on the scala vestibuli side is mesodermal in origin; these cells are large, flat and elongated.

Stria vascularis: The outer vertical wall of the triangle of the cochlear duct formed on its other two sides by Reissner's membrane and the basilar membrane is the stria vascularis. Under the light microscope, lightly staining basal cells and darkly staining epithelial-like marginal cells can be recognized.

Basilar membrane structures (Figure 1.24): The spiral prominence is a bulge of connective tissue covered by epithelial cells which lies at the outer end of the basilar membrane over the spiral ligament. The outer hair cells are present in rows which, in the human organ of Corti, vary from three to five. They are separated from the single row of inner hair cells by the pillar cells which enclose the tunnel of Corti. Supporting cells separate outer hair cells. The spiral limbus is a bulge of periosteal connective tissue in the upper surface of the osseous spiral lamina. The fibres of this structure show a vertical arrangement of fibres to produce the 'auditory teeth of Huschke'. Epithelial cells on the upper margin of the spiral limbus, the interdental cells, secrete the tectorial membrane, a linear bundle of amorphous protein in which hairs of the outer hair cells lie.

Vestibular structures

Sensory areas of ampullae: The epithelium of the floor of the three ampullae is formed into a transverse ridge, the crista, and is their sensory epithelium. A viscous protein polysaccharide formation, known as the cupula, rests above each crista. The remainder of the ampullary and semicircular duct lining is formed by flattened cells.

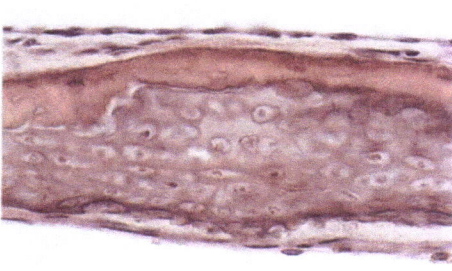

Figure 1.15 Stapes footplate. Beneath the cuboidal epithelium of the middle ear above, there is a thin layer of bone. Below this, the footplate consists of cartilage and there is a basal flattened layer of cells comprising the lining of the vestibule.   H & E (B)

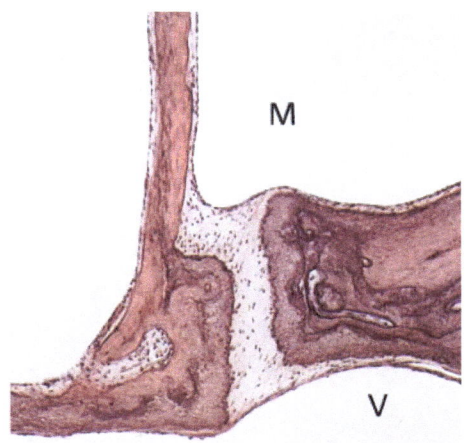

Figure 1.16 Stapediovestibular joint, part of footplate of stapes, adjacent bony labyrinthine wall and crus of stapes The footplate shows a lamina of cartilage on its vestibular surface, which is continuous with the cartilage of the stapediovestibular joint
M: middle ear cavity; V: cavity of vestibule.   H & E (A)

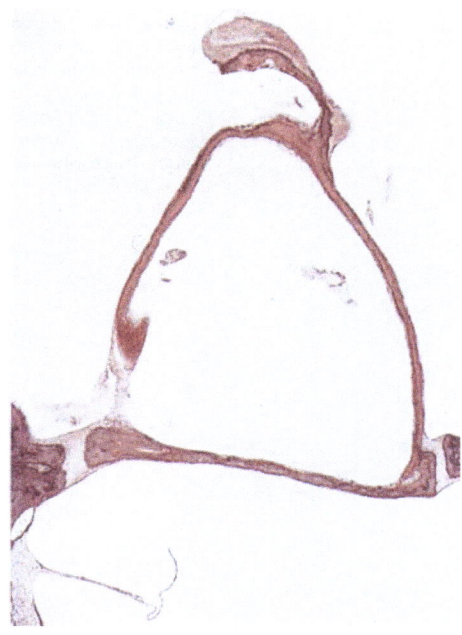

Figure 1.17 Stapes showing two crura and footplate below. Note the stapedio-vestibular joints adjacent to the footplate on each side. H & E (A)

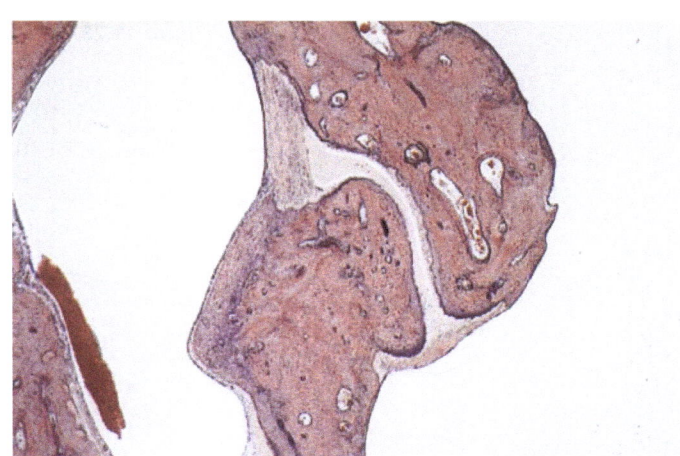

Figure 1.18   Malleo-incudal joint. Note the joint capsule at each end of the joint. The joint space is occupied by the fibrocartilage of the articular disc.   H & E (A)

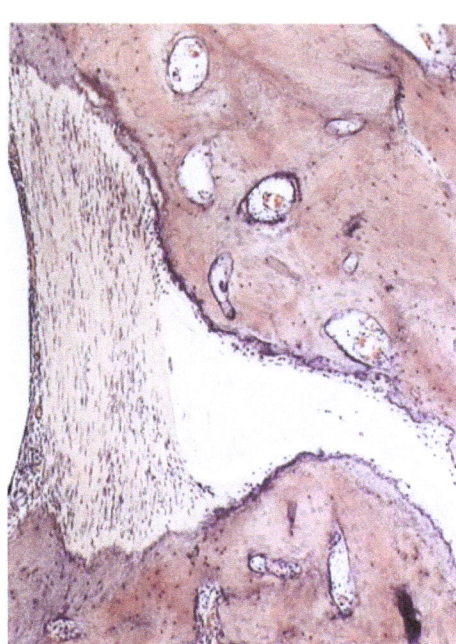

Figure 1.19 Higher power of part of Figure 1.18. Note joint capsule and articular disc.   H & E (B)

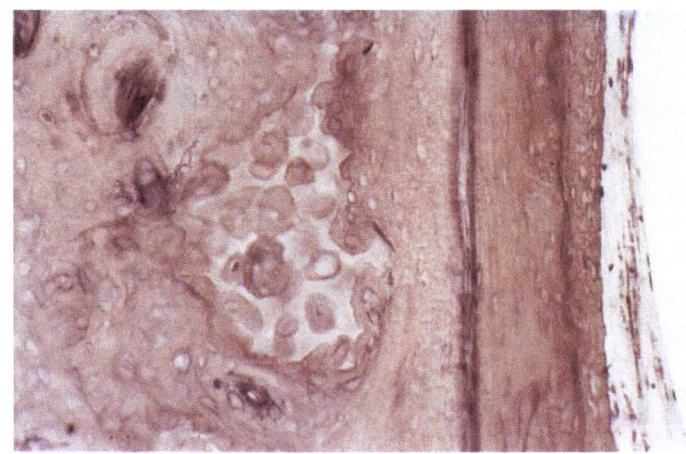

Figure 1.20 Globuli ossei (left) and endosteum (right) of cochlea.   H & E (B)

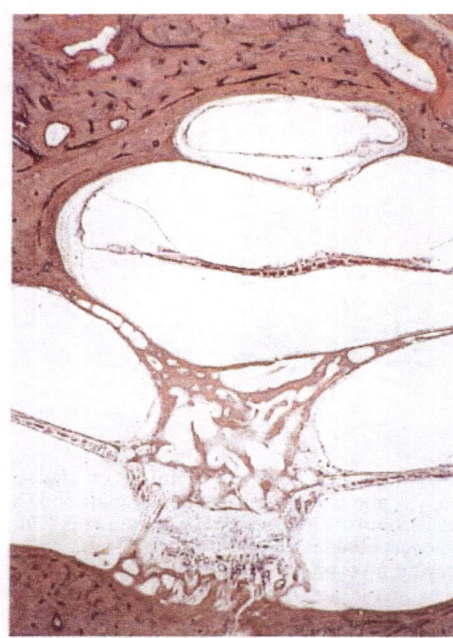

Figure 1.21 Modiolus and basal, middle and apical coils of the cochlea. H & E (A)

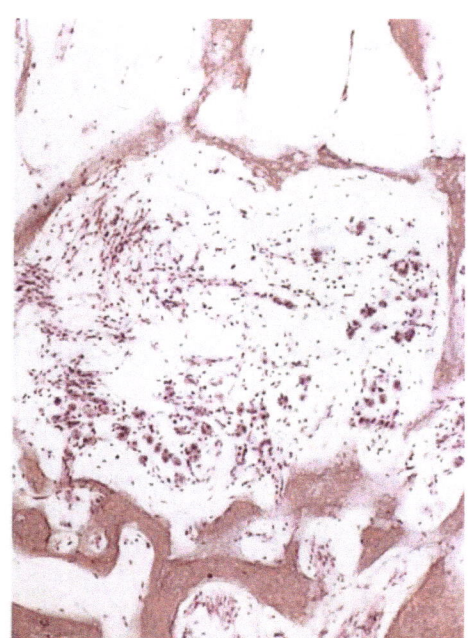

Figure 1.22 Higher power of part of Figure 1.21 showing spiral ganglion cells and nerve fibres in modiolus. H & E (B)

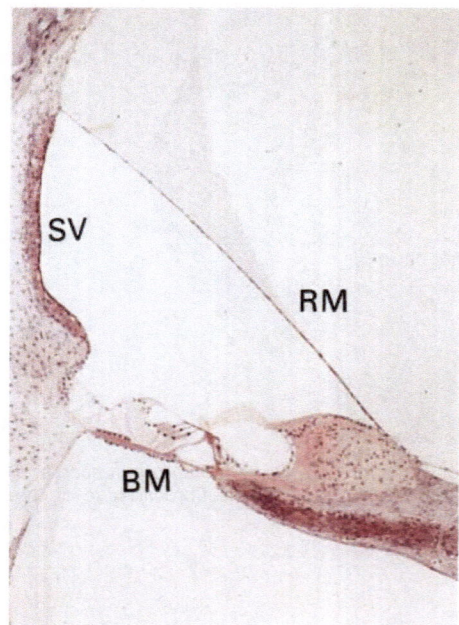

Figure 1.23 Scala media of cat. BM: basilar membrane; RM: Reissner's membrane; SV: stria vascularis. H & E (B)

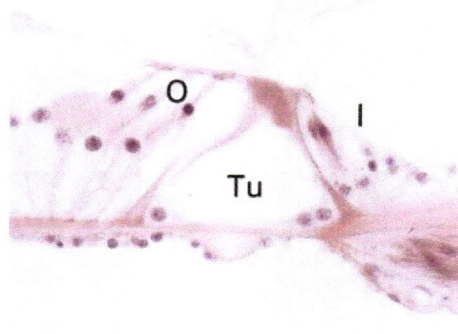

Figure 1.24 Higher power of organ of Corti from Figure 1.23. I: inner hair cells; O: outer hair cells; Te: tectorial membrane; Tu: tunnel of Corti. H & E (C)

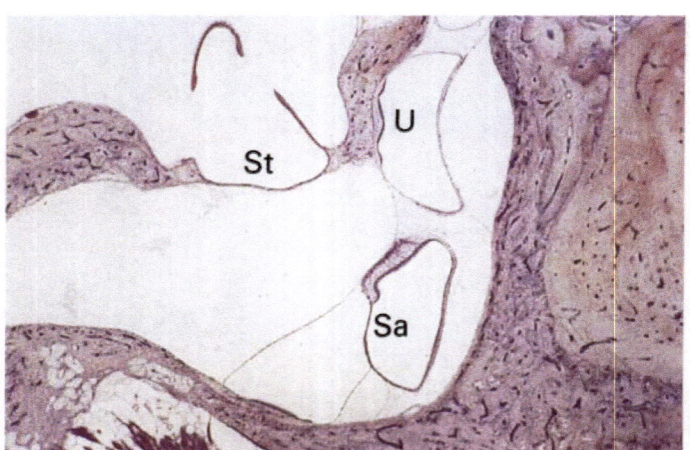

Figure 1.25 Ventricle of cat showing utricle (U) and saccule (Sa). St: stapes. H & E (A)

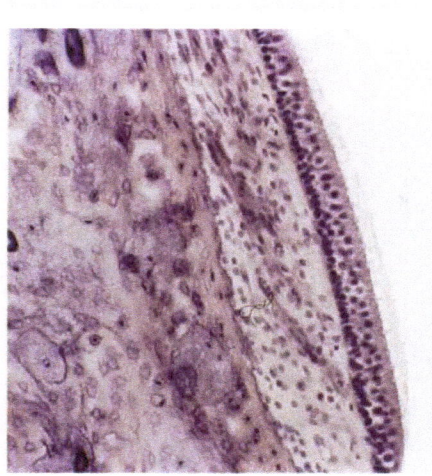

Figure 1.26 Higher power of part of Figure 1.25, showing macule of saccule. H & E (B)

Sensory areas of utricle and saccule (Figures 1.25 and 1.26): A large proportion of the two main membranous structures of the vestibule, the utricle and saccule, have a lining of sensory epithelium, the macula. Overlying the hairs of the sensory cells of the maculae are large numbers of crystalline bodies, known as otoliths, which are composed of a mixture of calcium carbonate and a protein, suspended in a jelly-like polysaccharide.

References

1. Michaels, L., Wells, M. and Frohlich, A. (1983). A new technique for the study of temporal bone pathology. *Clin. Otolaryngol.*, **8**, 77–85

2. Iurato, S., Bredberg, G. and Bock, G. (1982). *Functional Histopathology of the Human Audio-vestibular Organ. Euro-data Hearing Project.* (Commission of the European Communities)

3. Johnson, L. G. and Hawkins, J. E. (1967). A direct approach to cochlear anatomy and pathology in man. *Arch. Otolaryngol.*, **85**, 599–613

4. Michaels, L. (1989). The biology of cholesteatoma. *Otolaryngol. Clin. N. Am.*, **22**, 869–881

5. Sade, J. (1966). Middle ear mucosa. *Arch. Otolaryngol.*, **84**, 137–143

6. Lim, D., Jackson, D. and Bennett, J. (1975). Human middle ear corpuscles – a light and electron microscopical study. *Laryngoscope*, **85**, 1725–1737

Non-neoplastic Conditions of the External and Middle Ear

2

Malformations of the External Ear

The auricle develops from six knob-like protuberances, arising from the first and second branchial arches, which fuse to form auricular components, such as the helix, antihelix and tragus. The external auditory meatus is derived from the first branchial groove, a depression of the ectoderm between the first (mandibular) arch and the second (hyoid) arch. The deep extremity of this groove meets the outer epithelium of the corresponding first pharyngeal pouch, separated from it by only a thin layer of connective tissue. The point of meeting produces the tympanic membrane.

Malformations of the external ear include:

1. Partial or complete absence of the auricle.
2. Accessory auricles.
3. Preauricular sinus. This frequently shows a squamous epithelial lining (though a respiratory one may sometimes occur) deep to which the connective tissue is chronically inflamed. There is often elastic cartilage in the deep wall of the sinus (Figure 2.1).
4. Atresia of the external auditory meatus, which may present as a blind protrusion or may be completely absent.
5. Abnormalities of the shape and size of the auricle. These may be ascribed to defects of fusion of the knob-like protrusions and flaws in the hollowing-out of the first branchial groove.

Inflammatory Lesions of External Ear

The external ear is subject to a wide variety of inflammatory lesions. Some of these are identical to those occurring elsewhere on the skin. Others are specific to, or most common in, the region of the external ear and only these will be presented.

Diffuse external otitis

This is a common condition which affects the external auditory meatus. *Pseudomonas aeruginosa* is most commonly recovered from the inflammatory exudate. The skin of the ear canal is erythematous and oedematous and gives off a greenish discharge. Histological examination of the epidermis reveals marked acanthosis, hyperkeratosis and an acute inflammatory exudate in the dermis, particularly around apocrine glands.

Malignant otitis externa

This is defined as a severe infection of the external auditory canal, usually in elderly diabetics, resulting in purulent discharge, the formation of granulations in the ear canal and invasion of cartilage, bone and nerve tissue[1,2]. In my department, histopathological examination of temporal bones from three patients with that clinical condition showed thrombosis of the jugular bulb with surrounding inflammation. Severe otitis media was present in each case. It seems possible that the manifestations of 'malig-

nant otitis media' may be due to the spread of inflammation from the middle ear to the petrous apex via a thrombophlebitic jugular bulb.

Virus infection

Herpes zoster
Herpes zoster is caused by the virus of chicken pox which travels from the nerve ganglia to the skin along nerves. When the geniculate ganglion is affected, a vesicular eruption of the pinna, ear canal, postauricular skin, uvula, palate and anterior tongue is produced. When combined with disturbances of hearing and balance due to involvement of the ganglia of the eighth nerve, the condition is termed the Ramsay Hunt syndrome.

Non-infectious inflammatory lesions

Starch granuloma
Granulomatous inflammatory lesions, due to contamination by corn starch glove powder, have been commonly encountered in the peritoneum and pleura after surgery. Granulomatous inflammatory lesions in reaction to starch granules may also be seen in the ear canal and middle ear. The starch in the latter cases is derived, not from surgical glove powder, but from insufflations of antibiotic in which it is used as a vehicle. The antibiotic, with its base, is insufflated into the external ear in the treatment of external or middle ear otitis. Microscopically, there is an exudate of histiocytes and lymphocytes. Granules of starch are recognized as spherical or polyhedral basophilic bodies, $10-20\,\mu m$ in diameter, often within histiocytes. The granules show a Maltese cross birefringence and a brilliant red colouration after staining with periodic acid–Schiff reagent (Figures 2.2 and 2.3).

Hair granuloma
Biopsy sections taken from inflammatory lesions of the ear canal show quite commonly a granulomatous reaction of foreign body type with foreign body type giant cells surrounding and engulfing hair shafts (Figure 2.4). The hairs are derived from the patient's own hair, possibly by ingrowth from those near the orifice of the canal (in the same fashion as occurs in cases of pilonidal sinus of the sacro-iliac skin), or entry of small shafts after haircutting.

Keratin granuloma
Aural polyps frequently contain keratin with foreign body type giant cell granuloma in reaction to it. These are likely to be derived from a cholesteatoma of the middle ear[3] (Figure 2.5).

Relapsing polychondritis
Relapsing polychondritis is a disease characterized by recurring bouts of inflammation affecting cartilaginous structures and the eye. Although the cartilage of the external ear is most frequently involved, it is the inflammation with destruction of the cartilages of the respiratory

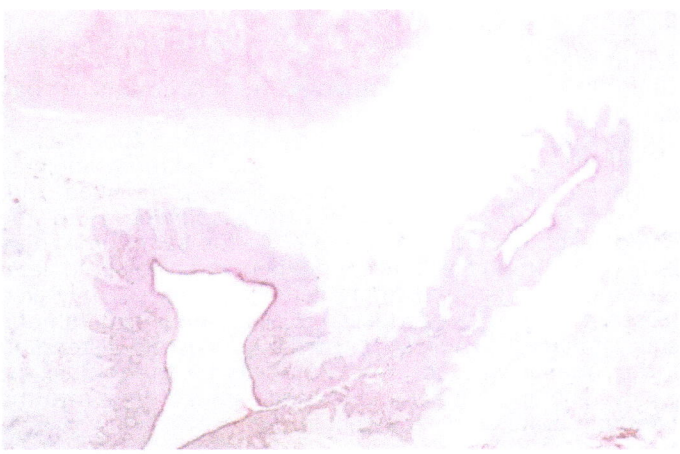

Figure 2.1 Preauricular sinus which is lined by stratified squamous epithelium and shows elastic cartilage in the adjacent connective tissue. H & E (A)

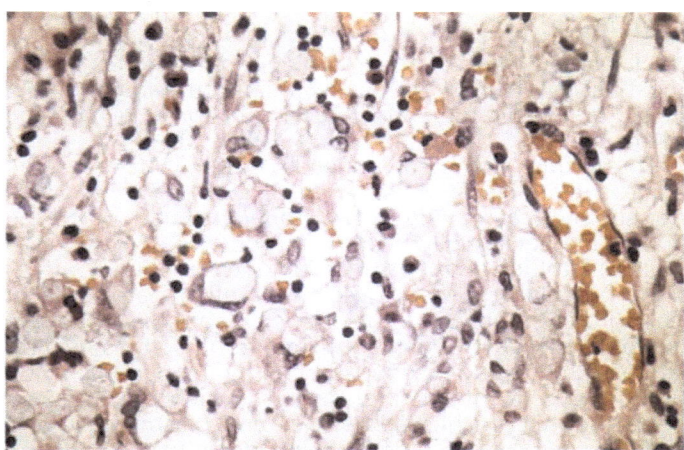

Figure 2.2 Starch granuloma of middle ear. There is a chronic inflammatory reaction with granules of starch phagocytosed by histiocytic cells. H & E (B)

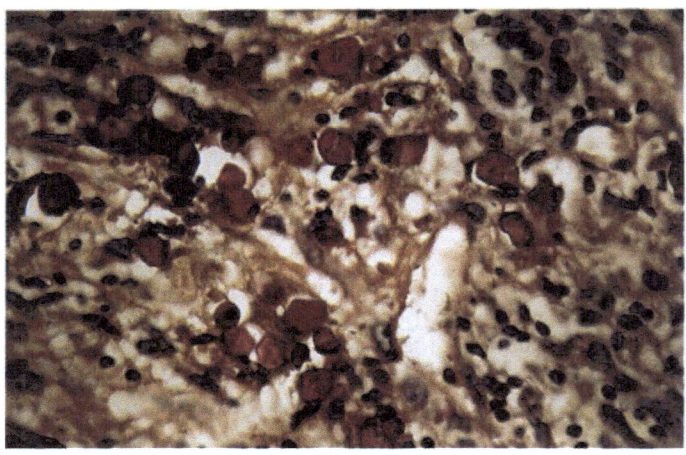

Figure 2.3 Starch granuloma of middle ear. The starch granules are stained red. Periodic acid–Schiff (B)

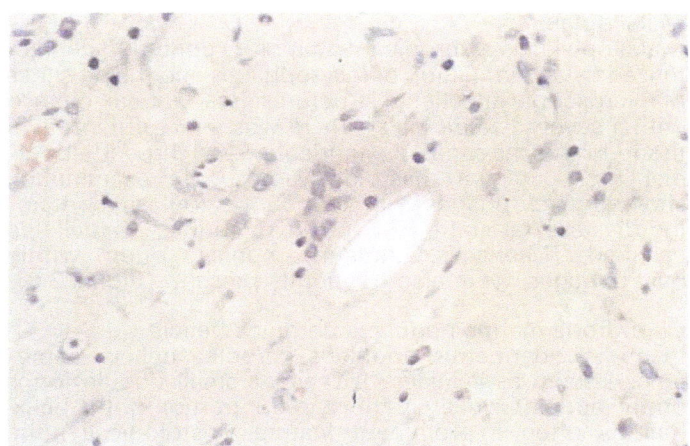

Figure 2.4 Hair shaft granuloma from ear canal. A hair shaft is engulfed by a foreign-body-type giant cell situated within chronic inflammatory tissue. H & E. Partially crossed polaroids (C)

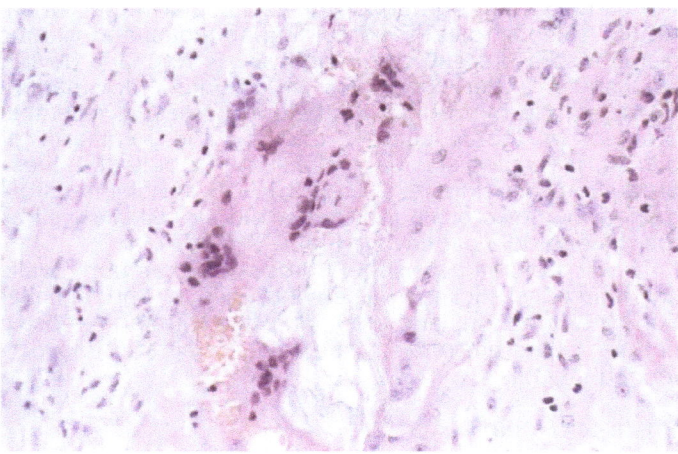

Figure 2.5 Keratin granuloma presenting in ear canal. Flecks of keratin are present within foreign-body-type giant cells. The keratin originated from a cholesteatoma of the middle ear. H & E (C)

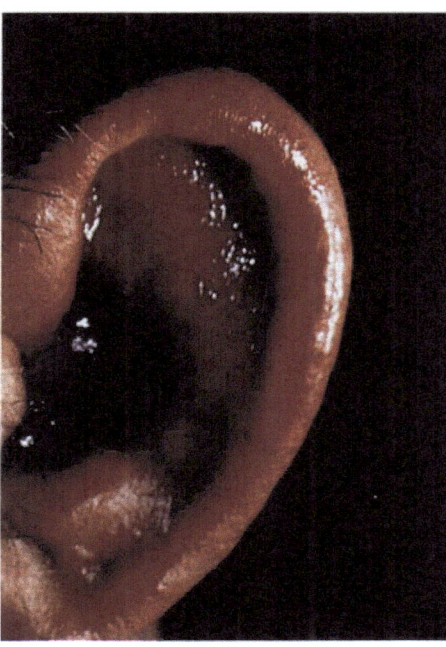

Figure 2.6 Acute stage of relapsing polychondritis showing swollen erythematous auricle

tract, particularly the larynx, which threatens life, and, in most cases where death has resulted from the condition, it is from respiratory obstruction due to such cartilage damage.

The lobule of the ear is usually normal. In the acute stage, the auricle is erythematous (Figure 2.6). The anterior surface may have a cobblestone appearance and the auricle may eventually become atrophic.

The histological appearances suggest a primary affection of cartilage prior to invasion by inflammatory tissue. The ground substance of the cartilage may become acidophilic (except for basophilia around some surviving lacunae), and show deeper staining by the periodic acid–Schiff method. Inflammatory tissue, which is composed of neutrophils in the early stages and plasma cells and lymphocytes later (Figure 2.7), invades into the cartilage from the perichondrium. Fibroblasts multiply, and eventually a dense poorly cellular scar results.

Lesions simulating neoplasms

A variety of lesions may be found in the external and middle ears which may show some similarity to neoplasms.

Malakoplakia

Malakoplakia is a chronic inflammatory condition characterized by accumulation of macrophages and the presence of microscopic lamellated structures. In a 10-year-old boy with a seventh-nerve palsy, there was a mass of vascular tissue in the ear canal, postauricular swelling and abnormal tissue in the mastoid. Microscopic examination showed macrophages with abundant cytoplasm containing diastase-resistant, PAS-positive granules. Lamellated calcified (Michaelis-Gutmann) bodies, often within macrophages, were also frequently present[4] (Figure 2.8).

Chondrodermatitis nodularis chronica helicis

In chondrodermatitis nodularis chronica helicis, sometimes known as Winkler's disease, a small nodule forms on the auricle, usually in the superior portion of the helix. Pain is often a prominent feature. Histologically, the nodule usually shows ulceration with marked irregular acanthosis at its margins. The collagen in the centre shows increased eosinophilia, is often degenerated, and is surrounded by chronic inflammatory granulation tissue. The perichondrium adjacent to the lesion is usually involved by the inflammatory tissue and the elastic cartilage of the auricle is also often degenerated (Figures 2.9 and 2.10).

Benign angiomatous nodules of face and scalp (atypical pyogenic granuloma or Kimura's disease)

Benign angiomatous nodules may occur anywhere in the skin, especially on the scalp and face, but there is a particular predilection for the external auricle and external auditory meatus.

Grossly, there are sessile or plaque-like red or reddish-blue lesions from 2 to 10 mm in diameter. Microscopically, there is a mixture of two proliferated elements in the dermis: blood vessels and lymphoid tissue. The blood vessels are often lined by plump, sometimes multilayered, endothelial cells (Figure 2.11). Occasionally, an artery or vein showing intimal fibrous thickening is part of the vascular component. The lymphoid tissue may possess germinal centres. Eosinophils, mast cells and macrophages may also be prominent.

Inflammatory Lesions of Middle Ear

Bacterial otitis media

Infection of the middle ear causes, not only generally-known inflammatory changes, but also others peculiar to the site.

Acute otitis media

Children are more often affected by this condition than adults.

The mucosa of the middle ear, including the mastoid air cells is congested and oedematous. Haemorrhage may be severe and the mucosa and air cells are filled with neutrophils (Figure 2.12). Pus is associated with the osteoclastic destruction of bone. At the same time, new bone formation takes place, commencing as osteoid, later becoming woven and finally lamellar. Fibrosis may also be active, even in the acute stage. The tympanic membrane shows marked congestion, the dilated vessels distending the connective tissue layer. Pus cells fill the middle ear cavity. The acute inflammation may spread deep into the temporal bone as osteomyelitis.

Chronic otitis media

An important feature of the gross appearances of chronic otitis media is the variation in the degree and extent of the inflammation. The tubotympanic region is the most frequently involved and mastoid air cells may also be affected. Mucopurulent material often fills the middle ear space in the tubotympanic region and may also be seen within mastoid air cells. In the inflamed areas, the mucosa is thickened and congestion may be severe. Granulation tissue formation may be extensive, showing as red thickened areas, particularly on the promontory, in the epitympanum, in the round and oval window niches and in the mastoid. The granulation tissue on the promonotory mucosa may be of sufficient thickness to protrude through the perforation in the tympanic membrane. Such a lesion is the common aural polyp presenting clinically in the external ear canal.

A variable degree of loss of ossicular bone may be observed. The most frequently affected ossicle is the incus, particularly in the region of its long process.

Cholesterol grauloma and cholesteatoma are frequently present in association with chronic otitis media (see below).

Microscopically, chronic inflammatory leukocytes and granulation tissue make up the composition of aural polyps. They are usually covered by columnar epithelium, which is often ciliated. Sometimes the epithelium is stratified squamous (Figures 2.13 and 2.14). If cholesteatoma is also present, foreign-body-type giant cells and keratin squames are usually abundant in the inflammatory tissue and polyps[3].

Unlike other parts of the respiratory tract, including the cartilaginous portion of the Eustachian tube, where tubulo-alveolar glands containing mucous and serous elements are present, the middle ear is normally devoid of glands. Under conditions of chronic inflammation, however, the middle ear epithelium comes to resemble the rest of the respiratory tract by the formation of glands. They consist usually of a simple tubule of mucus-producing cells (Figures 2.15 to 2.17). Glandular transformation may take place in the mastoid air cells as well as the main middle ear cavity (Figure 2.18).

The mastoid air cells show fibrosis and their bony walls are markedly thickened. Cement lines in the lamellar bone are numerous and irregular, often forming a mosaic pattern. There are often cystic cavities representing distended air cells.

Cholesterol granuloma

Yellow nodules are found in the tympanic cavity and mastoid in many cases of chronic otitis media. These are composed microscopically of cholesterol crystals (dissolved away to leave empty clefts in paraffin-embedded histological sections), surrounded by foreign-body-type giant cells and other chronic inflammatory cells (Figure 2.19). Such cholesterol granulomas are almost always

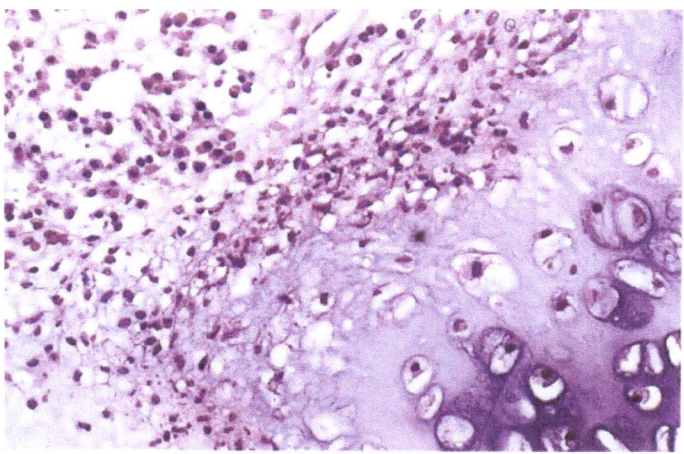

Figure 2.7 Cricoid cartilage biopsy in a case of relapsing polychondritis. The edge of the cartilage is eroded by inflammatory cells. There is pale staining of the cartilage near the interface with the inflammation. H & E (C)

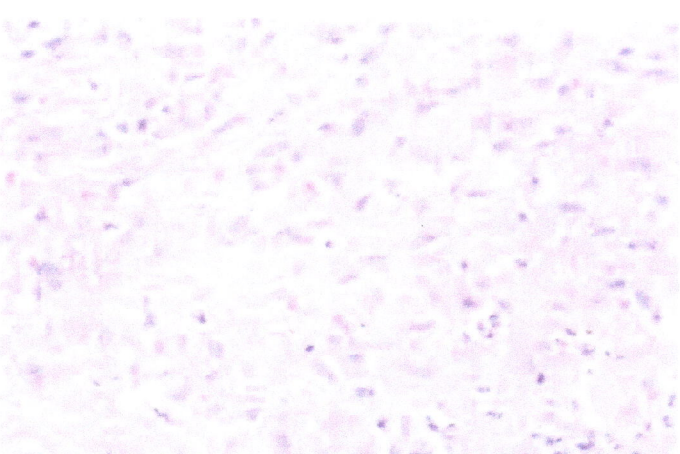

Figure 2.8 Malakoplakia of the middle ear. The tissue is composed of macrophages with abundant granular cytoplasm. Note also numerous calcified Michaelis–Gutmann bodies staining red. Periodic acid–Schiff (C)

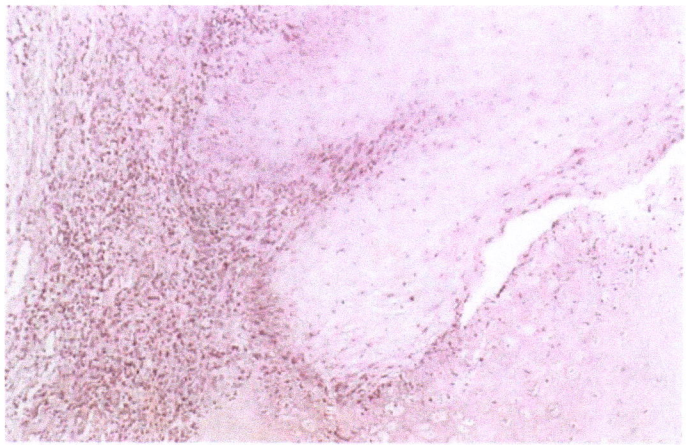

Figure 2.9 Chondrodermatitis nodularis chronica helicis. There is acanthotic squamous epithelium which extends to the cartilage of the pinna at the bottom right hand corner. H & E (B)

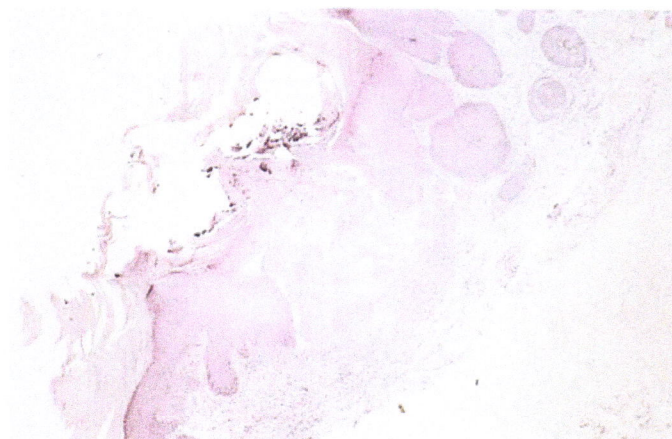

Figure 2.10 Chondrodermatitis nodularis chronica helicis. There is an irregular acanthosis at the margins of an ulcer, the crater of which is occupied by necrotic eosinophilic material. Inflammation extends down into the cartilage of the pinna. H & E (A)

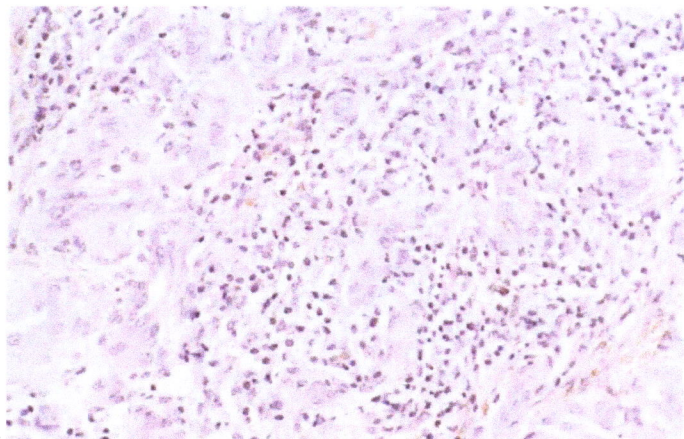

Figure 2.11 Benign angiomatous nodules (Kimura's disease) of external ear. The dermis of the skin around the pinna shows an exudate composed of abundant capillaries lined by plump endothelial cells and lymphoid tissue. H & E (B)

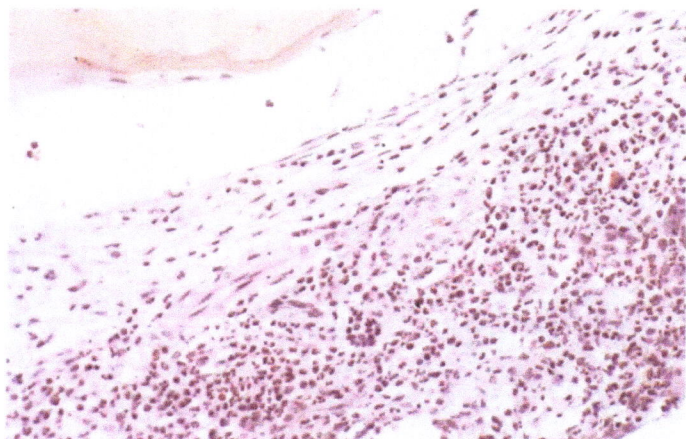

Figure 2.12 Acute inflammation of mastoid air cell. There is infiltration of the mucosa of the air cells by neutrophils. H & E (B)

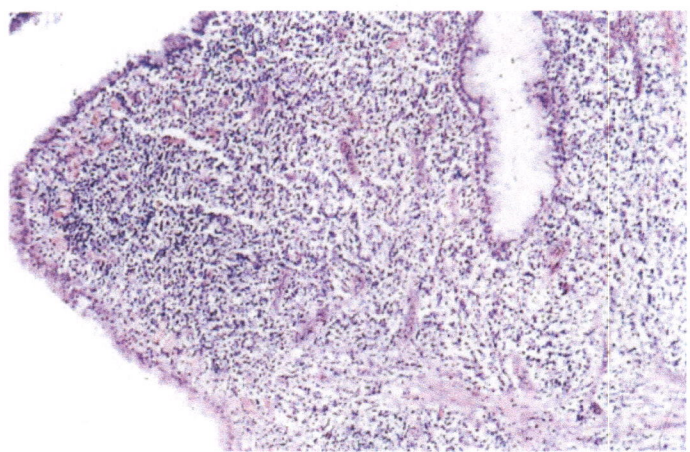

Figure 2.13 Aural polyp. This is composed of chronic inflammatory granulation tissue and is covered by columnar epithelium. Note the mucous gland within the polyp. This has been produced as a result of chronic inflammation in the middle ear.   H & E (B)

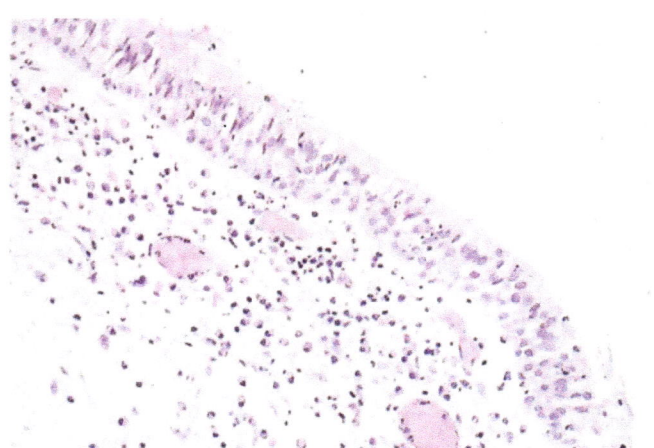

Figure 2.14 Aural polyp composed of chronic inf ammatory tissue and covered by ciliated columnar epithelium.   H & E (B)

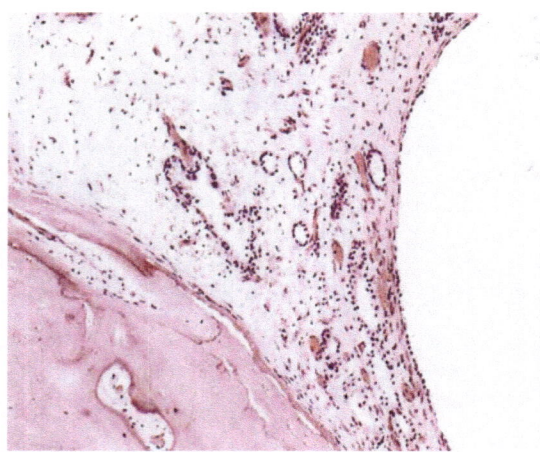

Figure 2.15 Glands formed in mucosa of middle ear in chronic otitis media. Bony wall of middle ear at bottom right.   H & E (B)

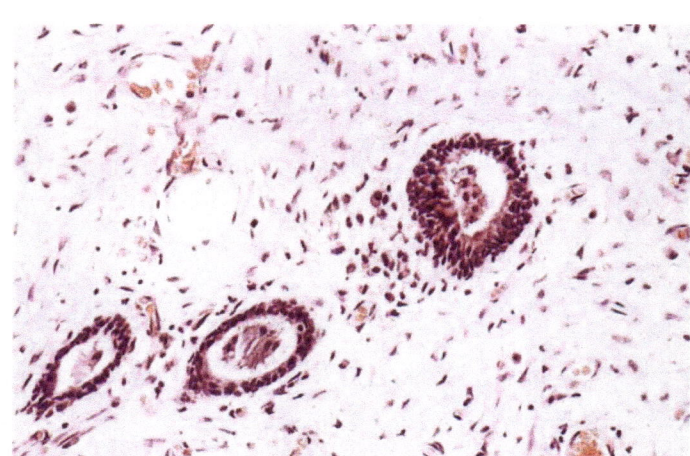

Figure 2.16 Middle ear mucosal glands in chronic otitis media.   H & E (B)

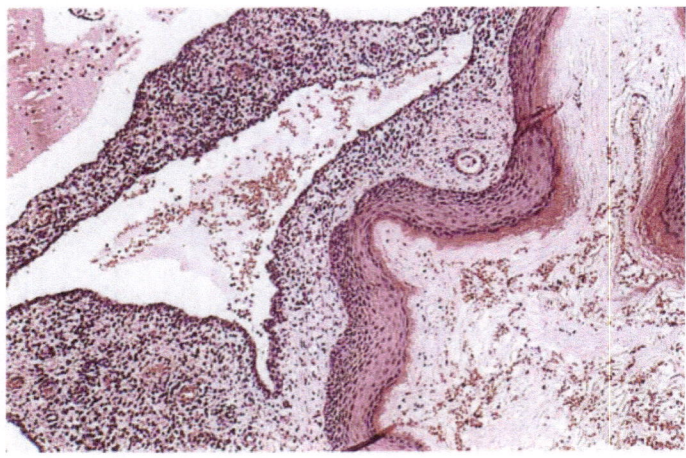

Figure 2.17 Middle ear gland in association with cholesteatoma.   H & E (B)

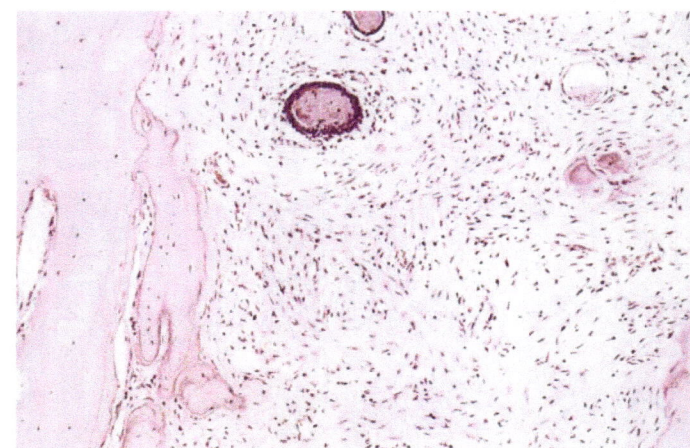

Figure 2.18 Glands formed in mastoid air cell in chronic mastoiditis. Bone of mastoid on right.   H & E (B)

found in the midst of haemorrhage in the middle ear mucosa. It seems likely that cholesterol granuloma is an end-product of haemorrhage.

Tympanosclerosis

Tympanosclerosis is a special form of fibrosis which is often encountered in chronic otitis media. Deposits of dense white tissue are laid down in the middle ear mucosa, not only on the tympanic membrane, which is particularly likely to occur in otitis media with effusion, but also, following chronic suppurative otitis media, on the crura of the stapes, within the tympanic cavity and sometimes in the mastoid. On dissection, the tympanosclerotic deposit may show a lamellated onion-skin-like structure.

Microscopically, the material is composed of hyaline collagen deposited in the mucosa. Deposits of calcium salts, appearing as basophilic dust-like areas, are irregularly distributed through the collagen. A multilayered structure corresponding to the gross appearance of lamellation is frequently observed. Bone is also often present in tympanosclerotic plaques (Figure 2.20).

There may be an autoimmune factor in the development of tympanosclerosis which leads to the degeneration of collagen. This is possibly enhanced by trauma, as in the use of ventilating tubes, which have been observed to lead to the development of tympanosclerosis of the tympanic membrane[5].

Cholesteatoma

Cholesteatoma is a pathological condition comprising the presence of stratified squamous epithelium within the middle ear cavity. It may be 'closed', in which a cystic squamous mass is present, or 'open', in which the keratin squames are shed directly into the middle ear cavity[6], 'congenital' or 'primary', in which a cyst is present behind an intact tympanic membrane, or 'acquired', in which there is a perforation of the tympanic membrane.

Congenital cholesteatoma

The congenital (primary) form of cholesteatoma appears as a cyst in the mesotympanum and is not related to the pars flaccida of the tympanic membrane. In the majority of cases, it is situated in relation to the upper anterior portion of the tympanic membrane in a space bounded by the handle of the malleus, the tensor tympani muscle and the processus cochleariformis. In some cases, it has been found to be occluding the Eustachian tube[7]. The term congenital cholesteatoma is also applied to a squamous epithelial cyst arising deep in the temporal bone and elsewhere, which causes damage by erosion of the skull. This is quite a different entity from the middle ear cholesteatoma.

Microscopically, the congenital form of cholesteatoma is usually a closed epidermoid cyst. The epithelium comprises only about four layers, the rest of the material of the cyst being composed of keratin squames (Figure 2.21).

The origin of congenital cholesteatoma in the majority of cases is likely to be from a cell rest that I described in the developing middle ear[8]. This was seen in most fetal ears up to 33 weeks' gestation. It is always in the same position – in the epithelium of the middle ear adjacent to the anterior limb of the osseous tympanic ring. The cell rest is plunging or spherical in most cases. Occasionally, it is composed of stratified squamous cells which are flattened on the epithelial surface (Figures 2.22 and 2.23). These two forms are likely to be precursors of the closed and open forms of cholesteatoma, respectively.

Acquired cholesteatoma

This form is much more frequent and is usually situated in the upper part of the middle ear cleft, usually with a perforation of the pars flaccida of the tympanic membrane through which the lesion discharges. The cholesteatoma usually has a lobulated outline, comprising, in most cases, the open form of the condition.

Under the microscope, the pearly material of the cholesteatoma, as in the congenital variety, consists of dead, fully differentiated, anucleate keratin squames. The capsule, often called the matrix, is composed of differentiated squamous cell epithelium, resting on connective tissue. There is a substantially greater thickness of the matrix in the case of the acquired variety as compared with the congenital variety. The cells are, moreover, larger with nuclei that show prominent nucleoli (Figure 2.24).

Chronic inflammatory changes are always present. Aural polyps, composed of inflammatory tissue, may be the first presenting feature of cholesteatoma. When examined histologically, they usually show a foreign-body giant-cell reaction to keratin squames (see above). In most cases of acquired cholesteatoma, at least one ossicle is seriously damaged, so interrupting the continuity of the ossicular chain.

Migration of stratified squamous epithelium from the outer surface of the tympanic membrane (see Chapter 1) is the currently favoured explanation for the invasion of squamous epithelium into the middle ear from the outer layer of the tympanic membrane to produce acquired cholesteatoma[9].

References

1. Cohen, D., Friedman, P. and Eilon, A. (1987). Malignant external otitis versus acute external otitis. *J. Laryngol. Otol.*, **101**, 211–215
2. Cohen, D. and Friedman, P. (1987). The diagnostic criteria of malignant external otitis. *J. Laryngol. Otol.*, **101**, 216–221
3. Milroy, C. M., Slack, R. W. T., Maw, A. R. and Bradfield, J. W. B. (1989). Aural polyps as predictors of underlying cholesteatoma. *J. Clin. Pathol.*, **42**, 460–465
4. Azadeh, B. and Ardehali, S. (1983). Malakoplakia of middle ear: a case report. *Histopathology*, **7**, 129–134
5. Poliquin, J. F., Catanzaro, A., Robb, J. and Schiff, M. (1981). Adaptive immunity of the tympanic membrane. *Am. J. Otolaryngol.*, **2**, 94–98
6. Politzer, A. (1891). Das Cholesteatom des Gehororgans von anatomische und klinischen Standpunkten. *Wien. Med. Woch.*, **8**, 331–334
7. Levenson, M. J., Parisier, S. C., Chute, P., Wenig, S. and Juarba, C. (1986). A review of twenty congenital cholesteatomas of the middle ear in children. *Otolaryngol. Head Neck Surg.*, **94**, 560–567
8. Michaels, L. (1986). An epidermoid formation in the developing middle ear: possible source of cholesteatoma. *J. Otolaryngol.*, **15**, 169–174
9. Michaels, L. (1989). The biology of cholesteatoma. *Otolaryngol. Clin. N. Am.*, **22**, 869–881

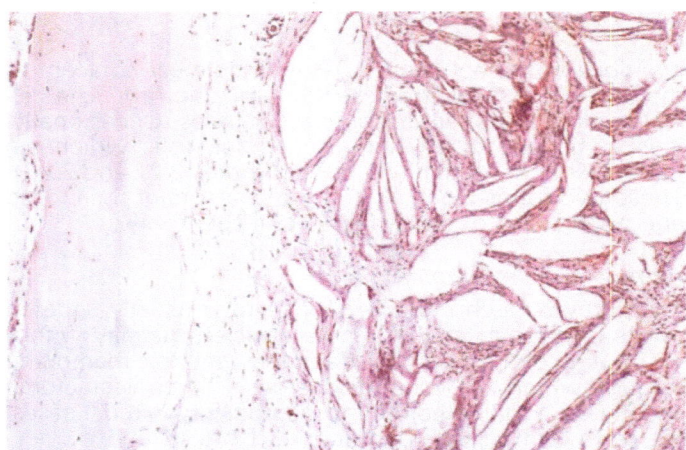

Figure 2.19 Cholesterol granuloma of middle ear. The lesion is composed of cholesterol clefts surrounded by foreign body giant cells and other chronic inflammatory cells.   H & E (B)

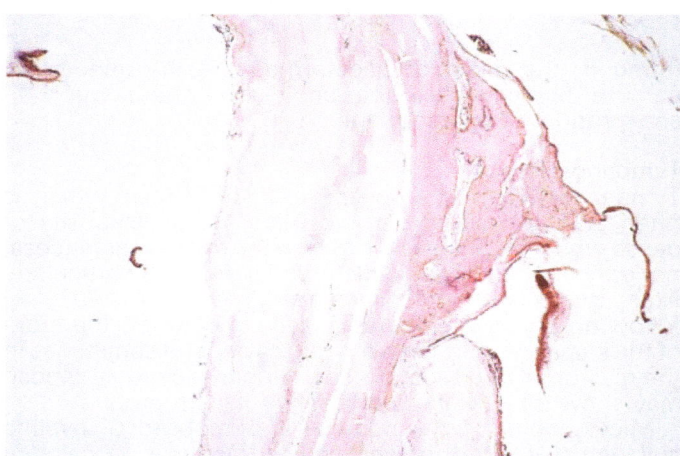

Figure 2.20 Tympanosclerotic plaque of middle ear mucosa. Layers of hyaline poorly cellular collagen thicken the mucosa on the left. The darker areas in the pale collagen represent zones of calcification. An area of ossification is seen on the right. The latter change is not uncommon in tympanosclerosis.   H & E (A)

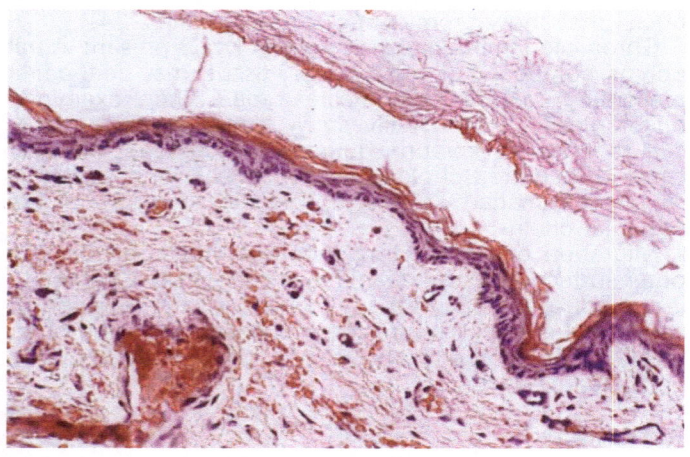

Figure 2.21 Congenital cholesteatoma showing thin-walled epidermoid cyst.   H & E (B)

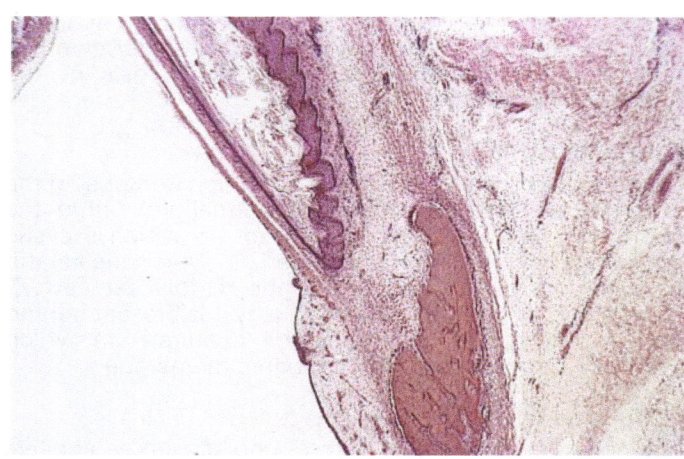

Figure 2.22 Epidermoid cell rest (arrow) in middle ear mucosa, just anterior to tympanic membrane in a fetus of 26 weeks gestation. The adjacent bone is the anterior limb of the tympanic ring. An additional epidermoid formation is present just anterior to it. The two apparently discrete structures fuse together in serial section.   H & E (A)

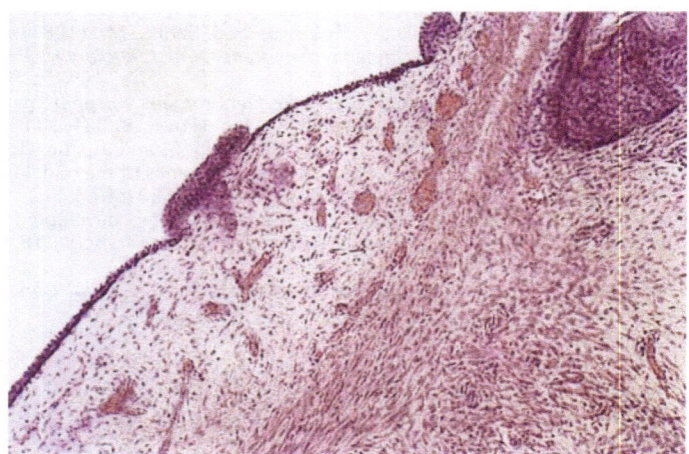

Figure 2.23 Higher power of epidermoid cell rest and similar adjacent structure from Figure 2.22.   H & E (B)

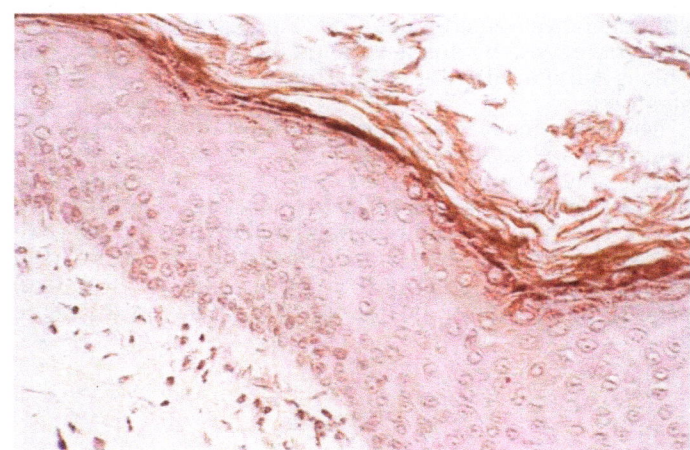

Figure 2.24 Acquired cholesteatoma. The stratified squamous epithelium shows prickle, granular and cornified layers. The epithelium is much thicker than that of the congenital cholesteatoma shown in Figure 2.21.   H & E (B)

Neoplasms of the Ear

3

Choristomas of the Middle Ear

Choristomas (developmental overgrowths of tissues not normally present in that particular part of the body) are occasionally seen in the middle ear. They are composed of either salivary gland or glial tissue.

Salivary gland choristomas consist, as a rule, of mixed mucous and serous elements, like the normal submandibular or sublingual gland, but unlike the parotid gland (which, because of its proximity to the ear, might be expected to contribute to such a new formation)[1] (Figures 3.1 and 3.2).

Glial masses are composed largely of astrocytic cells (Figures 3.3 and 3.4), the identity of which may be confirmed by immunochemical staining for glial acidic fibrillary protein.

Neoplasms of External Ear

The external ear is subject to a wide variety of neoplasms. Only those which are specific for the area will be dealt with.

Ceruminal gland neoplasms

External ear neoplasms derived from ceruminal glands are very uncommon. They can be benign or malignant (Table 3.1).

Ceruminoma

Ceruminomas (adenomas of the ceruminal glands) usually present with a blockage of the lateral part of the external auditory meatus, often associated with deafness and discharge. An important part of the clinical investigation of all glandular neoplasms of the ear canal is to exclude an origin in the parotid gland.

Gross appearances are those of a superficial grey mass, up to 4 cm in diameter, which is covered by skin.

Microscopically, this neoplasm is composed of regular glands, often with intraluminal projections (apocrine or capitation secretion). The glandular epithelium is distinctly bilayered, the outer layer being myoepithelial, but this may not be obvious in all parts of the neoplasm (Figures 3.5 and 3.6). In some ceruminomas, acid-fast fluorescent pigment, which is similar to that found in normal ceruminous glands, may be found in the tumour cells[2].

The most frequent of the malignant ceruminal gland neoplasms is adenoid cystic carcinoma, which has the gross and microscopic features of the corresponding major or minor salivary gland neoplasm, including its tendency to invade along nerve sheaths (see Chapter 6). Relentless recurrence and eventual bloodstream metastasis is likewise a feature of this cancer.

Neoplasms of bone

Benign fibro-osseous lesion (fibrous dysplasia)
Fibrous dysplasia and ossifying fibroma are lesions of bone with well-defined characteristics when they are of

Table 3.1 Classification of ceruminal gland neoplasms

Benign
Adenoma (ceruminoma)
Syringocystadenoma papilliferans
Chondroid syringoma – mixed tumour
Malignant
Adenoid cystic carcinoma
Mucoepidermoid carcinoma
Adenocarcinoma

odontogenic origin[3]. In the external ear, as in the maxilla (see Chapter 7), a decision as to whether a lesion is fibrous dysplasia or ossifying fibroma is more difficult. It is useful in practice to employ the umbrella term 'benign fibro-osseous lesion' for neoplasms of woven bone and fibrous tissue unless there is a polyostotic condition or endocrine/pigmentary disturbance pointing to fibrous dysplasia[4].

In most cases, there is progressive bony occlusion of the external auditory meatus. X-ray examination reveals an enlargement of the temporal bone associated with sclerosis or a uniform 'ground glass' appearance of the swollen bone.

The gross appearance is one of yellowish-white resilient tissue, which occasionally includes small cysts filled with an amber-coloured fluid. The transition to normal bone is sharp. Microscopically, irregular trabeculae of woven bone are embedded in a connective tissue stroma. The bony trabeculae often lack osteoblasts around their periphery but this is by no means invariable (Figures 3.7 and 3.8).

The majority of patients with benign fibro-osseous lesion of the temporal bone require surgical removal of the abnormal bony tissue[5].

Neoplasms of the Middle Ear

The neoplasms which have been reported as growing in the middle ear are listed in Table 3.2.

Adenoma

A benign glandular neoplasm confined to the middle ear and originating from its epithelium was first described in 1976[6,7].

The neoplasm appears grey or reddish at operation and

Table 3.2 Neoplasms of the middle ear

Adenoma
Meningioma
Paraganglioma
Squamous cell carcinoma
Inverted papilloma
Papillary adenocarcinoma
Metastatic

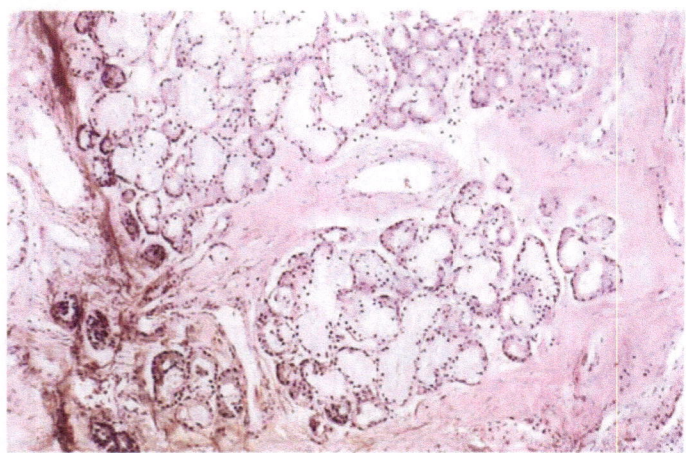

Figure 3.1 Salivary gland choristoma of middle ear. Lobules of salivary gland tissue are present in the mucosa.   H & E (A)

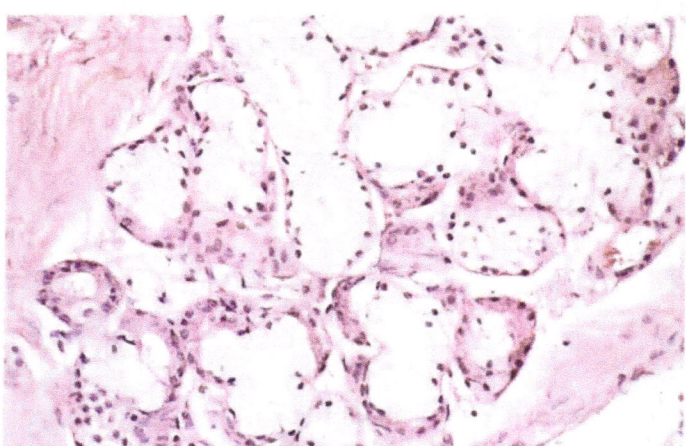

Figure 3.2 Higher power of part of Figure 3.1 showing acini composed of both mucous and serous glandular elements.   H & E (B)

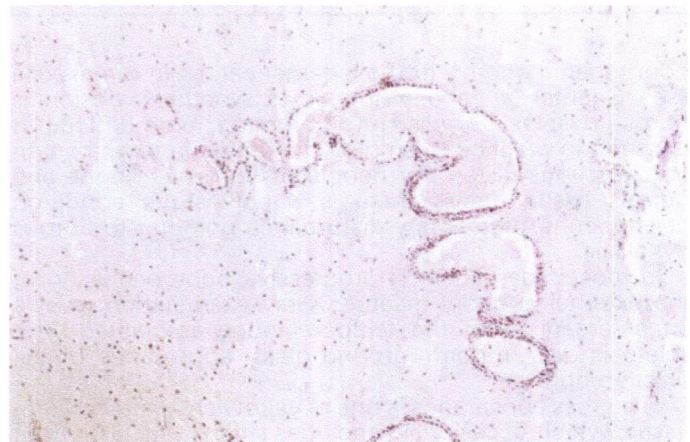

Figure 3.3 'Glioma' of middle ear. The tissue formation is composed of fibrillary astrocytes. Glands formed by 'irritated' middle ear mucosa are also present.   H & E (A)

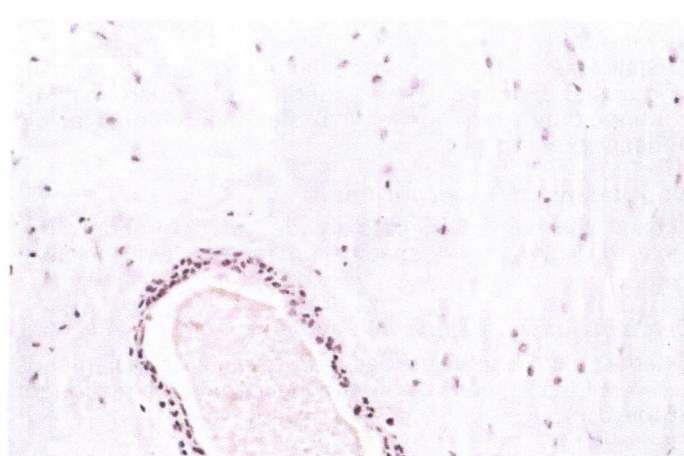

Figure 3.4 Higher power of part of Figure 3.3 showing fibrillary astrocytes and part of gland.   H & E (B)

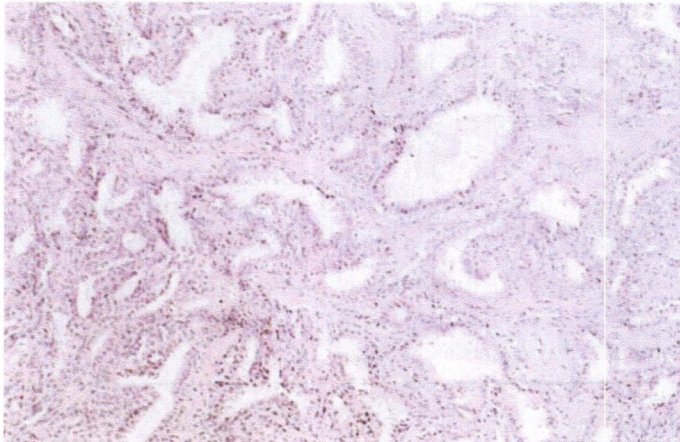

Figure 3.5 Ceruminoma of ear canal composed of regular glands with some intraluminal projections. The glands are separated from each other by a small amount of connective tissue.   H & E (B)

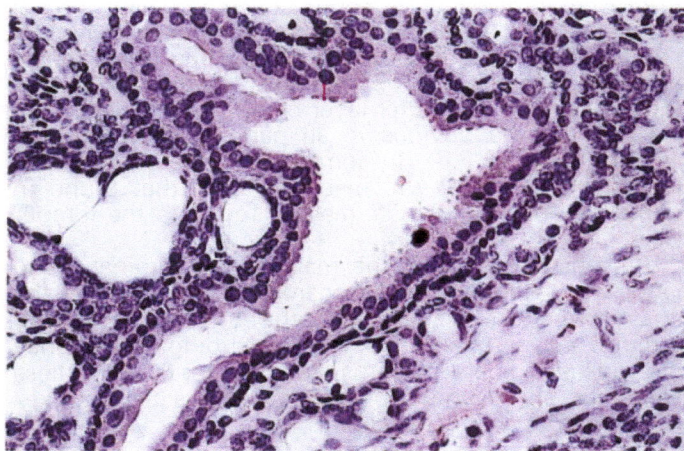

Figure 3.6 Ceruminoma showing intraluminal projections and bilayered epithelium.   H & E (C)

is not particularly vascular. It seems to peel away from the walls of the surrounding middle ear with ease, although ossicles may sometimes be entrapped in the tumour mass and may even show destruction.

Microscopically, adenoma is composed of closely apposed small glands with a 'back-to-back' appearance (Figures 3.9 to 3.11). In some places, a solid or trabecular arrangement is present (Figure 3.12). Sheet-like disorganized areas are seen in which the glandular pattern appears to be lost. This is probably artefactual and related to the effects of the trauma of the biopsy on the delicate structure of this neoplasm, but the appearance may lead one to suspect malignancy. The cells are regular and cuboidal and may enclose luminal secretion. No myoepithelial layer is seen.

Adenoma of the middle ear is a benign neoplasm. The treatment is by simple excision resulting, in the cases of Hyams and Michaels[6] for instance, in only a single recurrence.

Carcinoid tumour

Carcinoid tumours, diagnosed on the basis of cytoplasmic neuroendocrine granules on electron microscopy, have been reported in the middle ear[8]. Such neoplasms that I have seen not only showed those structures, but were also argyrophil and possessed immunochemical characteristics of a neuroendocrine lesion, namely the presence of neurone-specific enolase and protein gene product[9]. Apart from these features, the neoplasms are otherwise typical of adenoma as described above and there seems, at present, little justification for invoking the term 'carcinoid' with its suggestion of endocrine and a more aggressive behaviour, which these tumours did not possess.

Meningioma

Meningiomas are usually intracranial neoplasms. Extracranial meningiomas are, however, sometimes seen. Like the intracranial variety, they are thought to arise from arachnoid villi which may be formed at a number of sites in the temporal bone. Thus, meningiomas may arise from a wide area within the temporal bone itself[10]. The commonest temporal bone site for primary meningioma is in the middle ear cleft. Symptoms are usually those of otitis media; involvement of the chorda tympani and the facial nerve may also occur.

Gross appearances are those of a granular or even gritty mass. Microscopically, the neoplasm takes the same forms as any of the well-described intracranial types of meningioma. The commonest variety seen in the middle ear is the meningothelial type, in which the tumour cells are arranged in epithelioid groups of regular cells, often disposed into whorls (Figures 3.13 and 3.14). Fibroblastic and psammatous varieties are also sometimes seen in the middle ear.

There are indications that at least some of the meningiomas of apparently middle ear origin eventually manifest themselves as arising from outside the petrous bone, probably on its external surface, invading the middle ear secondarily. Such tumours do not necessarily present with the symptoms of a space-occupying intracranial lesion.

Jugulotympanic paraganglioma

Most jugulotympanic paragangliomas arise from the paraganglion situated in the wall of the jugular bulb; a minority of the tumours arise from the paraganglion situated near the middle ear surface of the promontory. The distinction between jugular and tympanic paragangliomas can easily be made radiologically. The jugular neoplasm shows evidence of invasion of the petrous bone. The tympanic neoplasm is confined to the middle ear.

The majority of patients with this neoplasm are females.

The mean age of onset is 50 years. The commonest symptom is hearing loss which is of conductive type. On examination, a red vascular mass is seen either behind the intact tympanic membrane or sprouting through the latter into the external auditory meatus. At operation, the tumour bleeds severely during removal.

The neoplasm is a reddish sprouting mass at its external canal surface. In the jugular variety, the petrous temporal bone is largely replaced by red firm material and the middle ear space is occupied by soft neoplasm as far as the tympanic membrane. The bony labyrinth is rarely invaded by paraganglioma.

The neoplasm in a typical section shows some resemblance to the carotid body tumour. Epithelioid uniform cells are separated by numerous blood vessels. The tumour cells often form clusters or 'Zellballen' (Figures 3.15 and 3.16). Nuclei are usually uniform and small, but diagnosis is sometimes made difficult by the presence of bizarre or multinucleate cells. These appearances do not denote a malignant origin (Figure 3.17). A fibrous stroma is sometimes encountered. Reticulin stain usually shows groups of tumour cells surrounded by reticulin, without reticulin fibres between the cells. Neurone-specific enolase and PGP 9.5[9], as demonstrated by the immunoperoxidase method, may be found in the cells of this neoplasm. Formalin-induced fluorescence, indicating significant catecholamine content, has been detected in paragangliomas of the middle ear by a touch technique[11]. Electron microscopic examination shows membrane-bound electron-dense granules in the cytoplasm of the tumour cells.

Jugulotympanic paraganglioma is a neoplasm of slow growth. The jugular variety infiltrates the petrous bone but distant metastasis is rare. Recurrence is stated to occur in from a third to a half of treated cases and the mortality is about 17%[12].

Squamous carcinoma

Squamous carcinoma is very uncommon but, nevertheless, is the most frequent of the neoplasms of the middle ear. There is an equal incidence between the sexes. The average age of occurrence is 60 years.

Aural discharge and conductive hearing loss are present in all patients. Pain in the ear, bleeding and facial palsy are common.

In microscopic sections, the tumour may be seen arising from surface squamous epithelium, itself metaplastic from cubical epithelium. In certain areas, an origin from the basal layer of cuboidal or columnar epithelium may be seen. The neoplasm shows a similar degree of keratinization and epithelial differentiation as neoplasms of the same histological type elsewhere in the upper respiratory tract.

The mode of spread of the neoplasm from the middle ear epithelium was ascertained in temporal bone autopsy sections by Michaels and Wells[13] and subsequently confirmed radiologically in living patients[14]. The carcinoma tends to grow into and erode the thin bony plate which separates the medial wall of the middle ear, at its junction with the Eustachian tube, from the carotid canal. Having reached the carotid canal the growth will extend rapidly along the sympathetic nerves and the tumour is then impossible to eradicate surgically. Another important method of spread is through the bony walls of the posterior mastoid air cells to the dura of the posterior surface of the temporal bone. From there it spreads medially, enters the internal auditory meatus and may then invade the cochlea and vestibule. Spread into the lamellar bone in both of these situations is along vascular channels between bone trabeculae. A similar type of bone invasion may also occur from other parts of the middle ear surface, such as in the region of the facial nerve. The special bone

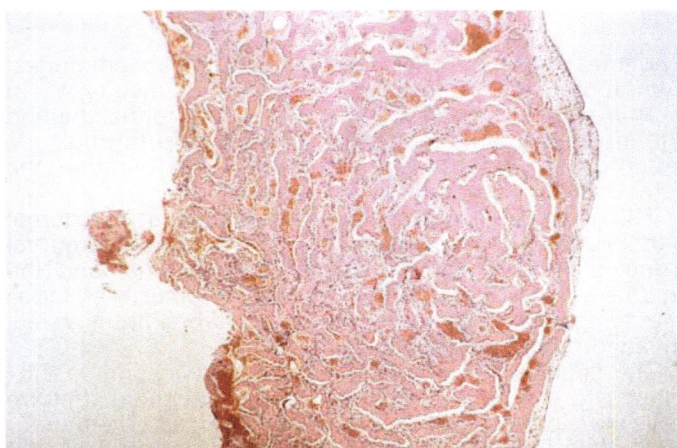

Figure 3.7 Benign fibro-osseous lesion in bone of ear canal. Trabeculae of woven bone are embedded in a connective tissue stroma. H & E (A)

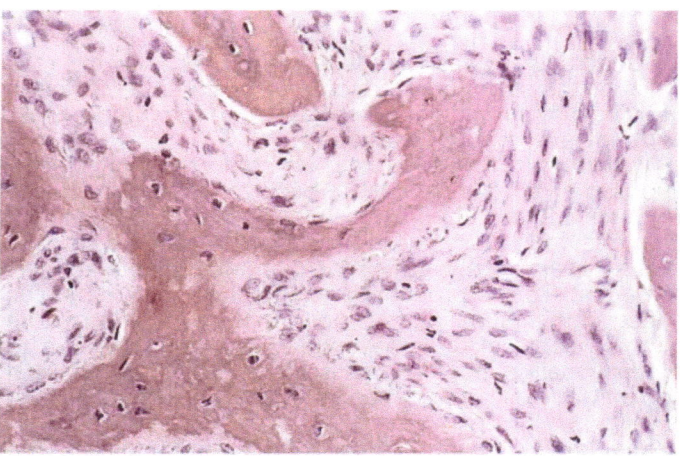

Figure 3.8 Higher power of benign fibro-osseous lesion of ear canal showing trabeculae of woven bone and intervening fibrous tissue with fibroblasts. H & E (B)

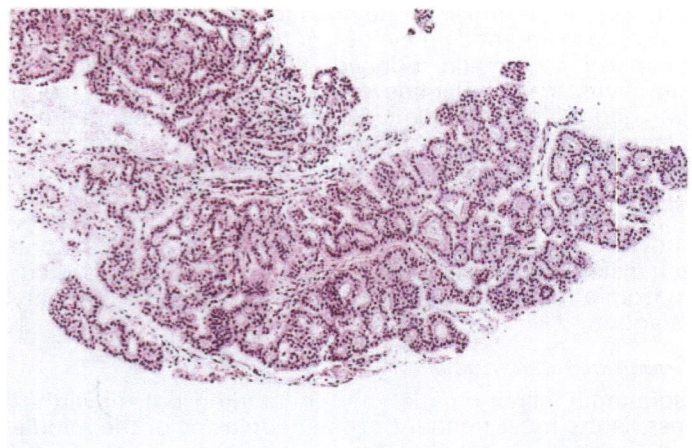

Figure 3.9 Adenoma of middle ear showing regular small glands. H & E (A)

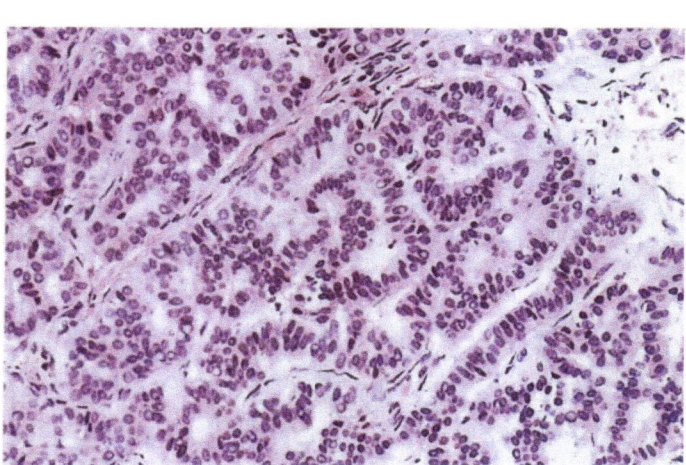

Figure 3.10 Adenoma of middle ear. The glands are closely packed in a 'back-to-back' arrangement. H & E (B)

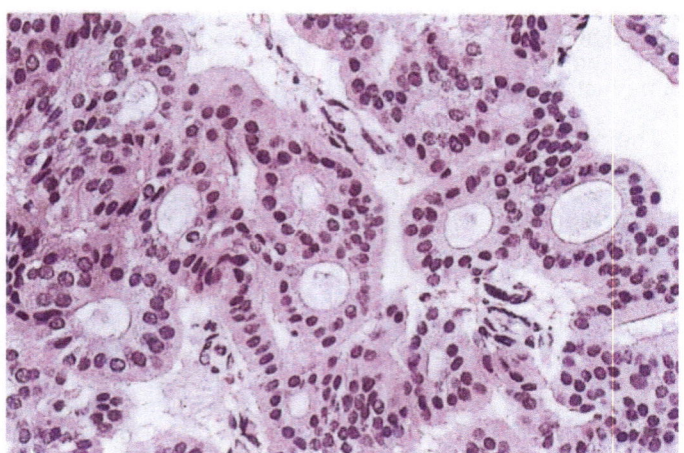

Figure 3.11 Adenoma of middle ear. The cells lining the glands are regular and cuboidal. H & E (C)

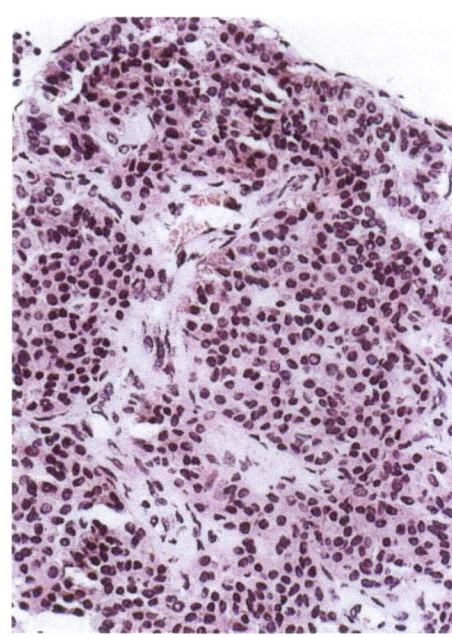

Figure 3.12 Solid arrangement of tumour cells in adenoma of middle ear. H & E (B)

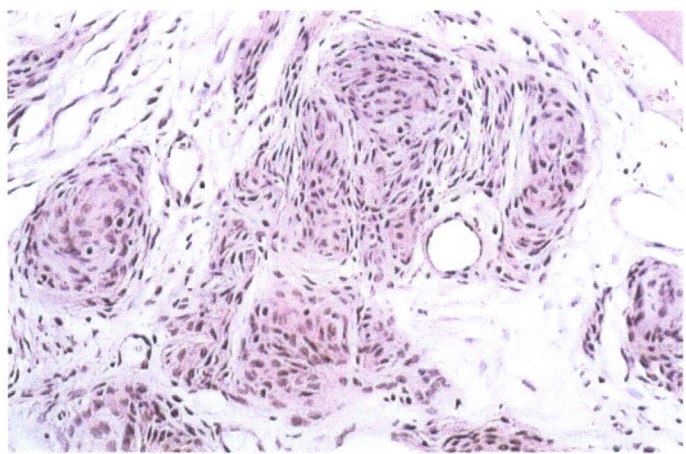

Figure 3.13 Meningioma of middle ear showing regular epithelioid groups with a slight tendency to a whorled arrangement. H & E (B)

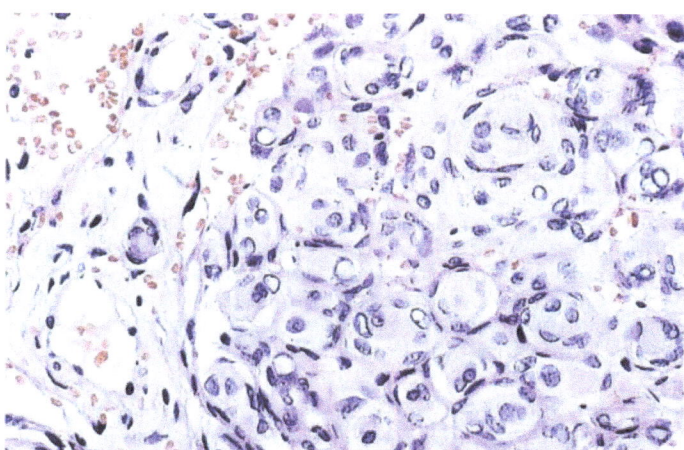

Figure 3.14 Meningioma of middle ear showing concentrically arranged whorls of epithelioid cells. H & E (B)

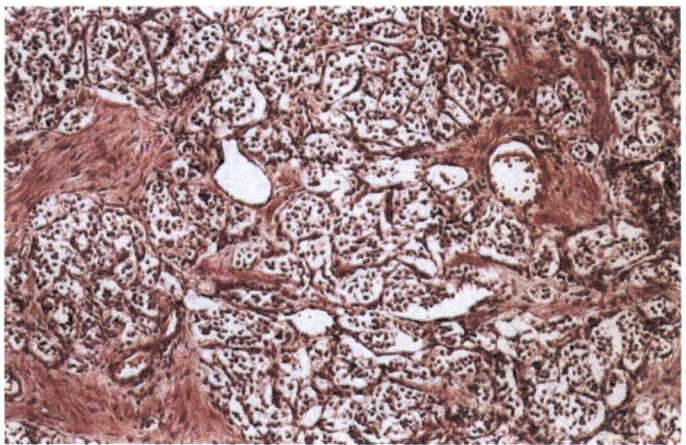

Figure 3.15 Jugular paraganglioma. The tumour cells form small clusters with numerous intervening blood vessels. H & E (A)

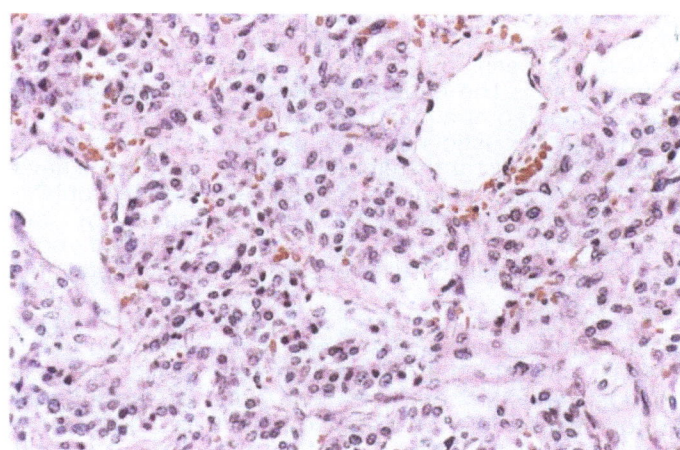

Figure 3.16 Higher magnification of jugular paraganglioma showing small regular cells in 'Zellballen' groups between blood vessels. H & E (B)

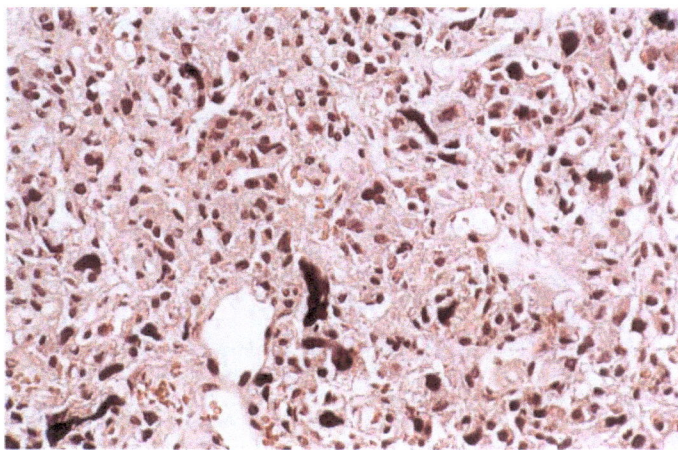

Figure 3.17 Paraganglioma of middle ear (tympanic type) showing bizarre and multinucleate cells. H & E (B)

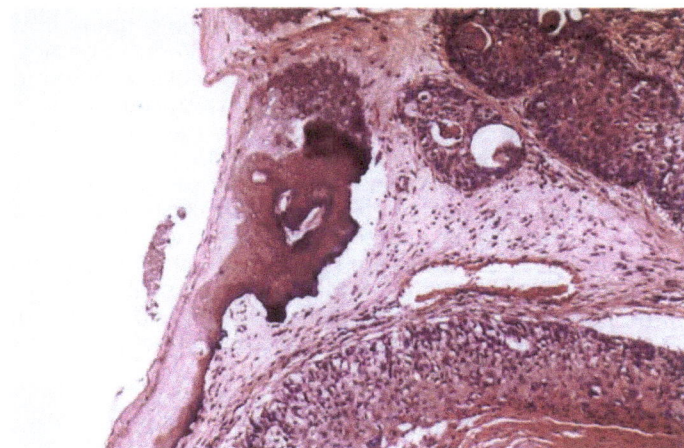

Figure 3.18 Squamous carcinoma of middle ear encroaching on, but not invading, footplate of stapes and annulus fibrosus. H & E (A)

of the osseous labyrinth is, on the other hand, peculiarly resistant to direct spread of growth from tumour within the middle ear; even the oval and round windows are not invaded (Figure 3.18). When invasion does occur, it takes place after entry of the tumour into the internal auditory meatus and penetration of the bone by way of the filaments of the vestibular and cochlear divisions of the eighth nerve. In the later stages, tumour grows extensively in the middle cranial fossa and may invade the condyle of the mandible. Lymph node metastasis is unusual and spread by the bloodstream even more so. Death is usually due to direct intracranial extension.

Invading from the nasopharynx

On rare occasions, tumours of the nasopharynx may occur in the middle ear which they appear to have reached by spread through the Eustachian tube. I have observed papillary adenocarcinoma, cylindric cell carcinoma and squamous cell carcinoma extending by this passage.

Neoplasms of Inner Ear

Acoustic neuroma

Acoustic neuroma, a schwannoma of the eighth cranial nerve, is the most frequent neoplasm of the temporal bone. It has been found at a frequency of four of 883 postmortems[15]. The neoplasm affects females in 64% of cases, appearing at a mean age of 45 years.

Although acoustic neuroma usually grows from the vestibular division of the eighth nerve, most patients have hearing loss and tinnitus at presentation, while only a few complain of vertigo. Defective function of both the cochlea and the labyrinth are, however, elicited more often by the sophisticated procedures of audiometry and caloric testing.

The neoplasm is of round or oval shape. The larger tumours often have a mushroom shape with two components, an elongated intratemporal stalk and an expanded extratemporal part. The bone of the internal auditory meatus is often widened funnelwise by the slow growth of the neoplasm. A fluid exudate may frequently be observed in the cochlea and vestibule (Figure 3.19).

Acoustic neuroma has the features of a neoplasm of Schwann cells or neurilemmoma with arrangement of the cells into a specific, almost organoid, pattern. It is customary to define the two areas of different appearance in neurilemmomas as Antoni A and Antoni B types. The tumour cells in both areas are Schwann cells or their derivatives. In the Antoni A areas, the spindle cells of the neoplasm are closely packed together and there is a tendency to towards palisading of nuclei. Verocay bodies, whorled formations of palisaded tumour cells resembling tactile corpuscles, may be present in Antoni A areas (Figures 3.20 to 3.24). The spindle cells frequently show a moderate degree of pleomorphism, with mitotic figures on rare occasions, but this does not denote a malignant tendency on the part of the neoplasm. Antoni B areas show a loose reticular pattern, sometimes with histiocytic proliferation. These areas are rarely prominent in acoustic neuromas. Homogeneous fluid exudate is usually present in the perilymphatic spaces of the cochlea and vestibule. This may arise as a result of pressure by neoplasm on veins in the meatus.

Bilateral acoustic neuroma

Bilateral acoustic neuroma is not associated with cutaneous neuromas and cafe-au-lait spots (von Recklinghausen's disease) but represents a separate hereditary condition – neurofibromatosis 2 – inherited as an autosomal dominant[16].

At postmortem, neural neoplasms are frequent in both eighth nerves and other central nerves (Figure 3.25). There are often many small schwannomas and neurofibromas growing on cranial nerves. Meningiomas, usually multiple, are also present in this condition. As well as the major acoustic tumours, meningiomas and neurofibromas of microscopic size may be present, the former on the meninges in the vicinity of the acoustic neuromas and sometimes even intermixed with them microscopically. The neuromas are histologically identical to those of the single acoustic tumours, but are more invasive in their behaviour, tending to involve the cochlea and vestibule[17].

Papilloma (adenoma) of endolymphatic system

There is a small literature indicating the occasional presentation of a papillary epithelial neoplasm arising from the epithelial covering of the endolymphatic system, sometimes associated with Meniere's disease[18].

Leukaemia

Leukaemia may be seen to involve the inner ear in two ways:

1. More frequently, haemorrhage may occur into the membranous spaces, perilymphatic and/or endolymphatic. If the patient survives long enough, the organ of Corti and spiral ganglion will become severely degenerated and connective tissue and bone will grow into the scalae.

2. In some cases of leukaemia, particularly those of chronic lymphocytic leukaemia, there is severe leukaemic infiltration of the perilymphatic spaces of the cochlea (Figure 3.26).

The symptom of hearing loss, often reversible, may also result from an increased concentration of plasma proteins which can occur in some lymphoreticular neoplasms, leading to an increased plasma viscosity[19].

Neoplasms Metastatic to Temporal Bone

The temporal bone is frequently the site of blood-borne metastasis for carcinomas originating in the following organs, in order of frequency: breast, kidney, lung, stomach, larynx, prostate and thyroid. Malignant melanoma may also be a common source of metastasis to this site[20]. The neoplasm may disseminate along vascular channels in the petrous bone and along nerves emanating from the internal auditory meatus into the labyrinthine structures and bone. I have seen a case of metastatic adenocarcinoma in which the neoplasm grew along the connective tissue of the tympanic membrane between the squamous and cuboidal epithelia (Figure 3.27).

References

1. Quaranta, A., Mininni, F. and Resta, L. (1981). Salivary gland choristoma of the middle ear. A case report. *J. Laryngol. Otol.*, **95**, 953–956
2. Cankar, V. and Crowley, H. (1964). Tumors of ceruminous glands: A clinicopathological study of seven cases. *Cancer*, **17**, 67–75
3. Pindborg, J. J. and Kramer, I. R. H. (1971). Histological typing of odontogenic tumours, jaw cysts and allied lesions. *International Histological Classification of Tumours. No. 5.* (Geneva: World Health Organization)
4. Dehner, L. P. (1973). Tumors of the mandible and maxilla in children. 1. Clinicopathologic study of 46 histologically benign lesions. *Cancer*, **31**, 364–384
5. Nager, G. T., Kennedy, D. W. and Kopstein, E. (1982). Fibrous dysplasia: a review of the disease and its manifestations in the temporal bone. *Ann. Otol. Rhinol. Laryngol.*, **91** [Suppl. 92]
6. Hyams, V. J. and Michaels, L. (1976). Benign adenomatous neoplasms (adenoma) of the middle ear. *Clin. Otolaryngol.*, **1**, 7–26
7. Derlacki, E. L. and Barney, P. L. (1976). Adenomatous tumors of the middle ear and mastoid. *Laryngoscope*, **86**, 1123–1135
8. Murphy, G. E., Pilch, B. Z., Dickersin, G. R., Goodman, M. C. and Nadol, J. B. (1980). Carcinoid tumour of the middle ear. *Am. J.*

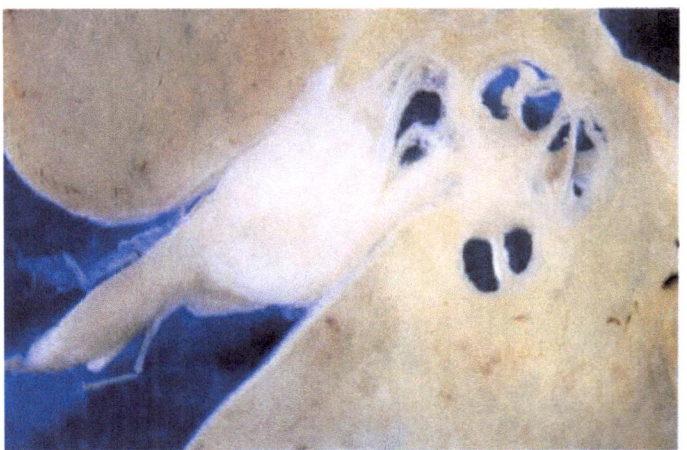

Figure 3.19 Acoustic neuroma in microsliced temporal bone. The neoplasm is arising from the vestibular division of the eighth nerve and compressing the cochlear division. Note the granular deposit lining the cochlea

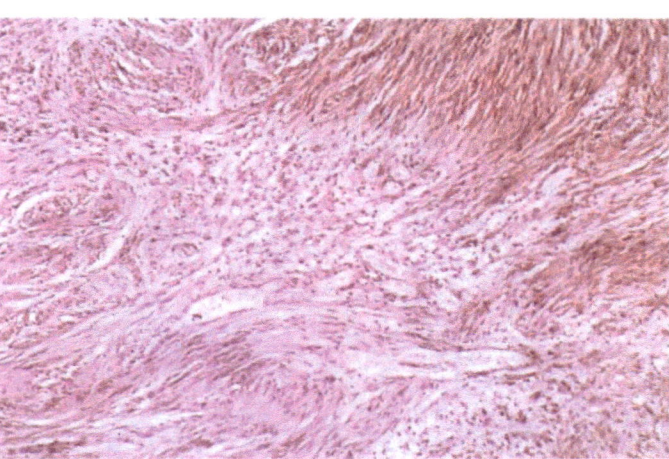

Figure 3.20 Acoustic neuroma. Both Antoni A and B appearances are present in this field.   H & E (A)

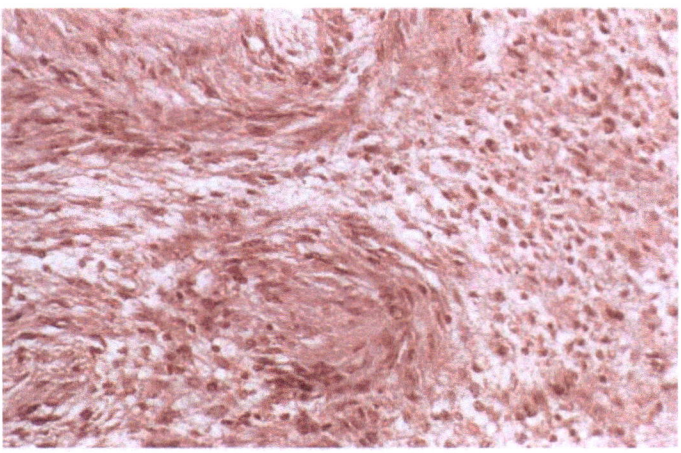

Figure 3.21 Acoustic neuroma showing Verocay body composed of whorled formations of palisaded tumour cells.   H & E (B)

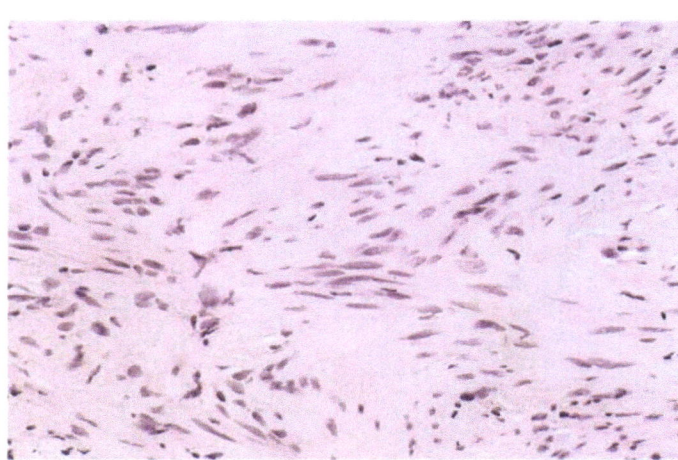

Figure 3.22 Antoni A area of acoustic neuroma showing palisading.   H & E (B)

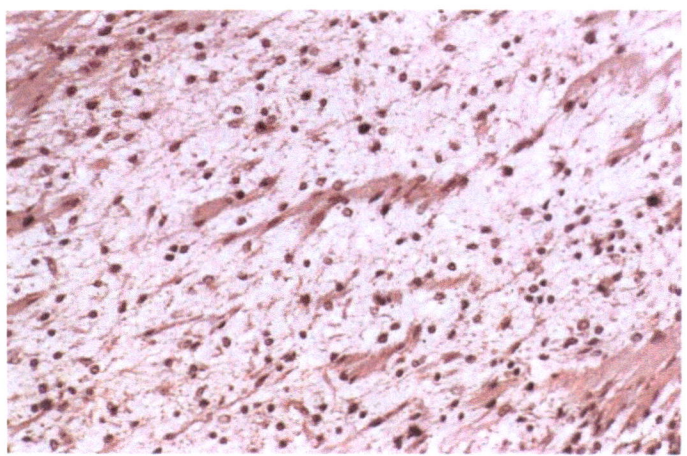

Figure 3.23 Acoustic neuroma showing Antoni B appearance characterized by loose reticular pattern.   H & E (B)

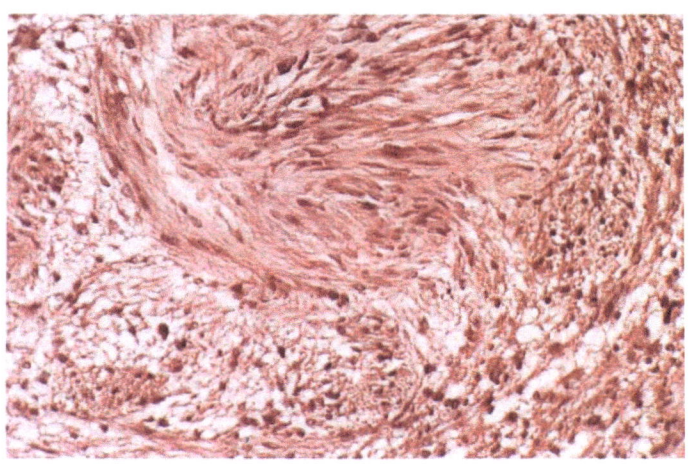

Figure 3.24 Acoustic neuroma showing Antoni A (palisading) and Antoni B appearances.   H & E (B)

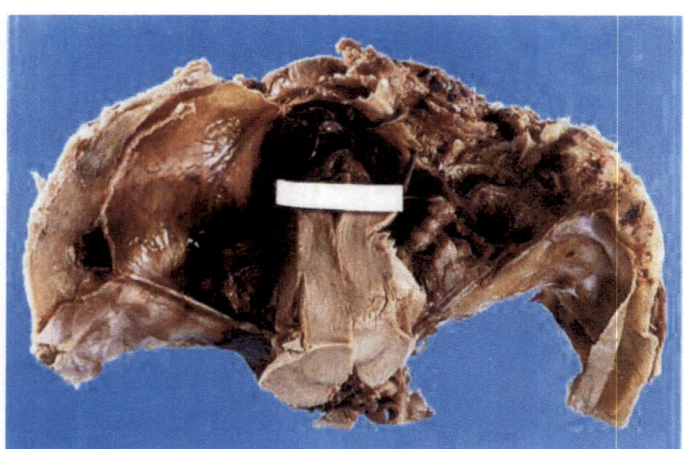

Figure 3.25 Bilateral acoustic neuroma in specimen composed of the two temporal bones with the medulla in the midline. Note that the tumours project from the posterior walls of the temporal bones

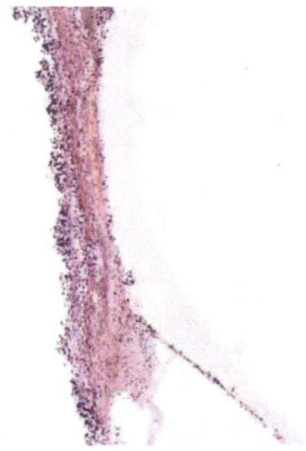

Figure 3.26 Cochlea in chronic lymphatic leukaemia. Numerous lymphoid cells are present in the scala tympani adjacent to the basilar membrane.   H & E (B)

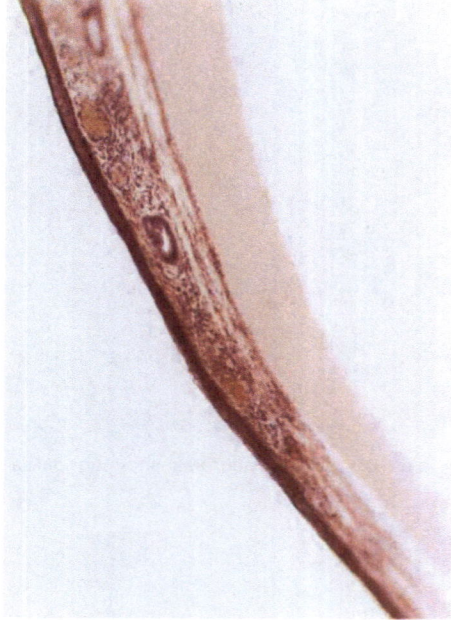

Figure 3.27 Metastatic adenocarcinoma of temporal bone. Section of tympanic membrane. Adenocarcinoma has grown from the bony tympanic ring into the connective tissue layer of the membrane.   H & E (A)

Clin. Pathol., **73**, 816–823

9. Rode, J., Dhillon, A. P., Doran, J. F., Jackson, P. and Thompson, R. J. (1985). PGP 9.5, a new marker for human neuroendocrine tumours. Histopathology, **9**, 147–158

10. Nager, G. T. (1963). Meningiomas Involving the Temporal Bone. (Springfield Ill.: Charles C. Thomas)

11. DeLillis, R. A. and Roth, J. A. (1971). Norepinephrine in a glomus jugulare tumor. Arch. Pathol., **92**, 73–75

12. Rosenwasser, H. (1973). Long-term results of therapy of glomus jugulare tumors. Arch. Otolaryngol., **97**, 49–54

13. Michaels, L. and Wells, M. (1980). Squamous cell carcinoma of the middle ear. Clin. Otolaryngol., **5**, 235–248

14. Phelps, P. D. and Lloyd, G. A. S. (1981). The radiology of carcinoma of the ear. Br. J. Radiol., **54**, 103–109

15. Leonard, J. and Talbot, M. (1970). Asymptomatic acoustic neurilemmoma. Arch. Otolaryngol., **91**, 117–124

16. Martuza, R. L. and Eldridge, R. (1988). Neurofibromatosis 2. Bilateral acoustic neurofibromatosis. N. Engl. J. Med., **318**, 684–688

17. Igarashi, M., Jerger, J., Alford, B. R. and Stasney, C. R. (1974). Functional and histological findings in acoustic tumor. Arch. Otolaryngol., **99**, 379–384

18. Hassard, A., Boudreau, S. F. and Cron, C. C. (1984). Adenoma of the endolymphatic sac. J. Otolaryngol., **13**, 213–216

19. Michaels, L., Wells, M. and Wells, D. G. (1977). Otolaryngological disturbances in Waldenstrom's macroglobulinaemia. Clin. Otolaryngol., **2**, 327–338

20. Jahn, A. F., Farkashidy, J. and Berman, J. M. (1979). Metastatic tumors in the temporal bone – a pathophysiologic study. J. Otolaryngol., **8**, 85–95

Inner Ear

4

Many pathological changes of the inner ear require the use of special postmortem techniques for their demonstration because of the poor fixation of the labyrinthine membranes during routine postmortem examination (see Chapter 1).

Ototoxic conditions

Ototoxic injury to the inner ear is the use of a variety of drugs. There are five classes of substances, the ototoxicity of which has been carefully investigated clinically and experimentally because they are so frequently used in clinical practice: aminoglycoside antibiotics, loop diuretics, salicylates, quinine and cytotoxic drugs used in the treatment of malignant disease. The structures in the inner ear which are particularly damaged by such drugs are the stria vascularis and the hair cells of the cochlea and the maculae and cristae of the vestibule. Drugs of the first two groups, being so important in treatment, constitute a serious hazard to the inner ear. Cytotoxic drugs have now become the standard therapy for the treatment of several malignant diseases and ototoxic effects are being noticed with increasing frequency. One such drug is cisplatin (*cis*-platinum; *cis*-dichlorodiammine-platinum). Changes are observed both in experimental animals and in humans to affect the whole length of the cochlea. Most pronounced alterations are present in the stria vascularis, the cells of which show degeneration and cystic change.

Viral infections

Infecting viruses reach the inner ear via the bloodstream and the nerves. There are four viral infections which are known to reach the labyrinth by the bloodstream: cytomegalovirus infection, measles, mumps and rubella. Little is known about the histopathological effects of these viruses on the inner ear. Changes have been detected in Reissner's membrane, the organ of Corti, the spiral ganglion, the tectorial membrane, stria vascularis and, in a very small number of cases, the vestibular structures (Figures 4.1 and 4.2). In rubella, we have noted a general retardation of development of the parts of the membranous labyrinth as well as a variety of malformations of those structures. The passage of virus particles along the seventh and eighth cranial nerves to reach the inner ear is characteristic of the virus of herpes zoster oticus (the varicella virus).

A condition which may be due to an as yet unidentified viral infection in the inner ear is that of Bell's palsy, which is manifest clinically as a peripheral facial paralysis. There have been a very small number of reports of temporal bone studies from patients with Bell's palsy. Serial sections of the temporal bone in a patient who came to postmortem in our centre 7 days after the onset of Bell's palsy showed osteoclastic resorption and inflammation of the region of the genu of the facial nerve (Figure 4.3). The descending part of the corresponding facial nerve presented swelling and vacuolation of myelin sheaths with some loss of axis cylinders. These findings suggest that the inflammation of the nerve, possibly of viral origin, led to compression of the nerve in its bony canal and its more distal degeneration.

Ménière's disease

Ménière's disease is an affection of both the hearing and balance organs of the inner ear characterized by episodes of vertigo, hearing loss and tinnitus. Its pathological basis has been established as hydrops, i.e. distension of the endolymphatic spaces of the labyrinth by fluid. The cause of the hydrops in Ménière's disease is unknown. There are, however, other diseases of known pathogenesis in which hydrops may be present as a complication. The common feature of these conditions is the presence of inflammatory or neoplastic involvement of the perilymphatic spaces. Thus, otitis media complicated by perilymphatic labyrinthitis, syphilitic involvement of the labyrinth or leukaemic deposits in the perilymph spaces may be associated with hydrops[1].

In hydrops, the cochlear duct and saccule are involved, but the utricular and semicircular ducts are usually not. In some cases, the cochlear duct alone is hydropic. Reissner's membrane, which is elastic, shows a variable degree of bulging. In the most severe cases, the membrane reaches the top of the scala vestibuli and may be in contact with a wide area of cochlear wall (Figure 4.4). In the apical region, it may bulge to such an extent that it fills the helicotrema. In this way, the distended scala media may even enter the scala tympani. The saccule swells up from its position on the medial wall of the vestibule and frequently touches the vestibular surface of the footplate of the stapes (Figure 4.5). The utricle may be compressed in the process. In some cases, the swollen saccule may herniate from the vestibule into the semicircular canals. There is often fibrosis of the vestibular aqueduct surrounding the endolymphatic sac (Figure 4.6). It has been suggested that the hydrops is caused by the resulting obstruction to drainage of endolymph.

Presbyacusis

Presbyacusis is a term in current use to denote the hearing loss in aged people which cannot be ascribed to any known cause other than old age. There has been a tendency in recent years to invoke degenerative changes in at least four different sites in the cochlea as pathological basis for different forms of this hearing loss, viz. hair cells, spiral ganglion cells (Figures 4.7 and 4.8), stria vascularis and basilar membrane[2]. The studies of Soucek et al.[3,4], however, which were based on electrophysiological, as well as pathological investigations, have indicated that it is the hair cells which are primarily responsible for the disorder. These studies, which were carried out on patients in geriatric wards of a hospital, showed that all subjects over 70 years of age have high-tone deafness with specific brain stem and electrocochleographic findings[3,4].

Surface preparations of perfused cochleas, stained for light microscopy by the method described in Chapter 1, showed atrophy of the outer hair cells and giant stereociliary degeneration in some of those outer hair cells which survived. A severe degree of loss of outer hair cells was present in all coils of all cochleas from the elderly patients. Approximate estimates of hair cell losses showed that the inner hair cells had sustained little loss, the first

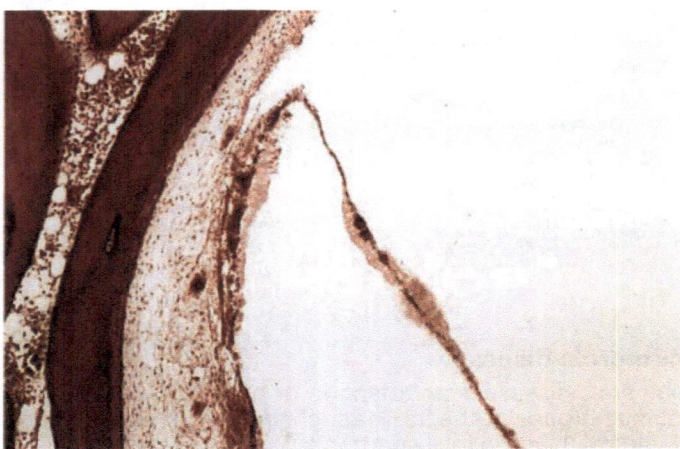

Figure 4.1 Cytomegalovirus infection in the cochlea of an infant. Note characteristic basophilic distension of nuclei and swelling of cytoplasm in cells of Reissner's membrane and stria vascularis. H & E (A)

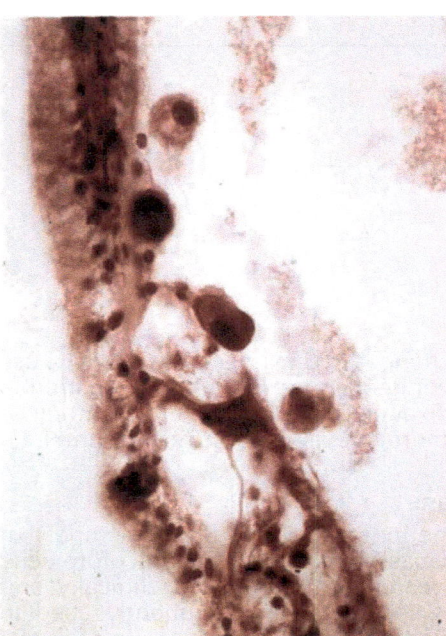

Figure 4.2 Higher power of stria vascularis region of Figure 4.1 showing appearance of cells infected with cytomegalovirus. H & E (C)

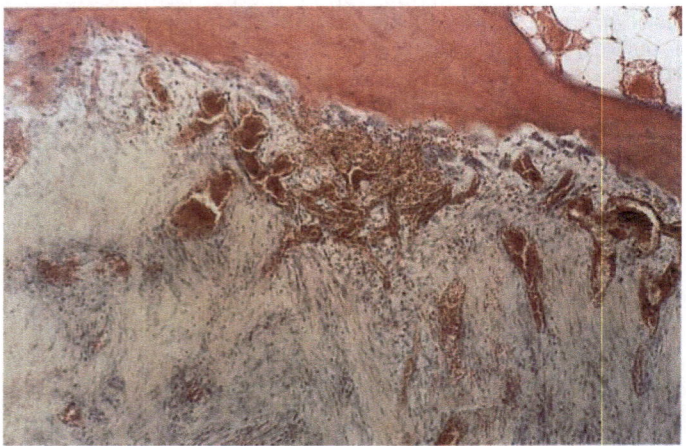

Figure 4.3 Horizontal section of temporal bone in genu region of facial nerve from a case of Bell's palsy in which death occurred from unrelated causes 1 week after onset. Interface between facial nerve and bone. Note inflammation and osteoclasts with evidence of bone resorption. H & E (A)

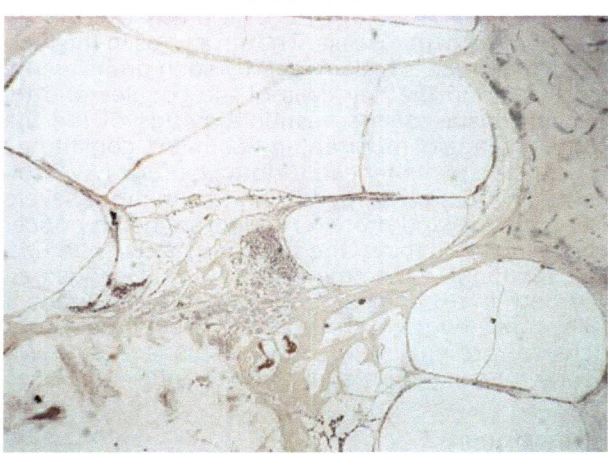

Figure 4.4 Cochlear hydrops in Ménière's disease. The distended Reissner's membrane reaches the top of the scala vestibuli. H & E (A)

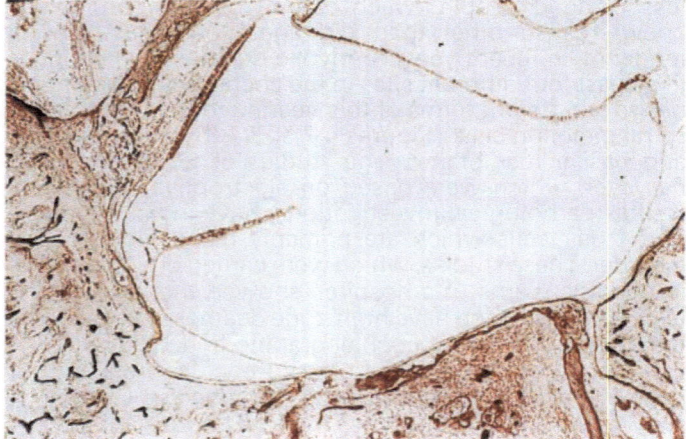

Figure 4.5 Hydrops in Ménière's disease involving vestibule. The saccule is distended to such a degree that it lines the base of the footplate of the stapes, which is artefactually fractured. A thin membrane, possibly the result of rupture, projects into the saccule. H & E (A)

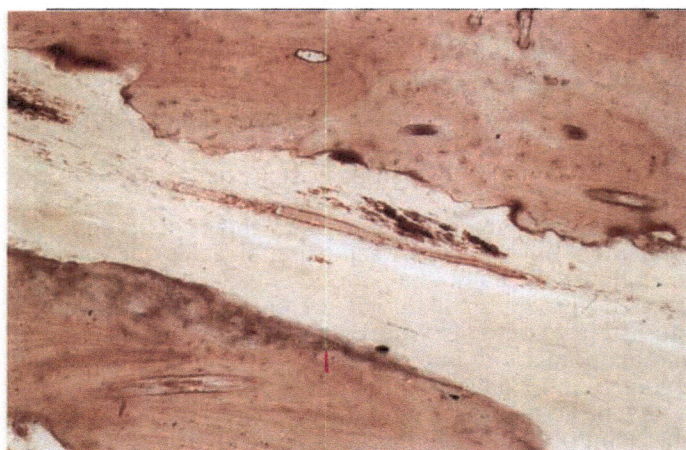

Figure 4.6 Fibrosis of endolymphatic duct in temporal bone from a case of Ménière's disease with hydrops. H & E (B)

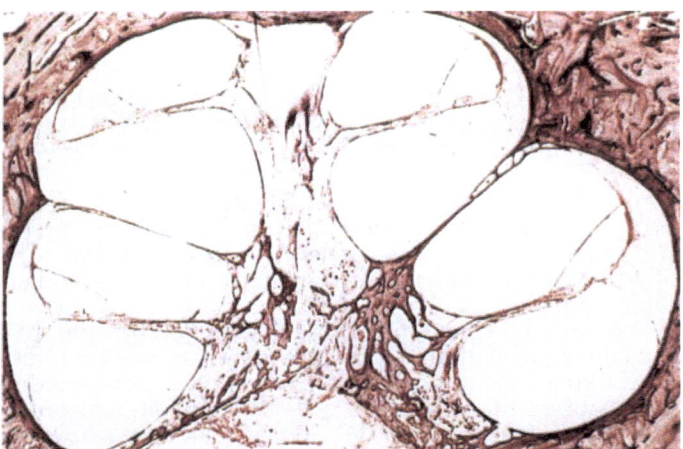

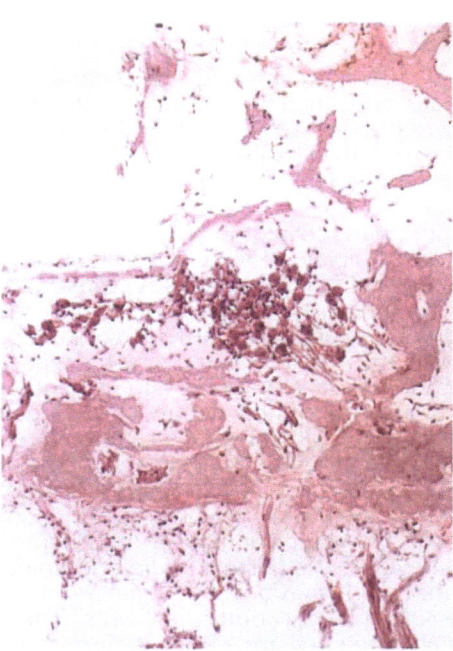

Figure 4.8 Higher power of Figure 4.7 showing but few spiral ganglion nerve in modiolar spaces. H & E (B)

Figure 4.7 Section of cochlea from 82-year-old man. Note paucity of spiral ganglion cells in modiolus. H & E (A)

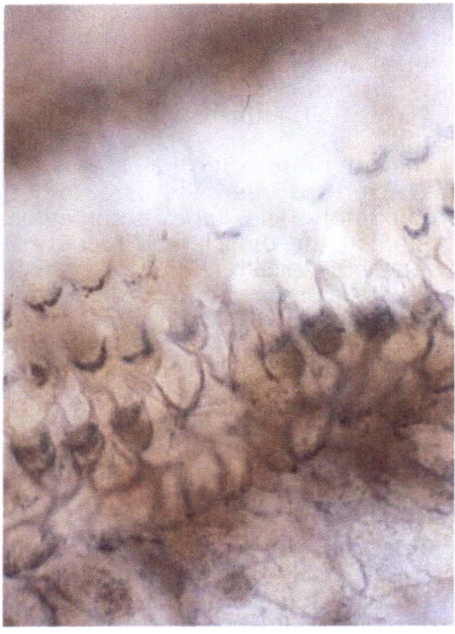

Figure 4.9 Surface preparation from basal coil in an 80-year-old man. The outer hair cells show gaps in each of the rows. Compare with normal surface preparation shown in Figure 1.8. Frohlich staining method (D)

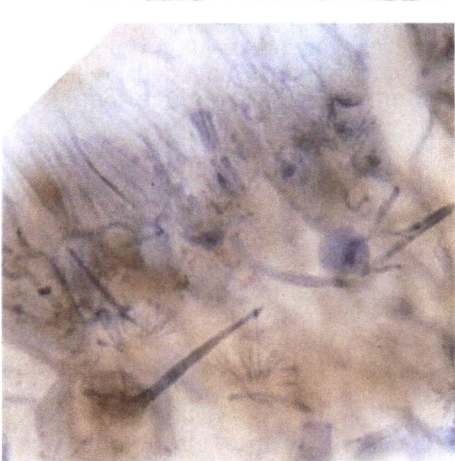

Figure 4.10 Surface preparation from middle coil of cochlea in a 76-year-old woman. Outer hair cells show giant stereocilia. Many hair cells are missing. Stereocilia in the middle coil are normally longer than in the basal coil (compare Figure 1.9). Frohlich staining method (D)

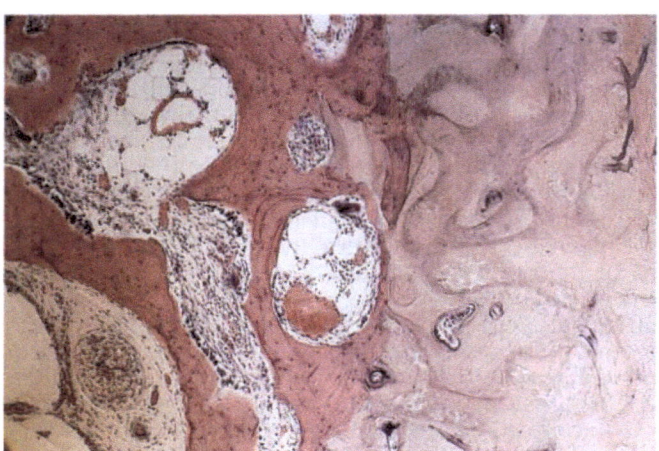

Figure 4.11 Paget's disease involving bony cochlea. There is a clear line of demarcation between pagetoid tissue and endochondral bone, the former staining deep red and showing marrow spaces and the latter staining pink and showing globuli ossei. H & E (A)

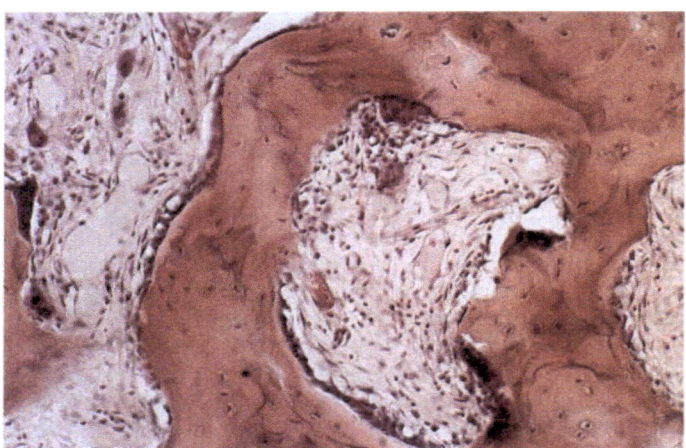

Figure 4.12 Paget's disease of bony cochlea, showing mosaic pattern of cement lines, osteoclastic giant cells, Howship's lacunae and chronic inflammatory tissue in marrow space. H & E (B)

row of outer hair cells had a greater loss, the second row loss was even greater and, in the third row, outer hair cells were very scanty or absent (Figure 4.9). In addition there was a complete loss of all hair cells of all rows, inner and outer, at the extreme lower end of the basal coil in every elderly cochlea.

The other important change was the presence of enormously lengthened and thickened stereocilia emanating from some surviving hair cells. These giant structures were found to measure as much as 60 μm in length. They overlapped many cells in the organ of Corti and sometimes covered the tunnel of Corti. The thickening in some places could be seen to be due to adhesion of hairs to each other as longitudinal lines were identified within an enlarged stereocilium (Figure 4.10). Giant stereocilia were found only in the outer hair cells of middle and apical coils, not in the outer hair cells of the basal coil (although loss of hair cells was just as advanced in this coil). Giant stereociliary degeneration was present to a mild degree in the inner hair cell layer of the basal, middle and apical coils. It is possible that giant stereociliary degeneration is a stage in the dissolution of the outer hair cells. There is evidence that giant stereociliary degeneration is an alteration that is slowly taking place throughout life, resulting eventually in presbyacusis, for it is not until the later years have been reached that hair cells will have been lost to a sufficient extent to produce significant deafness.

Bony Abnormalities

Paget's disease

In Paget's disease, the petrous apex, the mastoid and the bony part of the Eustachian tube are most frequently affected. The periosteal part of the bony labyrinth is the first to undergo pagetoid changes. The endochondral layer is also affected in many cases but the endosteal layer and modiolus infrequently (Figures 4.11 and 4.12). The internal auditory meatus may show protuberances of pagetoid tissue into its lumen[5]. In a few cases only the stapes may be tethered by pagetoid change of its footplate as in otosclerosis (see below). Fissure fractures, occurring during life, are more frequent in the temporal bone of patients with Paget's disease. Patients with Paget's disease are predisposed to neoplasms of bone, particularly osteosarcoma and fibrosarcoma. A spindle cell sarcoma of the temporal bone has been described in one of the cases of Paget's[6]. A similar case is also present in the files of my department.

Osteogenesis imperfecta

Osteogenesis imperfecta is a general bone disease with a triad of clinical features: multiple fractures, blue sclerae and conductive hearing loss. There is a congenital recessive form which is often rapidly fatal and a tardive one in adults which is inherited as a mendelian dominant and is more benign. The pathology is produced by a disturbance in the development of collagen; hence the thin (blue) sclerae as well as poorly formed bone tissue.

In the ear, the bony labyrinth is sometimes deficient in bone[7]. In the temporal bone of one infant with the congenital recessive form of osteogenesis imperfecta, X-ray of the bony labyrinth showed a sharply defined sieve-like pattern of the highly calcified, but poorly collagenized, endochondral bone. Histological examination indicated scanty periosteal and endosteal bony trabeculae (Figures 4.13 and 4.14). The ossicles in the tardive form are very thin and subject to fractures. The stapes footplate is also frequently fixed.

Osteopetrosis

Osteopetrosis (marble bone disease) is a rare disease of bone, in which there is a failure to absorb calcified cartilage and primitive bone. Recent evidence suggests that there is a deficient activity of osteoclasts. A relatively benign form, inherited as a dominant, presents in adults, and a malignant one, inherited as a recessive, in infants and young children. The patients with the benign form often survive to old age and present prominent otological symptoms[8].

The intermediate, endochondral portion of the otic capsule is swollen and appears as an exaggerated thickened form of the normal state. Globuli osse composed of groups of calcified cartilage cells are normally present in this region (see Chapter 1) and, in osteopetrosis, they are greatly increased in number and are arranged into a markedly thickened zone (Figures 4.15 and 4.16). The periosteal bone is normal. The organ of Corti is usually normal, but, in a few cases, has been said to be atrophied. The ossicles are of fetal shape and filled with unabsorbed calcified cartilage.

Otosclerosis

Otosclerosis is a common focal lesion of the otic capsule of unknown aetiology, which is found principally in relation to the cochlea and footplate of the stapes. Otosclerotic deposits, not associated with hearing loss, are found in about 10% of all adult temporal bones at autopsy of white people[9].

In cases with prominent otosclerotic involvement of the otic capsule, the lesion may be seen as a smooth prominence of the promontory. The stapes is sometimes fixed. The pink swelling of the otosclerotic focus may sometimes even be detected clinically through a particularly transparent tympanic membrane. In microsliced temporal bones showing otosclerosis, the focus appears well demarcated and pink. Blood vessels are prominent and evenly distributed. X-rays show the well-defined lesion as a patch of mottled translucency (Figures 4.17 to 4.19).

The histological characteristic of otosclerosis is the presence of trabeculae of new bone, mostly of the woven type (Figure 4.20). This contrasts with the well-developed bone under the outer periosteum, the endochondral middle layer and the endosteal layer of the otic capsule (see Chapter 1), a sharply demarcated edge between normal and otosclerotic bone being a prominent feature. Numerous blood vessels are always present. In a few places, the bone may be more mature and less cellular, and even lamellar bone may be found.

The commonest site for the formation of otosclerotic foci is the bone anterior to the oval window. The fissula ante fenestram, a normally appearing slit connecting middle ear with vestibule, is present in the same region (Figure 4.19) but this anatomical relationship does not necessarily denote any developmental connection. Cartilaginous rests are also normal in this area and may be seen nearby. Otosclerotic foci may also be seen in the bone near the round window membrane, in the inferior part of the cochlear capsule or in the bone around the semicircular canals.

In a surgical specimen of stapes, either the superstructure (the head and crura) alone may have been removed (Figure 4.21) or the whole ossicle, including the footplate, may have been excised. Otosclerotic bone will be seen only in the footplate because the fixat on causing deafness has occurred by extension of the otosclerotic process from the adjacent temporal bone. In many cases, not even the footplate will be affected because the otosclerosis has not extended to this structure, but has caused only distortion and narrowing of the oval window. Thus, the surgical specimen is frequently free from any structural changes.

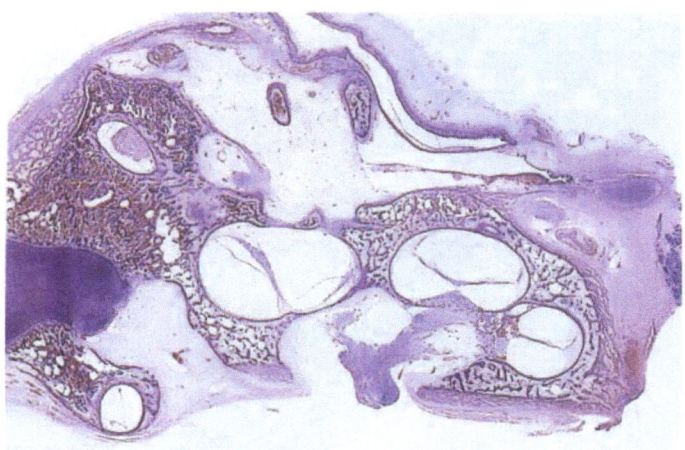

Figure 4.13 Osteogenesis imperfecta in cochlea of a stillborn infant of 26 weeks' gestation, showing bony trabeculae which are thin and highly calcified. H & E (A)

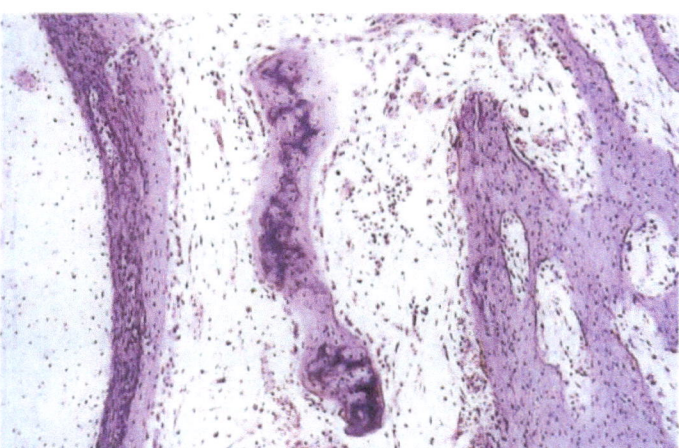

Figure 4.14 Osteogenesis imperfecta in same case as that shown in Figure 4.13 showing periosteal layer on left and highly calcified trabeculum of middle layer. Spiral ligament on the right. H & E (B)

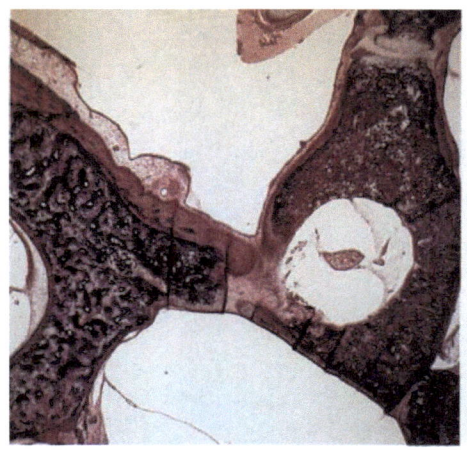

Figure 4.15 Osteopetrosis involving stapes and bony vestibule. H & E (A)

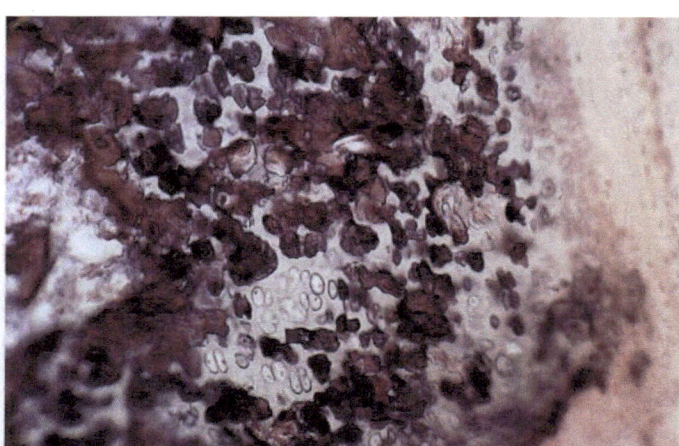

Figure 4.16 Higher power of osteopetrosis showing increased globuli ossei. H & E (C)

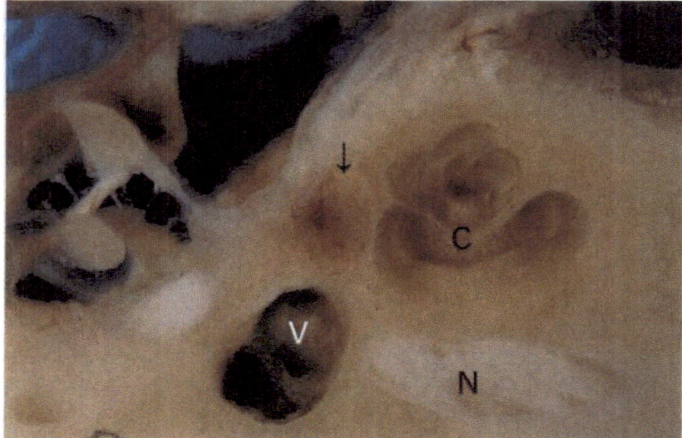

Figure 4.17 Microsliced temporal bone showing focus of otosclerosis (arrow). C: cochlea; N: eighth (cochleovestibular) nerve; V: vestibule

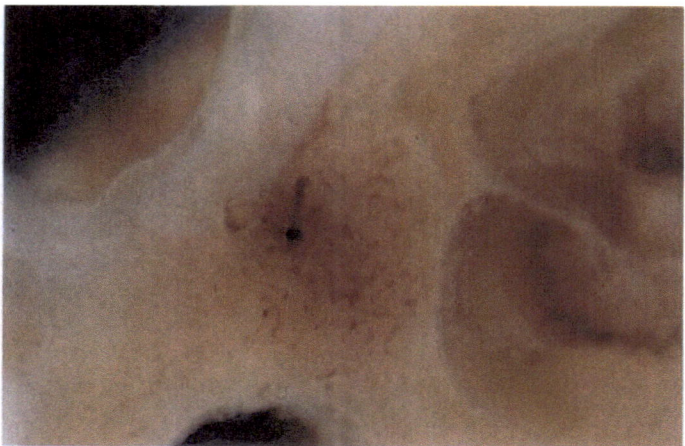

Figure 4.18 Higher power of area of otosclerotic focus in Figure 4.17. Note marked vascularity

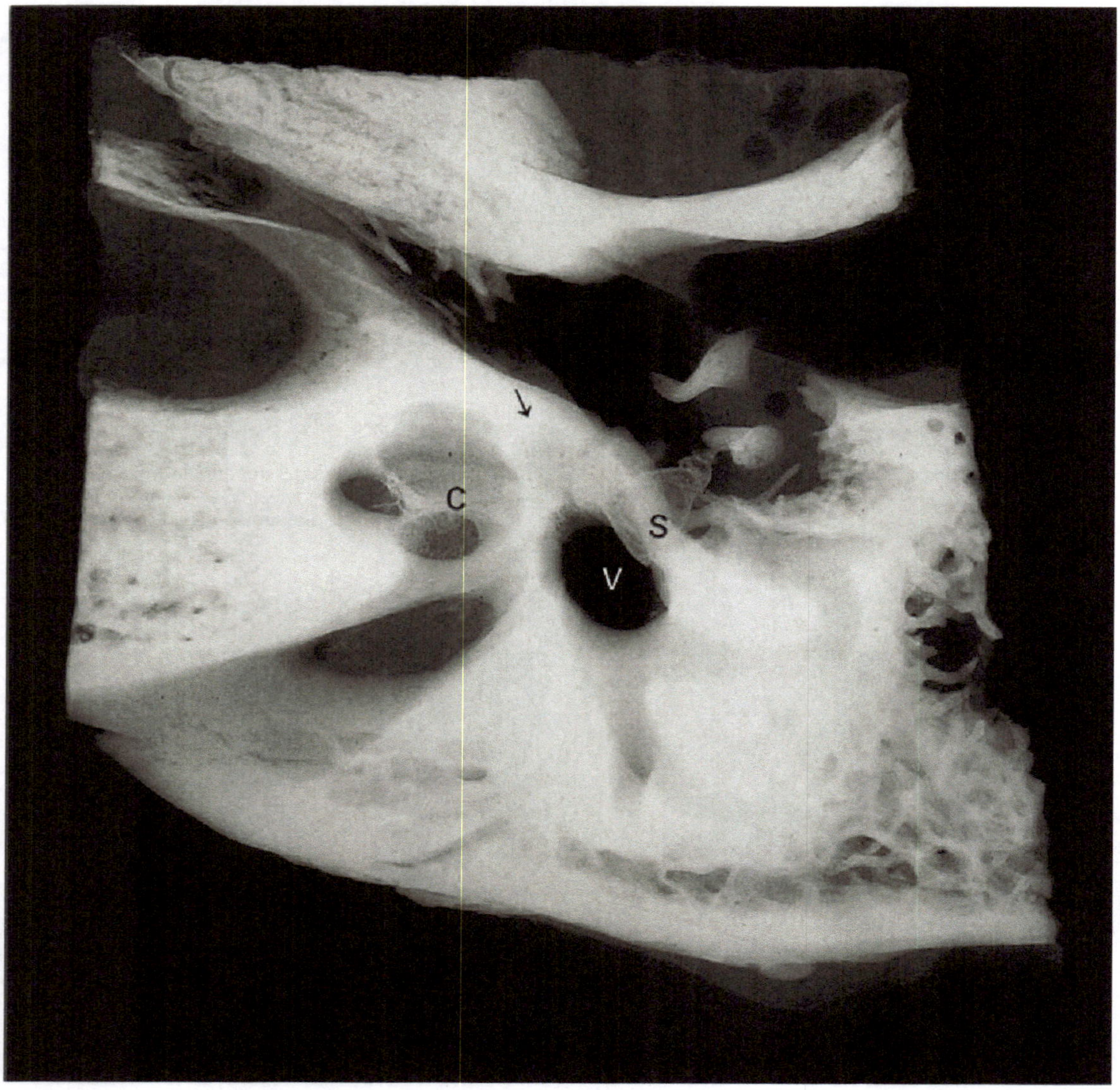

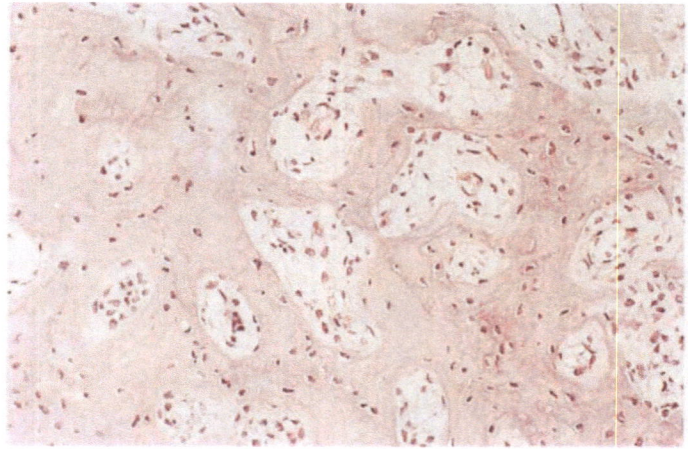

Figure 4.19 X-ray of microslice shown in previous two figures. The otosclerotic focus (arrow) appears as a mottled, translucent area. C: cochlea; S: stapes; V: vestibule. Note fissula ante fenestram between otosclerotic focus and middle ear surface

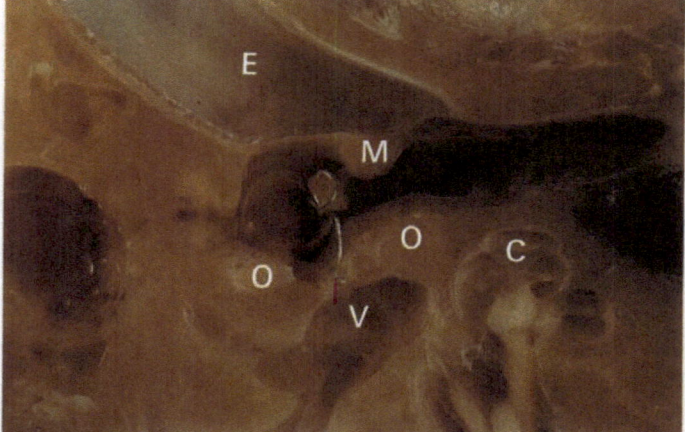

Figure 4.20 Focus of otosclerosis in temporal bone. It is composed of woven bone with numerous osteocytes and blood vessels in marrow spaces. H & E (A)

Figure 4.21 Temporal bone with foci of otosclerosis (O) adjacent to the vestibule (V) and anterior to the footplate of the stapes. The stapes with footplate has been removed and replaced by a metal prosthesis that has been tethered to the incus and to adipose tissue inserted into the opening of the vestibule made after removal of the stapes. C: cochlea; E: external auditory canal; M: handle of malleus

References

1. Lindsay, J. R., Kohut, R. I. and Sciarra, P. A. (1967). Meniere's disease: pathology and manifestations. *Ann. Otol. Rhinol. Laryngol.*, **76**, 5–22
2. Schuknecht, H. F. (1974). *Pathology of the Ear.* (Cambridge, Mass.: Harvard University Press)
3. Soucek, S., Michaels, L. and Frohlich, A. (1986). Evidence for hair cell degeneration as the primary lesion in hearing loss of the elderly. *J. Otolaryngol.*, **15**, 175–183
4. Soucek, S., Michaels, L. and Frohlich, A. (1987). Pathological changes in the organ of Corti in presbyacusis as revealed by microslicing and staining. *Acta Otolaryngol. (Stockholm)*, Suppl., 93–101
5. Davies, D. G. (1968). Paget's disease of the temporal bone. A clinical and histopathological survey. *Acta Otolaryngol. (Stockholm)* (Suppl), **242**, 1–47
6. Nager, G. T. (1975). Paget's disease of the temporal bone. *Ann. Otol. Rhinol. Laryngol.*, **84** (Suppl. 22), 3–32
7. Igarashi, M., King, A. I., Schwenzfeier, C. W., Watanabe, T. and Alford, B. R. (1980). Inner ear pathology in osteogenesis imperfecta congenita. *J. Laryngol. Otol.*, **94**, 697–705
8. Myers, E. N. and Stool, S. (1969). The temporal bone in osteopetrosis. *Arch. Otolaryngol. (Stockholm)*, **89**, 460–469
9. Guild, S. R. (1944). Histologic otosclerosis. *Ann. Otol. Rhinol. Laryngol.*, **53**, 246–266

Normal Histology and Inflammatory Conditions of the Nose and Paranasal Sinuses

5

Normal Histology

The vestibule, the anterior chamber of the nasal cavity, is lined by an internal extension of the integument of the external nose, including a keratinizing stratified squamous epithelial surface and an underlying dermis containing hair follicles, sebaceous and sweat glands. The degree of posterior extension of the vestibule varies with physiological conditions, races and individuals. The average depth is between 1 and 2 cm from the external rim of the nares. As the mucocutaneous junction (limen nasi) representing the anterior limits of the inner nasal cavity proper is approached, there is a gradual diminution and disappearance of the adnexa.

The nasal cavities are normally lined by ciliated pseudostratified columnar epithelium (Figure 5.1), designated as the 'Schneiderian membrane' to emphasize its origin from the ectoderm, as contrasted with a similar appearing epithelium of the larynx and lower respiratory tract which is of endodermal origin. In the sinuses, this epithelium is lower and sometimes is of a simple cuboidal type containing a few goblet cells. The tissue of the nasal cavity between bone and airway surface varies in thickness, being most pronounced over the inferior, medial and lateral portions of the middle and inferior turbinates, which represent the nasal surface most prominently exposed to inspired air (Figure 5.2). Immediately beneath the nasal cavity epithelium is a thin uniform zone of fibro-elastic tissue, the lamina propria. More deeply to this is a layer containing seromucinous glands and distinctive vascular structures; the glandular elements are situated more superficially (Figure 5.3). The majority of the blood vessels in the vascular tissue of the nasal cavity are capable of marked variation in luminal capacity (nasal 'erectile' tissue). This normal vascular pattern is, in its abundance, sometimes mistaken by pathologists for neoplasms such as haemangioma or angiofibroma (Figure 5.2). The paranasal sinus linings also contain some seromucinous glands, particularly in their ostial areas, but these are much fewer than in the nasal cavity. No prominent vascular network is present in the sinuses, the usual finding being only a thin submucosal fibrous layer adjacent to the periosteum.

The turbinate bones are scroll-like bony plates covered by mucosa, glandular and vascular tissue (Figure 5.2). The surface of the turbinate bones is irregular and frequently shows thin formations of osteoid, indicating recent bony deposition.

Olfactory epithelium

Olfactory epithelium is normally found in the superoposterior portion of each nasal cavity and is said to occupy an area of about 1.5 cm square[1]. The olfactory epithelium is composed of elongated sustentacular (supporting) cells, small basal cells and olfactory neural cells. The latter are bipolar structures with swellings protruding from their mucosal surfaces forming the olfactory vesicles. These give rise to cilia which project into the overlying mucus blanket (Figure 5.4). The central processes pass via the cribriform plate, as non-myelinated fibres to the olfactory bulb. Small simple serous-like Bowman's glands are located in the olfactory mucosa and their ducts open onto the surface. The columnar sustentacular cells rest on the basilar membrane and seem to act as supporting cells. The innermost polygonal basal cells perform as reserve replacements for both the sustentacular cells and the olfactory neural cells[2]. It may be of importance with regard to the pathogenesis of olfactory neuroblastomas that the olfactory epithelium is in a state of constant turnover, unlike any other peripheral nerve cell[3].

Infections

A large number of infectious agents have been identified as pathogens in the nose.

Scleroma

Scleroma (often termed 'rhinoscleroma') is a chronic inflammatory condition in which large deforming masses of tissue distend the nasal cavity. The disease is very common at present in Central and South America, in Egypt and some parts of Africa, the Middle East, India, the Philippines and some other areas of the Pacific, affecting impoverished people predominantly in rural areas.

Pathological appearances

In fully developed scleroma, there are large firm intramucosal masses with a coarsely granular surface. These lead to external expansion of the nose, particularly in the cartilaginous part. Scleromatous nodules may also be present under the skin adjacent to the nose (Figure 5.5). The cut surface of the affected tissue is pale grey. A progression of the gross changes of the disease from a 'rhinitic' stage, through an 'infiltrative' one to the nodular one described above is recognized[4].

The lesion is a thickening of nasal mucosa which usually retains its covering of respiratory epithelium. The inflammatory exudate, which characterizes the lesion, is a pleomorphic one. Plasma cells are prominent and Russell bodies are numerous. The specific cell of the lesion is the Mikulicz cell, which is large with clear cytoplasm containing bacilli (Figures 5.6 and 5.7). These almost certainly are *Klebsiella rhinoscleromatis*. The intracytoplasmic organisms are difficult to identify in conventionally stained sections, but may be displayed by silver impregnation stains, such as the Warthin–Starry stain, by Giemsa, by immunochemical methods using an antibody against *Klebsiella rhinoscleromatis*, or in 1 μm plastic sections.

Sarcoidosis

Sarcoidosis affects the nose fairly frequently. Lindsay and Perlman, in 1951, found nasal mucosal involvement in 18% of 50 patients with sarcoidosis[5].

Sarcoid lesions may affect the skin of the nose, the nasal bones or the nasal mucosa. The characteristic microscopic change is one of rather uniform tubercles composed of groups of epithelioid cells with no caseation (Figure 5.8) (although a limited degree of central necrosis

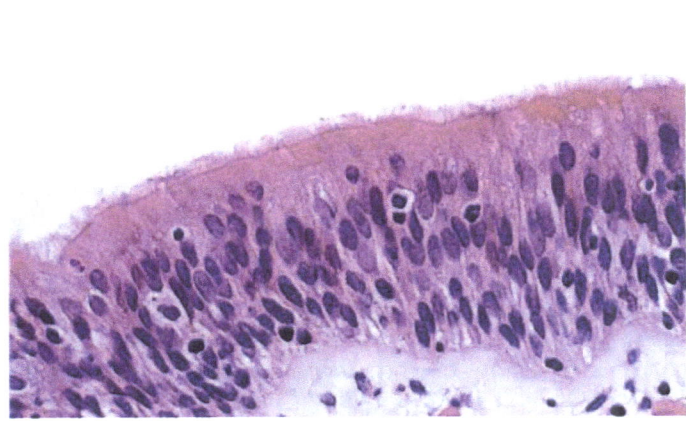

Figure 5.1 Normal pseudostratified (Schneiderian) columnar epithelium of nose. H & E (C)

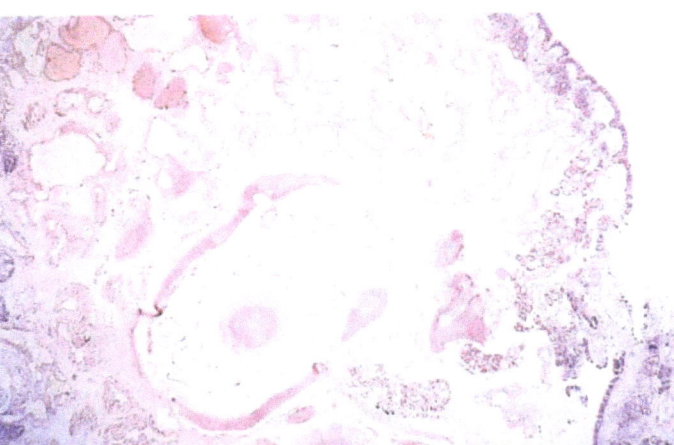

Figure 5.2 Normal nasal mucosa showing epithelium and seromucinous glands. Beneath the latter, lies the venous plexus and thin bony plate of the middle turbinate. H & E (A)

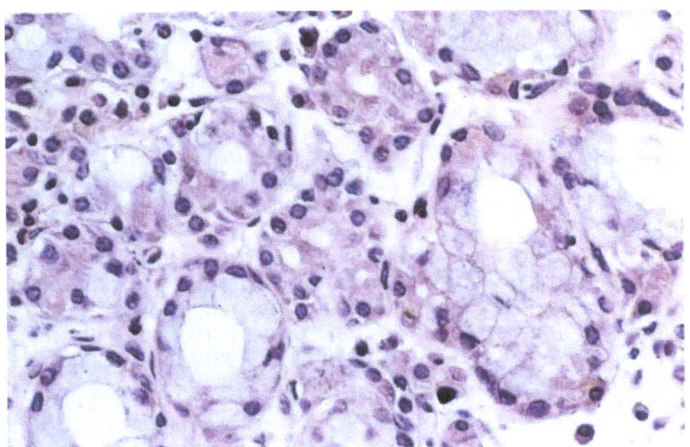

Figure 5.3 Normal seromucinous glands of nose showing both mucous and serous elements. H & E (B)

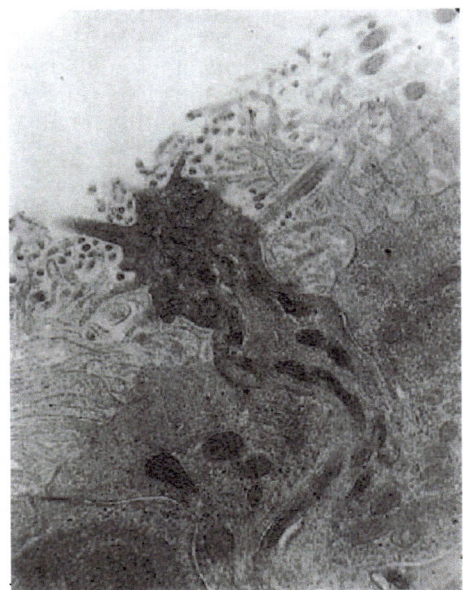

Figure 5.4 Olfactory epithelium. Electron micrograph showing an olfactory neural cell with projecting vesicle which is bearing cilia. The deep process from this cell is passing downwards to become a nerve fibre. The adjacent sustentacular cells show numerous microvilli on the surface. Guinea-pig preparation. × 27 300

Figure 5.5 Rhinoscleroma with large intramucosal mass projecting from left nostril, distortion of right nostril and a subcutaneous mass of inflammatory tissue beneath the latter

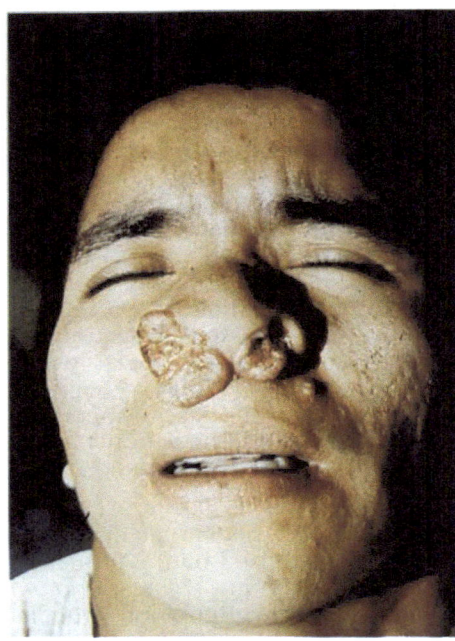

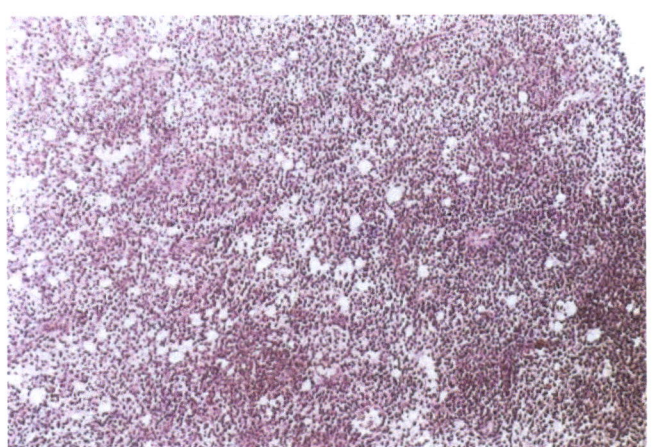

Figure 5.6 Rhinoscleroma showing pale Mikulicz cells and plasma cells in the exudate. H & E (A)

is often present). Foreign-body or Langhans-type giant cells are usually present and may contain a variety of crystalline, calcified or other inclusions. Fibrosis of the tubercle takes place around the periphery and grows to involve the whole of it. Later stages may be seen as a group of uniform round hyaline fibrous masses.

Non-sarcoid granulomas

It is important to note that the above features of the histology of sarcoidosis are non-specific. The diagnosis is essentially a clinical one. Tuberculoid granulomas are seen quite frequently in the nasal mucosa in which the characteristic histological features of sarcoid lesions are present, but in which investigation yields no systemic evidence of sarcoidosis and the patient does not develop clinical sarcoidosis subsequently. Such granulomatous foci usually present minor clinical disturbance or none and the lesions regress in the course of time, even without treatment.

Mycotic infections

The majority of mycotic infections of the nose and paranasal sinuses fall into one of the following clinical groups:

1. A low-grade infection with *Aspergilli*, taking the form either of a 'fungus ball' in the maxillary antrum accompanied only by a low-grade inflammation (aspergillosis) or of a polypoid sinonasal condition, allergic aspergillus sinusitis.

2. A slowly progressive disease process with much fibrosis involving the nasal and paranasal sinus mucosa and spreading externally into the subcutaneous tissues of the side of the nose and orbit (subcutaneous zygomycosis). This lesion is caused by a zygomycete, *Conidiobolus coronatus*.

3. A fulminating disease, usually occurring in diabetics, which spreads rapidly from the nose to the base of skull and brain (rhinocerebral zygomycosis or mucormycosis). This mycosis is caused by another zygomycete – *Rhizopus oryzae*.

4. A chronic granulomatous lesion of the nasal and conjunctival mucosae containing vast numbers of the sporangia of the fungus, *Rhinosporidium seeberi* (rhinosporidiosis).

The other mycotic infections of the nose are rare, the literature consisting of a few case reports only for each entity.

Fungi can usually be found in the diseased tissue on histological examination, and the type of the causal organism can, in most cases, be reasonably inferred. It is important, however, that, wherever possible, the fungus should be cultured in the laboratory from fresh tissue so that the diagnosis can be made as accurately as possible.

Aspergillosis

Aspergilli are naturally found as saprophytic organisms in soil.

The common non-invasive form or 'aspergilloma' usually affects the maxillary sinus. The patient has clinical features of a sinus affection, such as rhinorrhoea, nasal obstruction and pain, and the sinus is opaque to X-rays. The disease responds well to drainage of the sinus. The maxillary antrum is partially occupied by a 'fungus ball'. This is a soft mass of variable colour which lies within the lumen or is attached to the side wall of the antrum. Histologically, it is a tangled mycelium of aspergilli with a thin coating of inflammatory cells containing neutrophils, lymphocytes and multinucleate giant cells. The fungi are only faintly stained in haematoxylin and eosin sections,

are septate and branch at an acute angle of about 45° (Figures 5.9 and 5.10)[6].

Allergic aspergillus sinusitis affects young adults with asthma who develop a mucous exudate in the antrum. The histological features are those of inspissated eosinophilic or basophilic mucus in which sloughed respiratory epithelium, eosinophils and Charcot–Leyden crystals may be seen. Special staining for fungi, particularly using the Grocott silver stain, reveals small numbers of *Aspergillus* hyphae in the mucus[7].

A rare form of aspergillus infection, known as invasive aspergillosis, occurs in association with reduced immune reactions, e.g. in cases of treated malignant disease. There is invasion of the deeper tissues of the skull. Microscopically, the aspergilli are seen in giant cells with an active granulomatous reaction (Figure 5.11).

Infection by zygomycetes

Zygomycetes represent a class of fungi within the phylum of Zygomycota. Zygomycetes are characterized by a sparsely septate mycelium and spores borne in sporangia. Two main disease patterns are produced by these fungi:

1. Subcutaneous zygomycosis of the nasal mucosa and adjacent tissues produced by the species *Conidiobolus coronatus*, and

2. Rhinocerebral zygomycosis caused by *Rhizopus oryzae*.

Subcutaneous zygomycosis of the nasal mucosa and adjacent tissue: Patients with this mycosis have been reported from many tropical regions, principally Africa and Asia.

The infection commences in the nose and paranasal sinuses and then spreads into adjacent tissues of face and orbit. A large disfiguring mass is formed, which involves the nose, face and eyelids. Pale grey, hard tissue involves the mucosa of the nose and paranasal sinuses and widely infiltrates the tissues of the face and orbit.

Pathological appearances: The pathological tissue shows granulomatous inflammation with foreign-body giant cells, histiocytes, neutrophils and eosinophils. Fibroblasts and collagen are abundant. Fungal elements may be found only after a careful search. They are short poorly stained hyphae with thin walls. The fungi, *Conidiobolus coronatus*, may show irregular branching and very occasional septae. In many cases, but not all, the fungal fragments are embedded in an eosinophilic material, the Splendore–Hoeppli reaction (Figure 5.12).

Rhinocerebral zygomycosis (mucormycosis): Rhinocerebral zygomycosis is a fulminating infection which usually, but not always, occurs in uncontrolled, acidotic diabetics. The nasal turbinates and paranasal sinuses, including the sphenoid sinus, are the first sites of the disease, which rapidly spreads to involve the meninges and brain.

The bones of the nose show extensive necrosis and abscesses. The palatal bones may be affected as well as the lateral wall of the nose, maxilla and base of skull. Extensive necrosis and diffuse infiltration with polymorphonuclear neutrophils are characteristic features of the condition. Thrombosis due to invasion of blood vessels by the fungus is frequent and infarction is often prominent. The hyphae of *Rhizopus oryzae* of the class Mucorales, are broad, show infrequent septae and have non-parallel sides. They are often basophilic and stain deeply with haematoxylin (Figures 5.13 and 5.14).

Rhinosporidiosis: Rhinosporidiosis is a chronic disease of the nose and conjunctiva characterized by the formation of persistent polyps caused by a fungus, *Rhinosporidium seeberi*, which has not yet been cultured on artificial

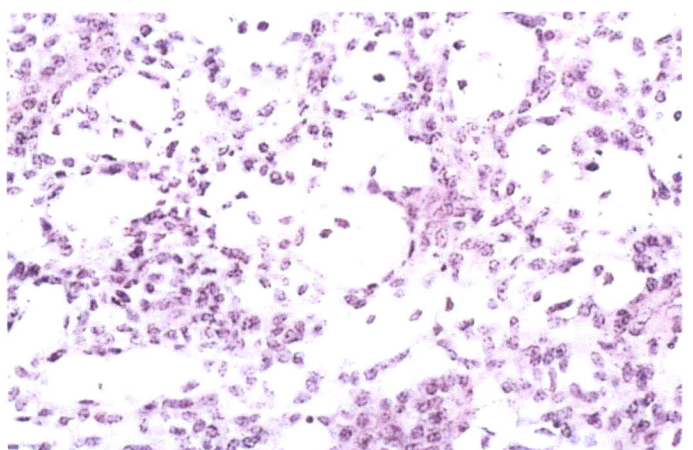

Figure 5.7 Higher power view of rhinoscleroma showing Mikulicz cells and plasma cells.   H & E (B)

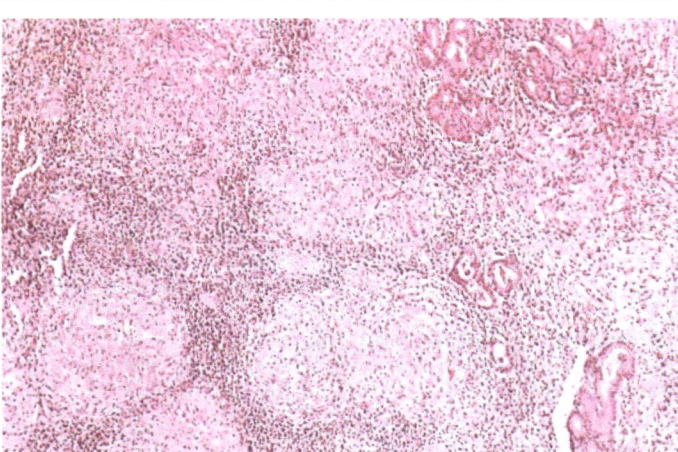

Figure 5.8 Sarcoid of the nose. Small round granulomas each surrounded by a cuff of lymphocytes infiltrate among the seromucinous glands of the nose.   H & E (A)

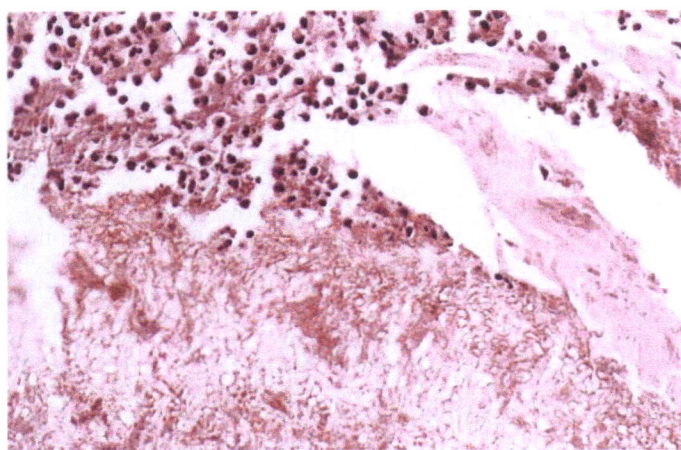

Figure 5.9 Aspergilloma of maxillary antrum. From a 'fungus ball'. The apergillus is seen as a tangled mass of septate hyphae. Inflammatory cells are present at the edge of the fungal mass.   H & E (B)

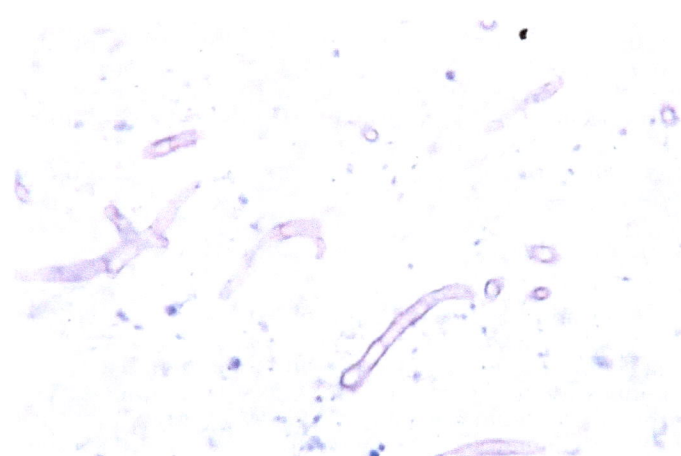

Figure 5.10 Hyphae of *Aspergillus* from nasal aspergillosis. The septate structures branch at about 45°. Periodic acid–Schiff (C)

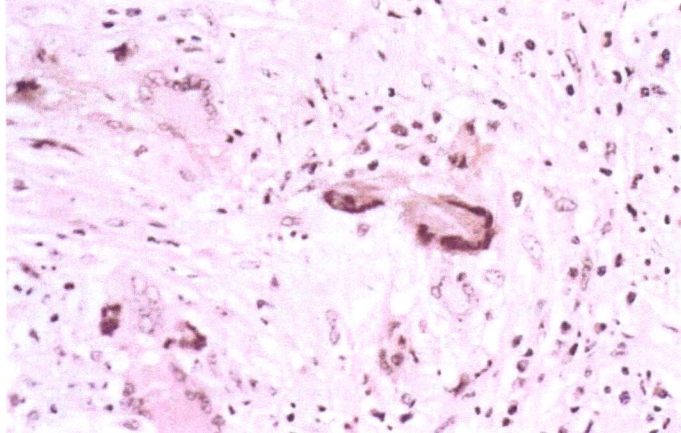

Figure 5.11 Invasive aspergillosis, a rare form of the nasal infection with this fungus, showing granuloma of histiocytes, lymphocytes, plasma cells and fibroblasts with hyphae in cytoplasm of giant cells.   H & E (B)

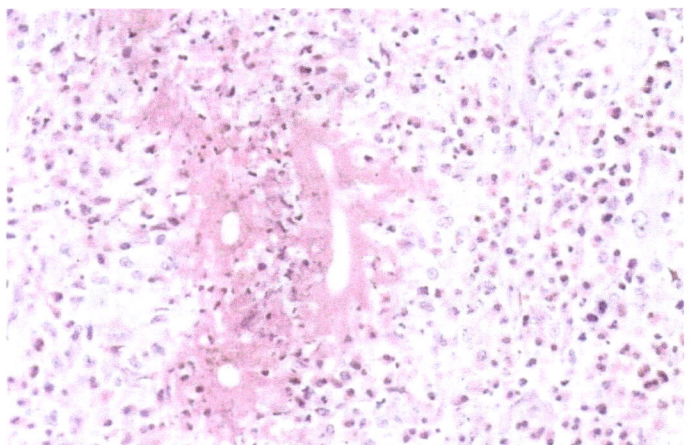

Figure 5.12 Granuloma of nasal tissue caused by *Conidiobolus coronatus*. Hyphae of the fungus are surrounded by eosinophilic amorphous material – the Splendore–Hoeppli reaction.   H & E (B)

media. The disease is seen in many countries, but most cases have been identified in the Indian subcontinent and Sri Lanka.

The lesions are rough, corrugated polyps affecting the nasal mucosa and sometimes the conjunctivae. The polyps may be single or multiple and pedunculated or sessile. The organism starts its life cycle in the tissues as a parasite measuring 6–8 μm. It then grows by repeated division into a sporangium measuring 200–300 μm, which contains thousands of spores. The latter develop independently after rupture of the sporangium. The tissue reaction is a chronic inflammatory one with numbers of giant cells of Langhans type in reaction to the sporangia (Figure 5.15)[8].

Myospherulosis

Myospherulosis is not a fungus infection, but represents the development of sac-like structures containing globules which occur in the paranasal sinuses and are associated with a foreign-body reaction. Microscopically, the lesions are characterized by the presence of closely arranged spaces in the submucosa giving a 'Swiss cheese' appearance. Within the spaces are brownish sac-like structures containing spherules which gave the appearance of "partly filled bags of marbles" (Figure 5.16)[9]. Rosai[10] showed that the spherules stained positively for haemoglobin, peroxidase and lipofuscin, suggesting an origin from erythrocytes altered by a foreign substance. Similar formations were obtained artificially by the action of tetracycline ointment on a pure preparation of human erythrocytes.

Non-infective Inflammatory Conditions

Nasal and paranasal polyposis

Swelling and polyposis of the mucosa of the nose and paranasal sinuses are produced in many different pathological conditions, both benign and malignant. Histological investigation is essential for accurate diagnosis.

By far the commonest form of nasal polyposis is a chronic oedematous swelling of the mucosa and submucosa, which leads to nasal obstruction.

Gross appearances

The majority of nasal polyps present a soft lobular grey-to-pink translucent appearance, measuring up to 3 cm in diameter. The cut surface is moist and pale pink. A stalk, produced by pulling on the mucosa during removal, is sometimes present. The antrochoanal polyp is usually found in children. It originates from the mucosa of the maxillary sinus, extrudes through the ostium into the nasal cavity and, because of its size, bulges backwards through the posterior choana into the nasopharynx.

Microscopic appearances

There is marked oedema of connective tissue with prominent lymphatic dilatation. In some cases, the stroma resembles myxoid tissue with markedly oedematous fibrillar deposition and fibrocytes. The respiratory epithelium reveals intense goblet cell hyperplasia and mucinous glands are similarly active. The epithelial basement membrane is markedly thickened. Eosinophils infiltrate the subepithelial tissue in variable, frequently large, numbers (Figure 5.17). There is also a pronounced plasma cell infiltrate. Collections of large histiocytic cells in the deeper part of the polyp are common. The stroma may appear fibrous. This feature, in conjunction with the presence of numerous blood vessels, may arouse suspicion of a possible diagnosis of juvenile angiofibroma. Irritation to the surface of the polyp frequently gives rise to squamous metaplasia of the lining epithelium. In some nasal polyps, there is a mucous glandular hyperplasia, suggesting an adenomatous neoplasm (Figure 5.18). Rarely, benign metaplastic cartilage or bone has been identified in otherwise benign inflammatory polyps.

Antrochoanal polyps show chronic inflammation only, without the features of hypersensitivity seen in most other nasal polyps.

Nasal polyposis with stromal atypia

Polyposis with stromal atypia is occasionally seen in otherwise typical nasal polyps, mainly in young patients. Microscopically, stromal cells of varying sizes are seen in groups or scattered singly[11]. The atypical cells are characterized by large hyperchromatic, sometimes multilobulated, nuclei with nucleoli which are sometimes multiple and by cytoplasm that is granular or vesicular. The overall appearances of the cells often suggest large fibroblasts (Figure 5.19). Mitotic activity is absent. There are no cytoplasmic cross-striations and glycogen content is minimal. These appearances and the absence of destruction of nasal or paranasal structures should distinguish this benign process from an embryonal rhabdomyosarcoma, with which it is most often confused. Another atypical appearance is the presence of groups of small cells with multiple nuclei in the stroma of nasal polyps (Figure 5.20); these cells have, likewise, no malignant significance.

Inspissated mucus

Inspissated mucus represents a collection of impacted mucus and cellular debris in the nose or the paranasal sinuses. It affects young adults or children with a history of chronic rhinitis or sinusitis of any cause. Grossly, a firm, rubbery grey to pink translucent mass is seen filling the sinus. The mass is easily removed from the cavity with no evidence of bony destruction. Histological appearance may be mistaken for a pleomorphic adenoma of salivary gland type or even a malignant neoplasm because of the homogeneous chondroid-appearing mucin-positive material (Figure 5.21). It is important to examine the mucus for *Aspergilli* by use of the Grocott stain because the presence of inspissated mucus in the nose and paranasal sinuses may be a manifestation of allergic aspergillus sinusitis[7] (see above).

Cholesterol granuloma

Cholesterol granuloma is frequently encountered in the nose and paranasal sinuses, particularly in the maxillary antrum. Occasionally, it may affect the frontal sinus. The antrum is occupied by a bluish swelling of the mucosa, sometimes thought to be a cyst. Histologically, the changes are similar to those of cholesterol granuloma of the middle ear (see Chapter 2), i.e. haemorrhage, haemosiderin mainly in histiocytes and extensive cholesterol clefts with foreign-body type giant cell reaction (Figure 5.22)[12].

The cause of this common condition is not known. It seems likely that, as with cholesterol granuloma of the middle ear (see Chapter 2), haemorrhage into the mucosa of the sinus is the basic lesion.

Organizing haematoma

A mass of organizing haemorrhage in the nose has sometimes been mistaken for a malignant neoplasm of blood vessels. It follows intranasal bleeding, when a clot forms either within the mucosa or on its surface. Organization by granulation tissue then takes place.

Grossly, a sessile vascular or pale mass is present, usually on the lateral wall, and biopsy may be carried out with the impression that it is a neoplasm. A large swelling frequently develops and it may be removed with a clinical diagnosis of a vascular neoplasm. The cut surface shows deep red and greyish foci. Histologically, there are exten-

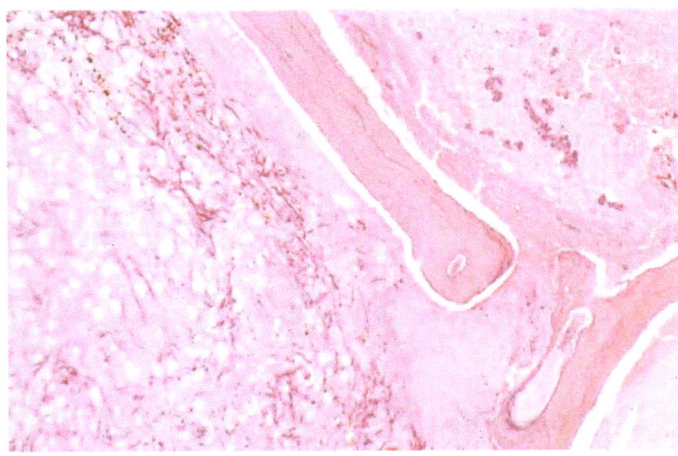

Figure 5.13 Mucor of nose showing a mass of fungal mycelium adjacent to bony trabeculae and necrotic tissue. H & E (A)

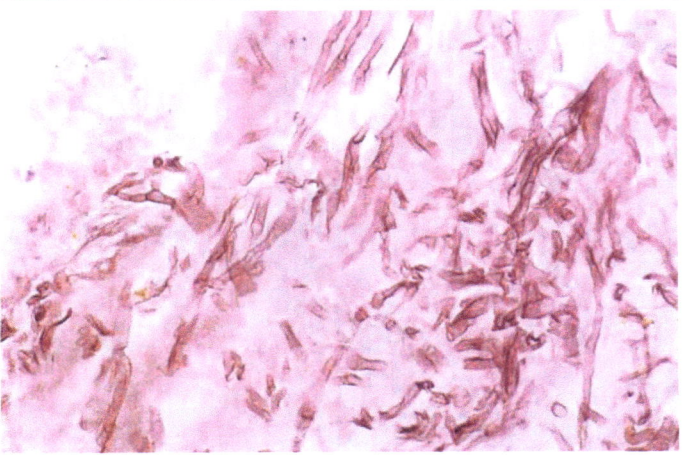

Figure 5.14 Higher power of mucor fungi which are septate and stain deeply with haematoxylin. H & E (B)

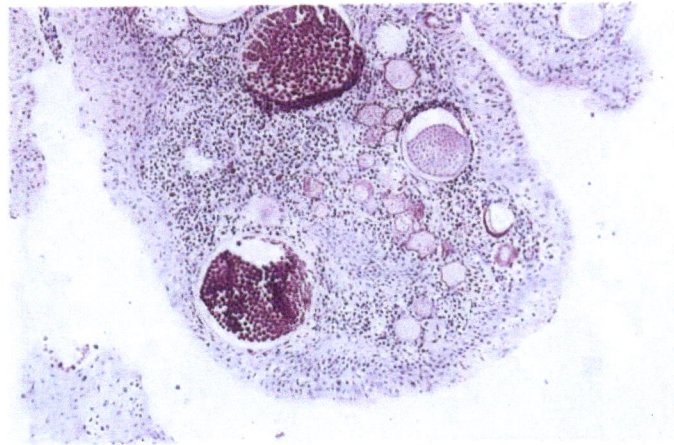

Figure 5.15 Rhinosporidiosis showing numerous sporangia, each containing numerous spores, in nasal mucosa. Periodic acid–Schiff (B)

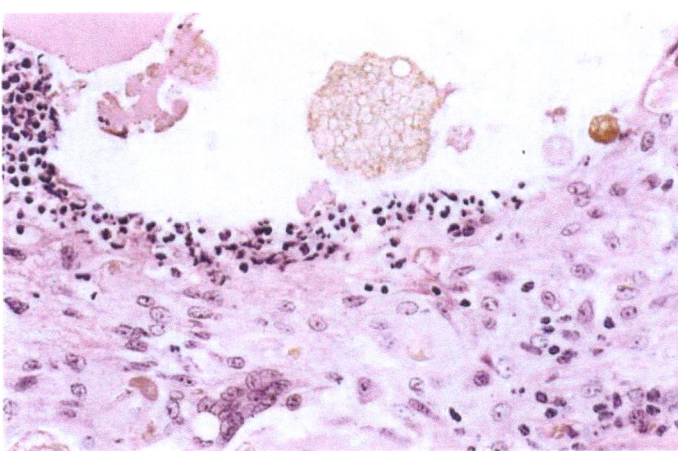

Figure 5.16 Myospherulosis of subcutaneous tissue of maxillary region. Sac-like structures containing brown spherules are present. H & E (B)

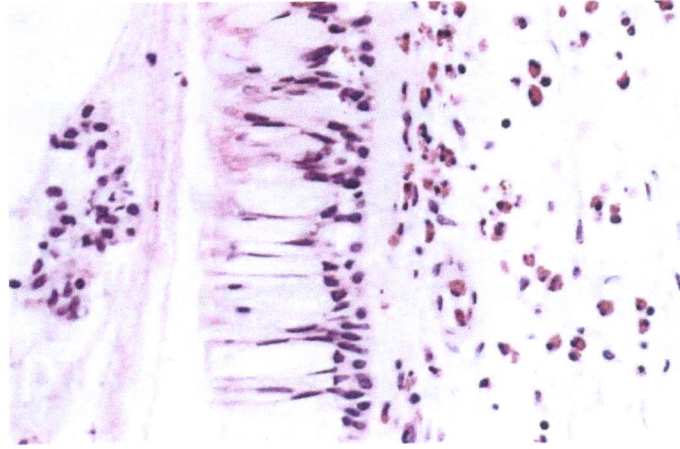

Figure 5.17 Surface of nasal polyp showing goblet cell hyperplasia, basement membrane thickening and numerous eosinophils and plasma cells in the lamina propria. H & E (C)

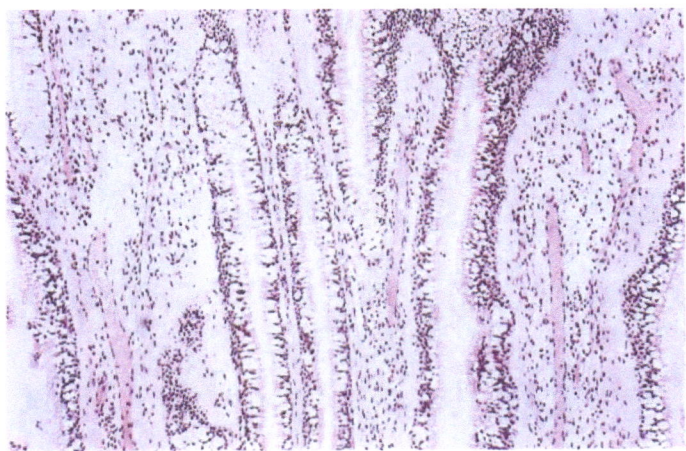

Figure 5.18 Hypertrophy and hyperplasia of mucous glands in nasal polyp. H & E (B)

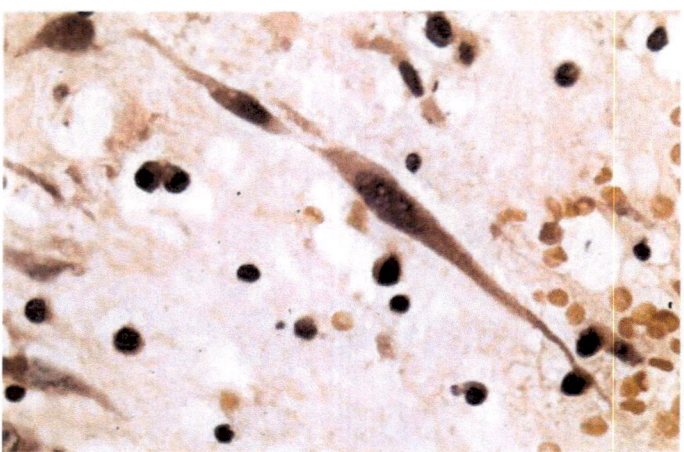

Figure 5.19 Nasal polyposis with stromal atypia showing large hyperchromatic nuclei. H & E (C)

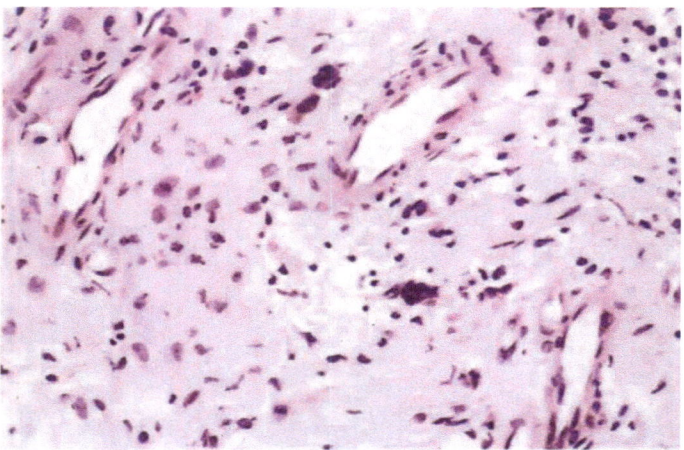

Figure 5.20 Nasal polyp with multinucleate cells containing small regular nuclei. H & E (B)

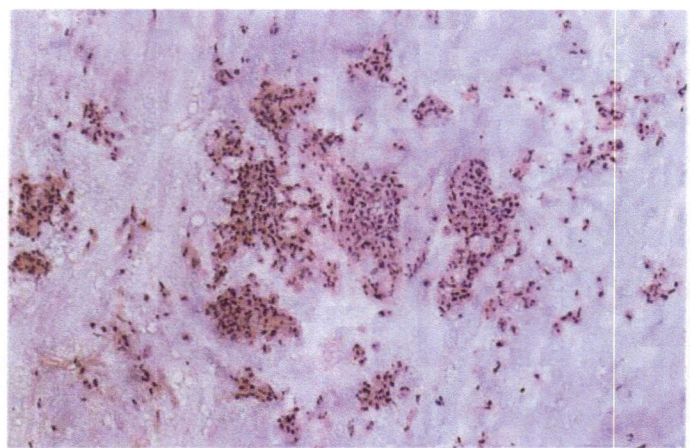

Figure 5.21 Inspissated mucus in maxillary sinus showing homogeneous bluish-pink staining substance containing groups of degenerate cells. H & E (B)

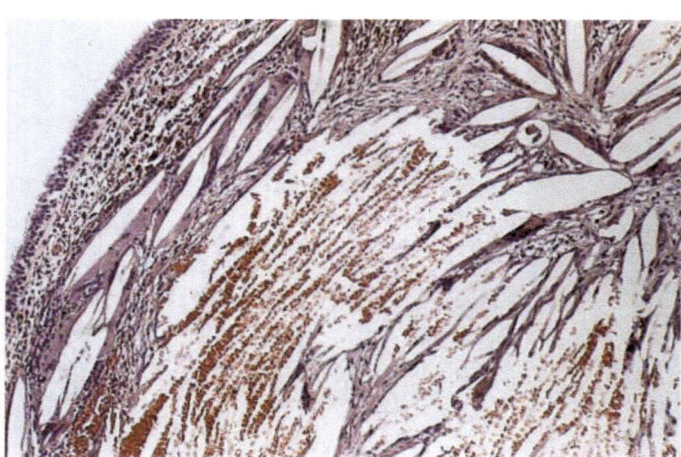

Figure 5.22 Cholesterol granuloma of maxillary antrum showing numerous clefts in mucosa with foreign-body giant cells and much haemorrhage. H & E (A)

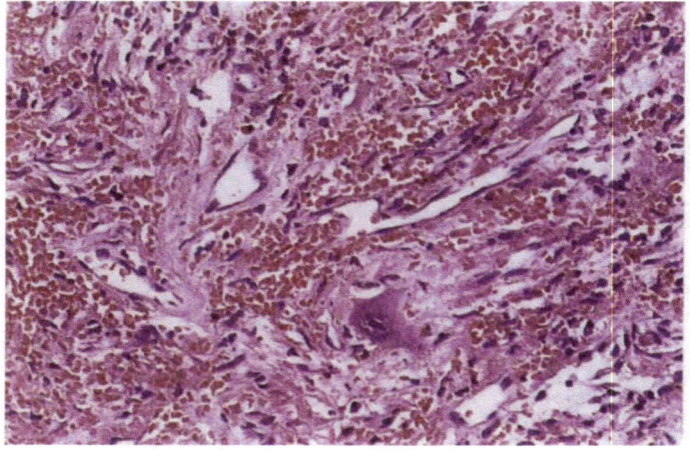

Figure 5.23 Organizing haematoma of nasal cavity showing haemorrhage and numerous small blood vessels accompanied by some atypical fibroblasts. H & E (B)

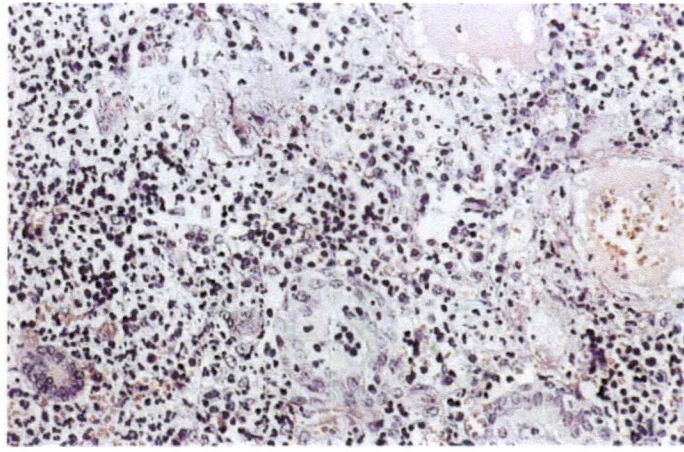

Figure 5.24 Wegener's granulomatosis showing acute inflammatory infiltration with some eosinophils and giant cells. H & E (B)

sive areas of irregular blood vessels often lined by bizarre endothelial cells, which may be mistaken for a malignant vascular neoplasm. Fibroblasts are numerous and fibrosis may be extensive. Large areas of fresh or partially degenerated blood which is becoming organized by granulation tissue are also present (Figure 5.23).

The source of the intranasal hemorrhage may be a neoplasm, such as an angiofibroma of the nasopharynx. Biopsy material may be taken from the organizing haematoma alone so that no evidence of the underlying neoplasm would be seen in the biopsy.

Wegener's granulomatosis

Wegener's granulomatosis is a systemic inflammatory condition affecting the nose (often with the paranasal sinuses), lungs and kidneys in all cases and other organs in some cases. Carrington and Liebow[13] have suggested that a limited form may affect the lungs only. The relationship of this entity to the systemic variety is not clear and the possibility of involvement of the nasal passages alone has not been clarified. In the light of present knowledge, I would suggest that only those cases in which the kidney is involved as well as the nose should be accepted as Wegener's granulomatosis.

Gross appearances

In the nose and sinuses, there is marked thickening of the mucosa by oedema and accumulation of pus in the maxillary antrum. Partial destruction of bony confines may be present, but the inflammatory process rarely, if ever, erodes through palate or face.

In the lungs, the lesions take the form of sharply circumscribed inflammatory masses in the parenchyma. Sometimes haemorrhagic infarcts caused by thrombosed arteritic vessels are present.

Kidneys are enlarged and show fine punctate haemorrhages and infarcts of the cortex[14].

Microscopic appearances

In biopsy sections of the nose and paranasal sinuses, vasculitis and necrosis may be present, but frequently only one of the two changes is seen in the limited material available with such biopsies. Indeed, in many nasal biopsies of definite Wegener's granulomatosis, I have been able to identify only a non-specific chronic inflammatory infiltration of the nasal mucosa with some necrosis, Langhans and foreign-body giant cells and a moderate infiltration of eosinophils (Figures 5.24 and 5.25).

The characteristic feature of the renal changes in Wegener's granulomatosis is one of segmental necrotizing glomerulonephritis. This lesion is generally focal (Figure 5.26). There is evidence of glomerular thrombosis, with or without necrosis. Weiss and Crissman[15] failed to demonstrate evidence of an immune complex pathogenesis for this condition in the renal glomeruli and suggested that glomerular thrombosis and necrosis are the prime findings. Serum autoantibodies against neutrophils and monocytes have recently been discovered as specific to Wegener's granulomatosis and they are stated to provide an accurate marker of disease activity[16].

Midline granuloma

I do not believe that midline granuloma exists as a pathological entity. Lymphoma is one of the many pathological conditions that may give rise to ulceration of the nose.

Patients with nasal ulceration should be investigated by the standard clinical, laboratory and radiological methods. Biopsy sections should be examined with care for evidence of lymphoma and other neoplastic conditions (Figure 5.27). If chronic inflammation or necrosis only is found, the pathologist should admit that no specific diagnosis can be made. In a few cases, ulceration continues in the absence of diagnostic features in the biopsy. Under these conditions, further biopsy material should be obtained.

Perforation of nasal septum

In cases of inflammatory non-specific perforation of the nasal septum, biopsy often shows widespread squamous metaplasia, hyperplasia and dysplasia of stratified squamous epithelium of adjacent tissue. In such cases, these changes should be recognized as having no neoplastic connotation (Figure 5.28).

References

1. Anson, B. J. (1966). *Morris' Human Anatomy. A Complete Systemic Treatise*, 12th Edn. (New York: McGraw-Hill)
2. Jafek, B. W. (1983). Ultrastructure of human nasal mucosa. *Laryngoscope*, **93**, 1576–1599
3. Matulionis, D. H., Breipohl, W. and Bhatnagar, K. P. (1982). Degeneration and regeneration of olfactory epithelium in the mouse. A scanning electron microscopic study. *Ann. Otol. Rhinol. Laryngol.*, **91** (Suppl. 89), 1–12
4. Reyes, E. (1946). Rhinoscleroma; observations based on study of 200 cases. *Arch. Dermatol.*, **54**, 531–537
5. Lindsay, J. R. and Perlman, H. B. (1951). Sarcoidosis of upper respiratory tract. *Ann. Otol. Rhinol. Laryngol.*, **60**, 549–566
6. Chandler, F. W., Kaplan, W. and Ajello, L. (1980). *A Colour Atlas and Textbook of the Histopathology of Mycotic Diseases.* (London: Wolfe Medical)
7. Katzenstein, A. A., Sale, S. C. and Greenberger, P. A. (1983). Pathologic findings in allergic aspergillus sinusitis. *Am. J. Surg. Pathol.*, **7**, 439–443
8. Khaleque, K. A. (1963). Interesting findings in rhinosporidiosis. *Am. J. Med.*, **35**, 566–568
9. McClatchie, S., Warambo, M. W. and Bremner, A. D. (1969). Myospherulosis. A previously unreported disease? *Am. J. Clin. Pathol.*, **51**, 699–704
10. Rosai, J. (1978). The nature of myospherulosis of the upper respiratory tract. *Am. J. Clin. Pathol.*, **69**, 475–481
11. Compagno, J. and Hyams, V. J. (1976). Nasal polyposis with atypical stroma. *Arch. Pathol. Lab. Med.*, **100**, 224–226
12. Graham, J. and Michaels, L. (1978). Cholesterol granuloma of the maxillary antrum. *Clin. Otolaryngol.*, **3**, 155–160
13. Carrington, C. B. and Liebow, A. A. (1970). Pulmonary veno-occlusive disease. *Hum. Pathol.*, **1**, 322–324
14. Godman, G. C. and Churg, J. (1954). Wegener's granulomatosis; pathology and review of the literature. *Am. Med. Assoc. Arch. Pathol.*, **58**, 533–553
15. Weiss, M. A. and Crissman, J. D. (1984). Renal biopsy findings in Wegener's granulomatosis: segmental necrotizing glomerulonephritis with glomerular thrombosis. *Hum. Pathol.*, **15**, 942–956
16. van der Woude, F. J., Rasmussen, N., Lobatto, S. *et al.* (1985). Autoantibodies against neutrophils and monocytes: tool for diagnosis and marker of disease activity in Wegener's granulomatosis. *Lancet*, **1**, 425–442

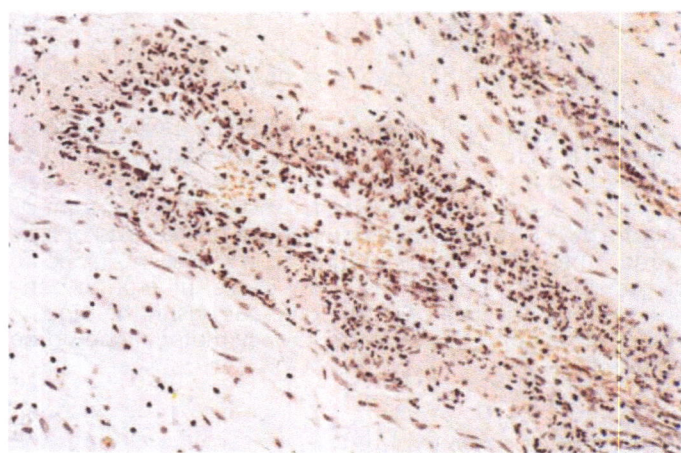

Figure 5.25 Wegener's granulomatosis. Biopsy of nose showing acute vasculitis. H & E (B)

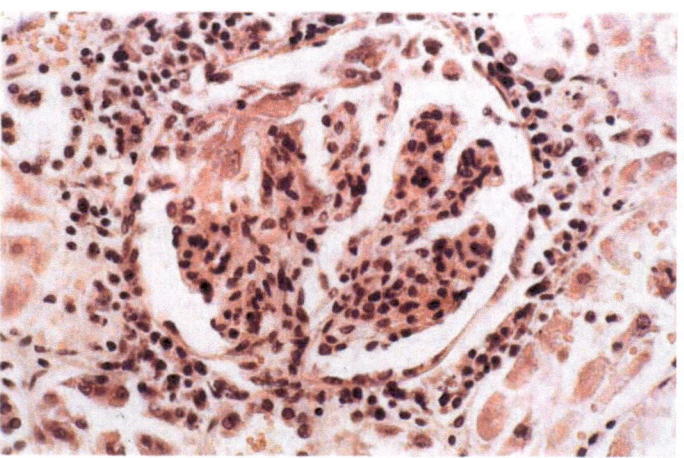

Figure 5.26 Kidney in Wegener's granulomatosis showing segmental deposition of fibrin and necrosis in glomerulus. H & E (C)

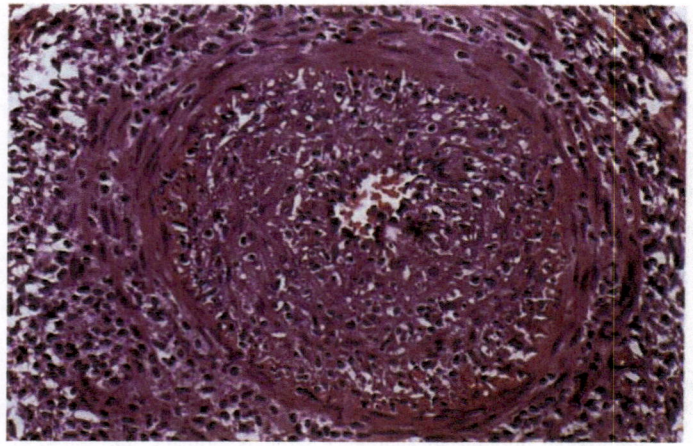

Figure 5.27 T-cell lymphoma of nose showing infiltration of arterial wall by atypical lymphoid cells. The patient's nasal biopsy showed extensive necrosis. H & E (B)

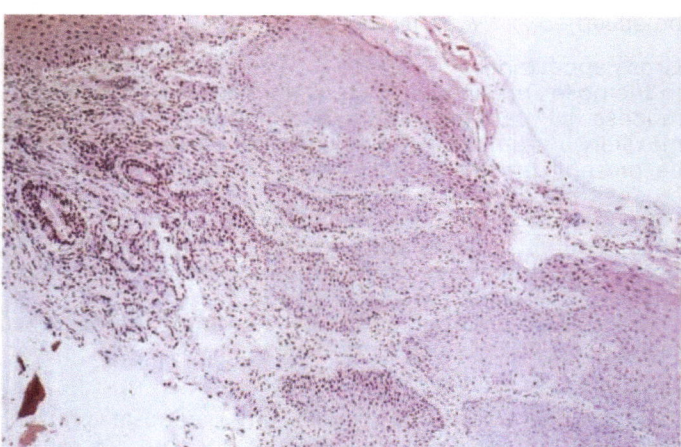

Figure 5.28 Epithelium at edge of nasal septal perforation showing dysplasia and hyperplasia. H & E (A)

Epithelial and Neuroectodermal Neoplasms of the Nose and Paranasal Sinuses

6

Papillomas

Three types of papilloma occur in the nasal cavity and paranasal sinuses. They are: inverted papilloma; fungiform or septal papilloma; cylindric cell papilloma.

Inverted papilloma

Inverted papilloma is a benign neoplastic proliferation consisting of both squamous and respiratory columnar epithelium and having a mesenchymal stroma.

Gross appearances
Inverted papillomas may look grossly like allergic nasal polyps but are usually more opaque and are never removed with an elongated stalk. The surface is frequently corrugated and shows small pits, the sites of the mucosal sinus-like inversions (Figure 6.1).

Microscopic appearances
The stroma of a sinonasal papilloma of inverted type is composed of loose connective tissue, often with dilated lymphatic vessels and is similar to that of nasal polyps. It differs, however, from all other tumours of the upper respiratory tract by the presence of invaginations of sinus-like character which are lined by variable amounts of stratified squamous epithelium, alternating with, or even covered by, ciliated or goblet cell-forming respiratory epithelium. The appearances of these invaginations are suggestive of the development of patches of squamous metaplasia in the epithelium of the ducts of mucoserous glands. The squamous epithelium in the infoldings or on the surface often contains large amounts of glycogen giving a clear cell appearance. The production of keratin or intercellular bridges (prickles) by the heaped-up cells is infrequent. In some places, ciliated columnar cells appear to form a row, lining the inner surface of an epidermoid area (Figures 6.2 to 6.4). Papillae of respiratory epithelium are often seen in inverted papillomas, suggesting a relationship between the latter and cylindric cell papilloma. The connective tissue of the inverted papilloma contains acute and chronic inflammatory cells, together with nuclear debris derived from them. Such cells are always present in considerable numbers among the epithelial cells of the neoplasm.

Mitotic figures are common in the heaped-up epithelium of inverted papillomas, usually near the basal layers. Woodson et al.[1] found that, when mitotic figures were rare or absent, recurrence was at a rate of 37%. Up to two mitoses per high-power field was associated with 80% recurrence. Recurrence in those cases with more than two mitoses per high-power field was 88%. The latter lesions were associated with mitoses situated towards the epithelial surface. Thus, the tendency to recurrence may be assessed by the numbers of mitoses in the epithelium and their position[1].

Association with malignancy
The inverted type of sinonasal papilloma may be accompanied or followed by malignancy. The former is much more frequent; the subsequent development of malignancy in benign inverted papilloma is rare. The carcinoma is keratinizing or non-keratinizing squamous cell or of the cylindric cell variety (Figures 6.5 and 6.6 and see below). An intraepithelial carcinomatous change may be observed in the inverted papilloma or in the adjacent epithelium without frankly invasive carcinoma. It is important, in such a case, that all papillomas be removed and examined carefully for possible invasive carcinoma.

Everted squamous cell papilloma

This is a wart-like process that usually occurs on the nasal septum.

Pathological appearances
The lesion is a raised verrucous excrescence attached to the mucosa by a wide base. Microscopically, there are fingers of growth showing a connective-tissue core and a stratified squamous epithelial covering sprouting from the septal mucosa. Portions of the surface epithelial covering may be composed of respiratory epithelium, either of ciliated or of mucous type (Figure 6.7).

Cylindric cell papilloma

Cylindric cell papilloma is usually seen in the lateral wall of the nose as well as in the maxillary and ethmoidal sinuses. It has been known by a variety of names, including papillary adenoma, microcystic adenoma, Schneiderian papilloma and transitional papilloma of exophytic type. The term cylindric cell papilloma refers specifically to its origin from the pseudostratified respiratory epithelium of the sinonasal tract.

Pathological appearances
This neoplasm is grossly friable and opaque, without the smooth surface of an inverted papilloma, but rather with a finely granular surface.

Microscopically, it is characterized by an everted frond-like series of folds of mucosa covered by respiratory epithelium. The cilia of the lining epithelial cells are usually not seen. The luminal portion of the lining epithelial cells often shows an eosinophilic staining property resembling oncocytic change. Numerous cystic mucus-containing spaces are present among the epithelial cells (Figures 6.8 to 6.10). These are probably derived from intracytoplasmic lumina in respiratory epithelial cells[2]. In some cases, the numerous cysts may give rise to the possibility of the lesion being one of rhinosporidiosis (see Chapter 5). The distinction may be easily made since, in cylindric cell papilloma, the cysts are entirely in the thickened epithelium, while, in rhinosporidiosis, they are in the subepithelial tissues.

The lesion has a tendency to recur but is benign.

Squamous Carcinoma

Squamous carcinoma of the mucosae of the nose and paranasal sinuses is a rare neoplasm but is the commonest malignant tumour of the nasal region. It probably represents less than 1% of all malignant neoplasms. The mucosae of the nose and paranasal sinuses comprise a freely intercommunicating system of spaces lined by respiratory epithelium. Malignant change tends to affect

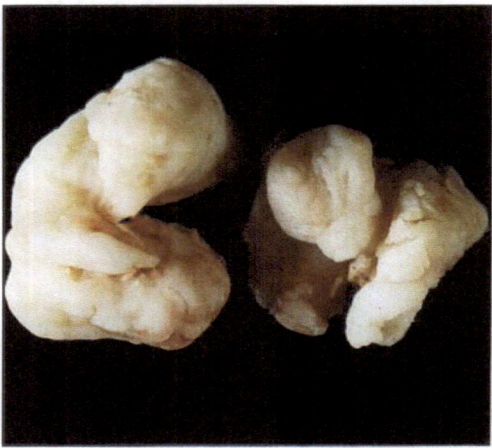

Figure 6.1 Inverted papilloma showing a lobulated mucosal-covered mass which is more opaque than the common nasal polyp and shows a corrugated surface with occasional small pits

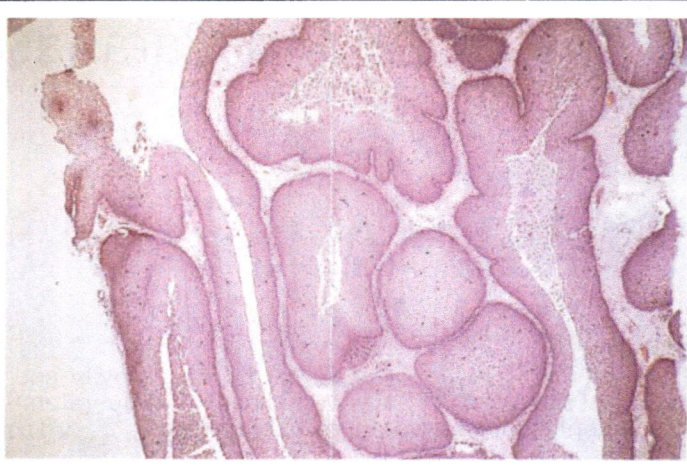

Figure 6.2 Inverted papilloma showing 'inverted' duct-like canals lined by metaplastic stratified squamous epithelium. Areas of the thinner respiratory epithelium can be seen in a few places. H & E (A)

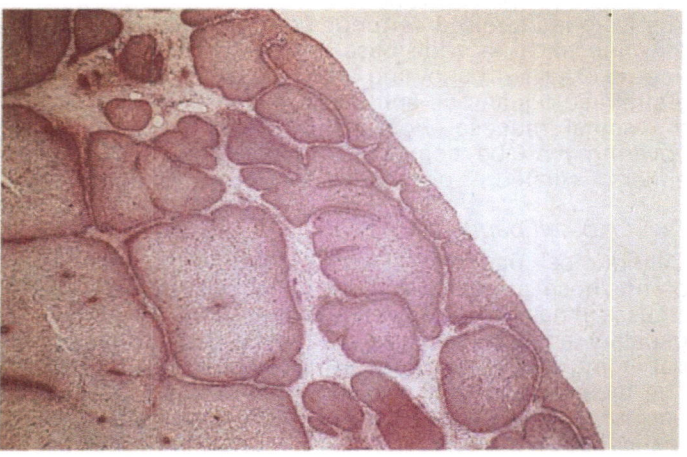

Figure 6.3 Inverted papilloma showing cluster of stratified squamous epithelial masses near surface. H & E (A)

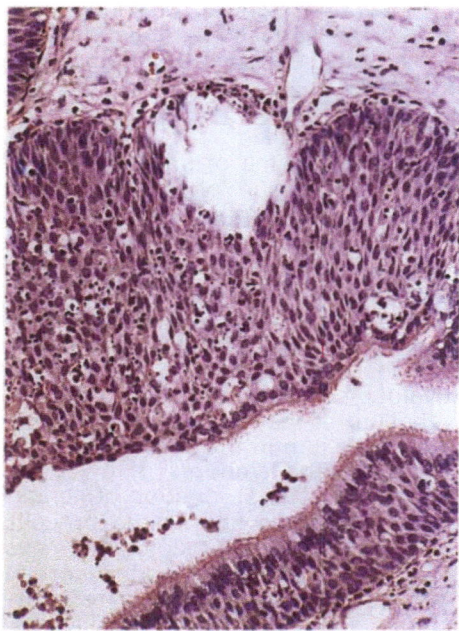

Figure 6.4 Deeper part of invagination of inverted papilloma showing non-keratinizing stratified squamous epithelium covered by ciliated respiratory epithelium. H & E (B)

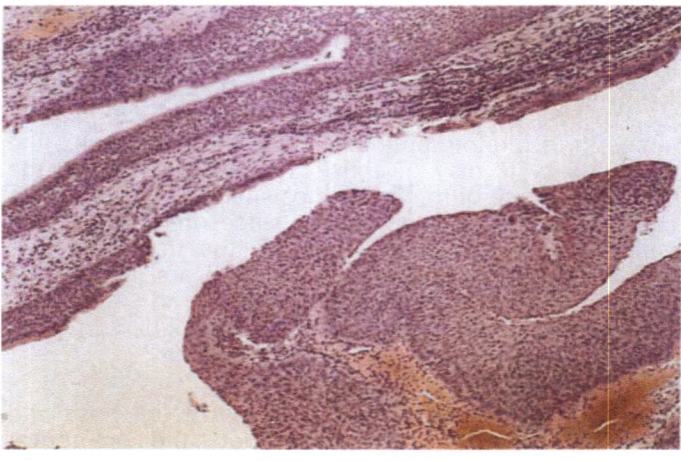

Figure 6.5 Inverted papilloma (top left) occurring in same specimen as cylindric cell carcinoma (bottom right). H & E (A)

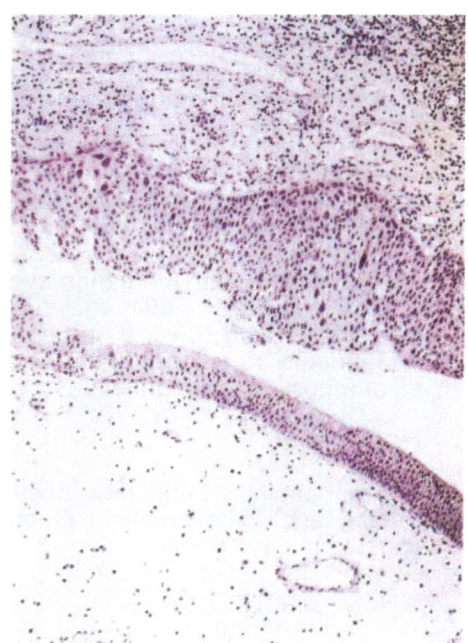

Figure 6.6 Inverted papilloma with an area of severe dysplasia (carcinoma in situ) shown in the upper horizontally displayed epithelium. H & E (B)

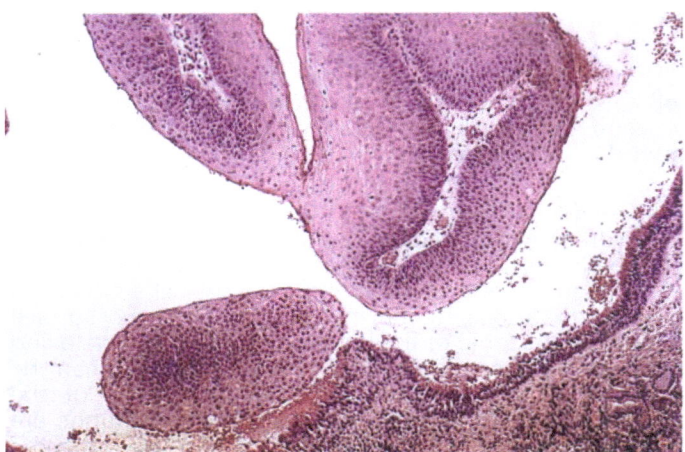

Figure 6.7 Everted papilloma of nasal septum. Fronds of squamous epithelium which arise from nasal lining epithelium. H & E (B)

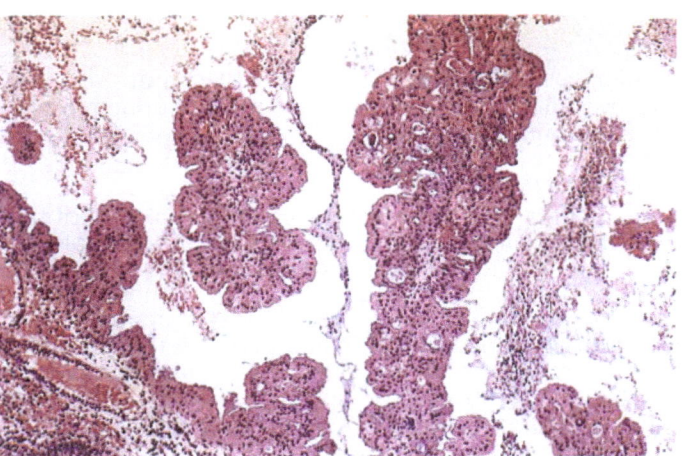

Figure 6.8 Cylindric cell papilloma showing papillary eversions of hyperplastic respiratory epithelium. H & E (B)

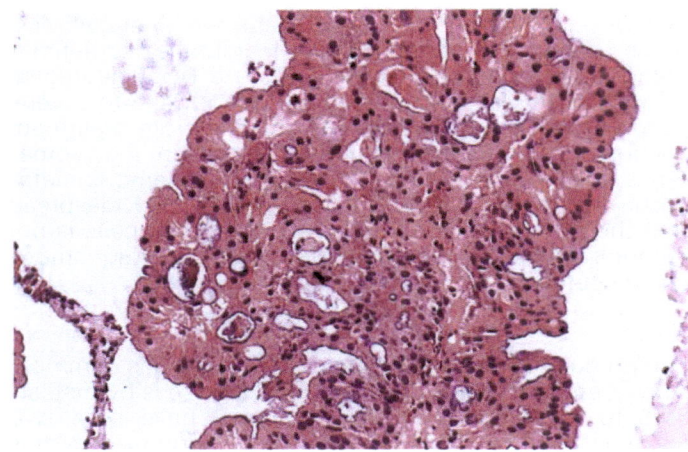

Figure 6.9 Cylindric cell papilloma showing some acini and numerous intracytoplasmic lumina. H & E (B)

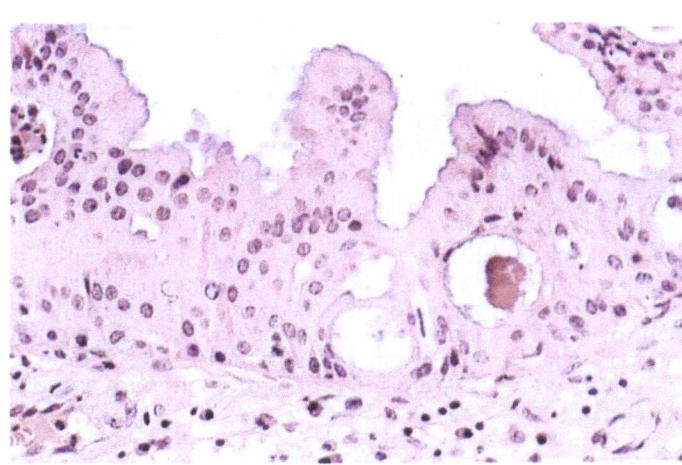

Figure 6.10 Cylindric cell papilloma showing intracytoplasmic luminae. There are no true cilia arising from the cell surfaces. H & E (C)

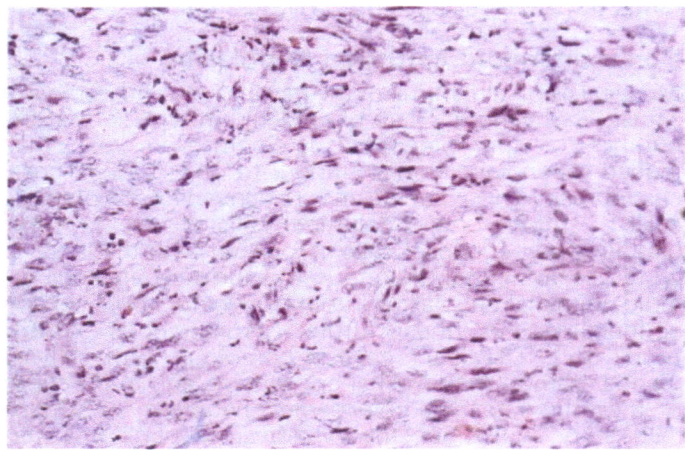

Figure 6.11 Spindle cell carcinoma of the maxillary antrum. H & E (C)

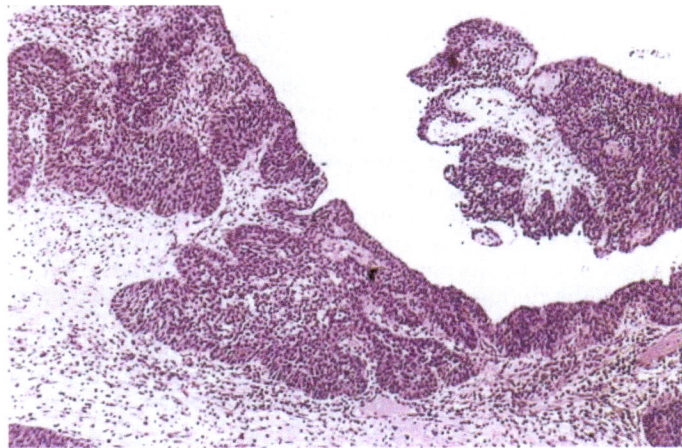

Figure 6.12 Cylindric cell carcinoma of nose. The surface is covered by malignant cylindric cell epithelium with downgrowths and shows also some papillae of cylindric cell epithelium. H & E (B)

the mucosae of several parts of the system at the same time; it is unusual for the neoplasm to be confined to one part of sinonasal system.

Gross appearances

In most cases, the growth involves the antral wall of the nose, the maxillary antrum and many of the ethmoid air cells. The frontal and sphenoidal sinuses are rarely affected. Spread of the neoplasm through bone to orbit, cranial cavity, oral cavity and zygoma is frequent. The neoplasm appears as a friable and papillary thickening of the mucosa, often with ulceration of the surface. The maxillary antrum becomes filled with tumour, producing a yellowish-grey mass in that location.

Microscopic appearances

In 80–85% of cases, the neoplasm shows keratinization, i.e. it is 'well' or 'moderately well' differentiated. Some well-differentiated but non-keratinizing carcinomas have been described as cylindric cell carcinoma or transitional cell carcinoma (see below).

Regions of carcinoma in situ may be seen at the edge of the invasive carcinoma and are sometimes present in biopsy material without invasive carcinoma. Carcinoma in situ may sometimes be seen in inverted papillomas as a manifestation of malignant change. Apart from this, carcinoma in situ is rare in the nasal cavity and paranasal sinuses (Figure 6.6). When present, a careful search for concomitant invasive carcinoma should be carried out.

Spindle cell carcinoma (Figure 6.11)

Spindle cell carcinoma is a squamous cell carcinoma at the other extreme of the spectrum of differentiation and is rare in the nose and paranasal sinuses. A definite diagnosis of this entity can only be made if squamous carcinoma in situ or invasive squamous cell carcinoma is present as well as the undifferentiated, malignant spindle cell tissue.

Spread

Cervical lymph nodes are involved in 17.6% of squamous cell carcinomas of the nose and paranasal sinuses. Disseminated metastases have been found in only 1.6% of all malignant neoplasms in that location[3].

Cylindric Cell Carcinoma

Cylindric cell carcinoma is a neoplasm which was well defined in the older literature and summarized by Ringertz[4], who also provided a careful description of his own experience with this cancer. The literature subsequent to Ringertz's account is, however, silent on this entity. The designation transitional carcinoma is applied to tumours with the features of cylindric cell carcinoma as well as to those with features of poorly-differentiated, non-keratinizing squamous carcinoma.

Although the respiratory epithelium of the nose resembles that of the larynx and lower respiratory tract microscopically, its development is from ectoderm while the latter is derived from entoderm. It would be expected that the nasal (Schneiderian) epithelium would have distinct attributes, particularly in its neoplastic form. Cylindric cell carcinoma is a tumour which is hardly ever found outside the nose and paranasal sinuses.

Gross appearances

Cylindric cell carcinoma has a tendency to exophytic growth from the mucosae of the nose and paranasal sinuses, producing protuberant areas with both papillary, i.e. finely corrugated, and polypoid, i.e. smooth-surfaced, appearances. Areas recognizable as oedematous nasal polyps may also be seen accompanying neoplastic formations, the latter being rougher and more friable in consistency. The maxillary antrum may be filled with solid yellowish-grey neoplasm. In most cases, areas of bone invasion and destruction, affecting particularly the maxillary bone, are observed.

Microscopic appearances

The microscopic characteristics of cylindric cell carcinoma were well described by Ringertz. The neoplasm is made up of interconnecting ribbons of tumour cells which, in some parts, appear to be invaginated from the surface epithelium. In some of the latter, a double layer enclosing a space (representing the invaginated crypt) can be recognized. Knob-like proliferations into some of the crypts are present. In other areas, the invaginations are filled up into solid columns. A further stage in some neoplasms is the confluence of the tumour columns. The stroma, which was external to the invaginations, now appears as isolated zones. In a few cases, there is necrosis of tumour cells distant from the stromal zones. The surface of the tumour shows papillary formations and is covered by malignant cylindric cell epithelium. The cells of the neoplasm are, for the most part, cylindrical, being set at right angles to the basement membrane on which they rest. Several layers of cells are present, the inner cells (i.e. those furthest from the basement membrane) sometimes being more rounded (Figures 6.12 to 6.14). The degree of nuclear atypia is variable, ranging from mild to severe. Mitoses are usually scarce. A transition from malignant cylindric cell epithelium to normal epithelium may sometimes be recognized. Foci of malignant squamous metaplasia are frequently present. This may be so widespread that the cylindric cell origin of the neoplastic cells is not recognized and the growth may be considered a squamous cell carcinoma.

Spread

Lymph node metastasis to the cervical region is common. A frequent termination of the clinical course is by metastases to the lung and other organs. I have seen two examples of metastatic cervical masses produced by this tumour, in which venous invasion was demonstrable grossly and confirmed microscopically.

Natural history

The natural history of cylindric cell carcinoma appears to be similar to that of squamous cell carcinoma, but further observation is required to determine possibly distinctive forms of behaviour possessed by this tumour.

Non-epidermoid Epithelial Neoplasms

Most cases of carcinoma of the nasal cavity and paranasal sinuses – a rare entity – are of epidermoid type so that the numbers of non-epidermoid carcinomas are very small indeed. Adenocarcinomas amount to only 6.2% of nasal carcinomas[5]. These neoplasms are derived from columnar cells of surface origin, columnar cells of seromucinous glands or myoepithelial cells associated with the latter. It would seem natural, therefore, to subdivide non-epidermoid epithelial neoplasms into those derived from surface epithelium and those from seromucinous glands (Table 6.1). The latter have a homology with salivary glands, both in their normal appearance and in the types of their tumours. The sole benign neoplasm of surface respiratory epithelium, the cylindric cell papilloma, has been described above. In the case of the malignant form of respiratory epithelium – adenocarcinoma – it is usually not possible to determine whether the neoplasm is derived from the surface cylindric cells or from the deeper glandular cells. Extremely well differentiated glandular neoplasms have sometimes been called adenoma, but, since an aggressive behaviour has on occasion been noted, they are best designated as low-grade adenocarcinomas[6].

Table 6.1 Non-epidermoid epithelial tumours of the nose and paranasal sinuses

Cells of origin	Neoplasm
Surface columnar	Cylindric cell papilloma
	Adenocarcinoma
Seromucinous glands: columnar cells	Adenocarcinoma
	Acinic cell carcinoma
	Oncocytoma
	Mucoepidermoid carcinoma
Myoepithelial cells	Pleomorphic adenoma
	Carcinoma ex pleomorphic adenoma
	Adenocystic carcinoma

Adenocarcinoma

The term adenocarcinoma covers a group of neoplasms composed of glandular structures with a range of patterns. My experience is similar to that of Heffner et al.[6] in that their most important feature for classification is the degree of differentiation of the glands and of the tumour cells. To make a distinction between a low-grade (better differentiated) and a high-grade (less differentiated) form of neoplasm is the first task of the pathologist after reaching a diagnosis of adenocarcinoma of the nose and paranasal sinuses.

Relationship to wood dust inhalation

An association between occupational exposure to wood dust and adenocarcinoma of the nose and sinuses was first reported from the High Wycombe area of England, where this disease was found to be 500 times more common among wood furniture workers than in the general population[7,8]. This association has been reported from many other countries, including the United States[9]. All reports are agreed that it is hard-wood dust, such as that of beech and oak, rather than soft-wood dust, such as that of pine, that is carcinogenic and that the characteristic neoplasm seen in the woodworkers is adenocarcinoma. Both low- and high-grade forms of adenocarcinoma are found in woodworkers.

Gross appearances

In some cases, the lesion is exophytic, producing a localized granular swelling which, histologically, is usually of a papillary appearance. In others, the tumour is deeply infiltrating and grossly represented by a pale-grey mass extending widely through the bony walls of the nose and sinuses.

Microscopic appearances

Low-grade adenocarcinoma: Low-grade adenocarcinomas are composed of uniform small glands lined by regular columnar cells with rare mitotic figures (Figures 6.15 and 6.16). An acinic cell carcinomatous appearance with the small acini showing cells containing granular basophilic cytoplasm and occasional foci of clear non-granular cells may often be seen[6]. Calcospherites or even larger areas of calcification may be present. A papillary pattern may be prominent in low-grade adenocarcinoma and the cases showing this are often grossly exophytic. The papillary appearance of low-grade adenocarcinoma should be distinguished from the more irregular colonic type of papillary pattern which occurs in high-grade carcinoma (see below).

It may be difficult to distinguish this tumour from cylindric cell papilloma. Microcysts in the epithelium are often prominent in the papilloma but are not found in adenocarcinoma. Papilloma also shows a more abundant, often myxoid, stroma.

High-grade adenocarcinoma: In this more-malignant form, there may be solid sheets of cells in many places. The papillary pattern, if present, is poorly defined and irregular. Nuclear pleomorphism is marked and mitotic figures are easily found (Figures 6.17 and 6.18).

Colonic type: A resemblance of some high-grade adenocarcinomas of the nose and paranasal sinuses to adenocarcinoma of the colon has been noted from time to time in the literature[10]. Papillary formations of tall columnar highly-atypical cells are characteristic. The cells are separated from the underlying stroma by a poorly defined basement membrane. There are numerous goblet cells. Argentaffin cells and Paneth cells may be present. In some cases, there is abundant mucus production and the cancer may then resemble colloid carcinoma of the colon.

Pleomorphic adenoma

Pleomorphic adenoma is a benign neoplasm with a mixed pattern combining epithelial and mesenchymal elements. It is generally believed that the latter stem from myoepithelial cells. While it is the commonest tumour of the parotid gland, it occurs but seldom in the nose and paranasal sinuses.

Site

Most nasal pleomorphic adenomas arise on the septum. Smaller numbers present on the lateral wall of the nose and even more unusual is the presentation of such a tumour in the mucosa of the maxillary antrum.

Pathological appearances

Pleomorphic adenomas are usually well demarcated with smooth lobulated surfaces. Their cut surfaces are greyish and usually homogeneous with a somewhat translucent appearance.

Both epithelial and mesenchymal formations of neoplastic cells should be present to allow a definite histological diagnosis of this entity. Epithelium is more prominent in nasal pleomorphic adenomas than in those tumours occurring in major salivary glands. The epithelial structures are mainly regular glands, often with secretion in their lumina. Areas of epidermoid cells are more prominent in nasal pleomorphic adenomas than in those seen elsewhere. The most usual mesenchymal feature in pleomorphic adenomas of the nasal passages is the filling of interglandular regions with loosely-arranged short spindle cells that appear to be in contiguity with, and of similar structure to, epithelial cells lining glands (Figures 6.19 and 6.20). Mucoid, myxoid and chondroid areas may also be present in which spindle cells of similar appearance are lodged within the particular ground substance. A fibrous capsule may sometimes be identified but is not usually so well defined as in the corresponding tumour of major salivary glands.

Acinic cell carcinoma

Acinic cell carcinoma is unusual in major salivary glands and rare in the nose and paranasal sinuses. Histologically there are nests of cells showing acinar and trabecular structure. Most tumour cells contain periodic acid–Schiff-positive diastase-resistant granules, resembling the parent acinic cells.

Clear cell carcinoma

Carcinomas formed by cells of clear cytoplasm which stain negatively for mucin are occasionally seen in the nose and paranasal sinuses (Figure 6.21). Some of these are acinic cell carcinomas with areas in which a clear cell appearance is produced as a result of an artefact in processing the tissue. In others, periodic acid–Schiff-positive granular cells cannot be found in any part of the neoplasm so that these cases cannot be considered to be acinic cell carcinomas. Glycogen may or may not be

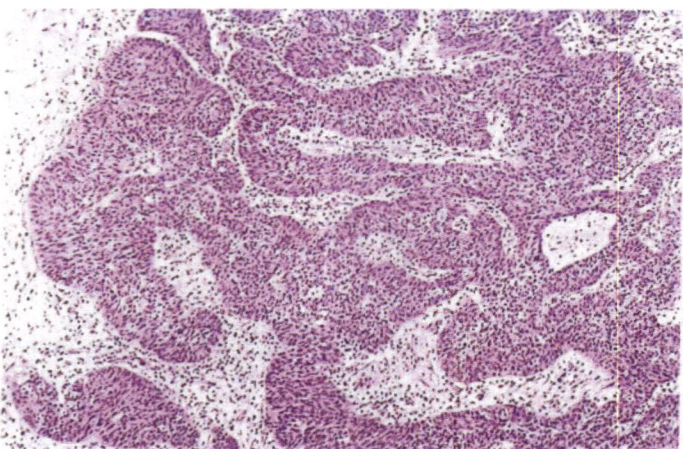

Figure 6.13 Cylindric cell carcinoma. The tumour is made up of invaginated ribbons of malignant cylindric cells.   H & E (B)

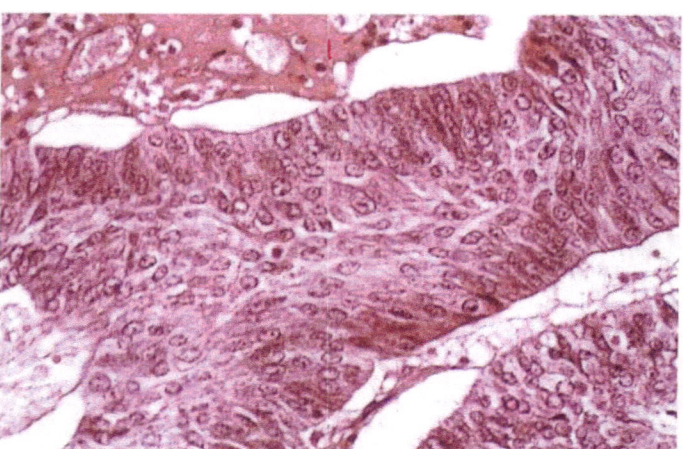

Figure 6.14 Higher power view of cylindric cell carcinoma showing basal tumour cells aligned at right angles to basement membrane.   H & E (C)

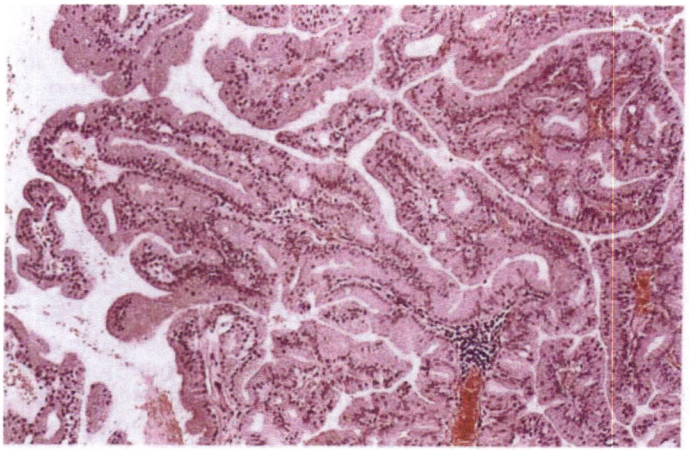

Figure 6.15 Low-grade adenocarcinoma of nasal cavity showing uniform small glands lined by regular columnar cells with areas of papilla formation.   H & E (B)

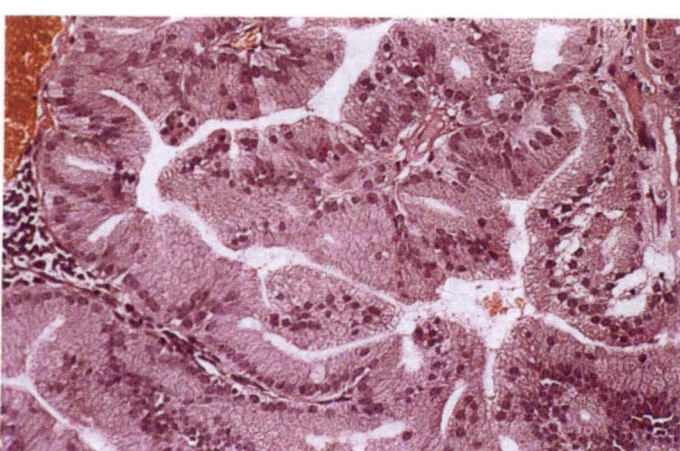

Figure 6.16 Higher power view of Figure 6.15 to show uniform appearance of nuclei.   H & E (C)

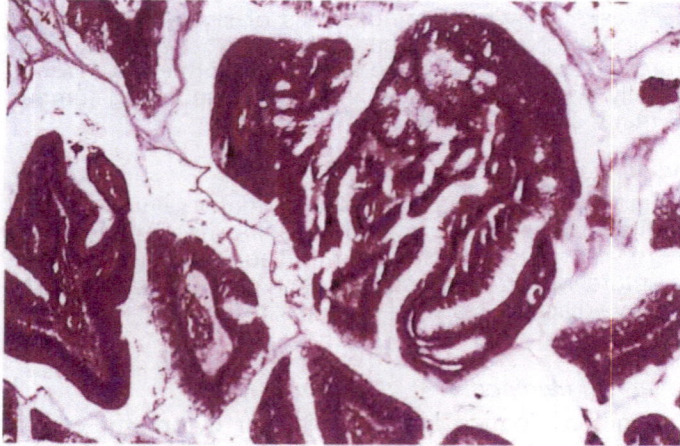

Figure 6.17 High-grade adenocarcinoma of nose showing papillae and lining of heaped-up highly atypical cells.   H & E (B)

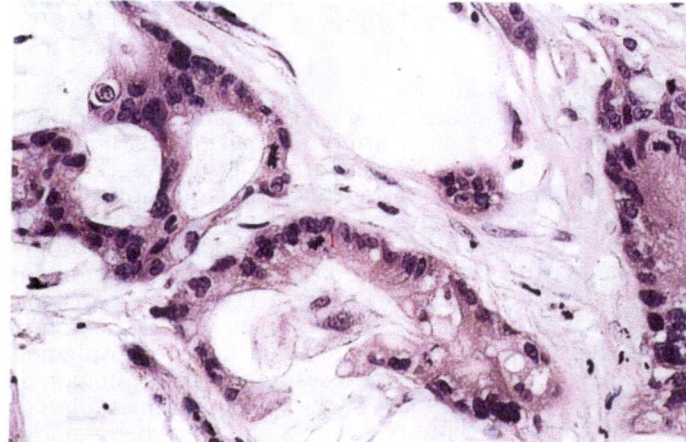

Figure 6.18 Woodworker's adenocarcinoma of nose showing highly atypical cells lining acini of tumour and pools of mucin.   H & E (C)

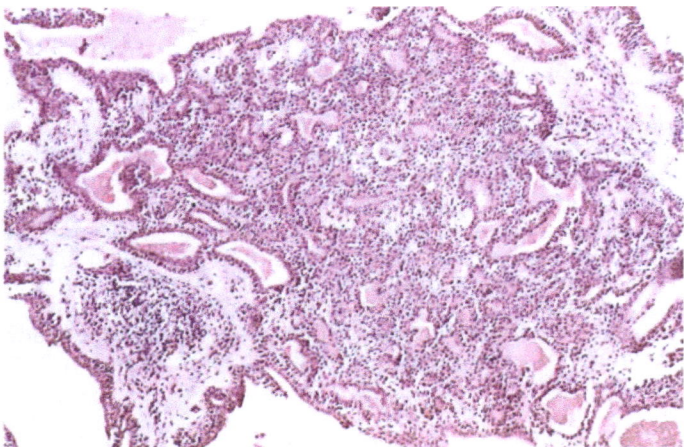

Figure 6.19 Pleomorphic adenoma of nasal septum. There are regular glands containing secretion and numerous cells in the interglandular areas. H & E (B)

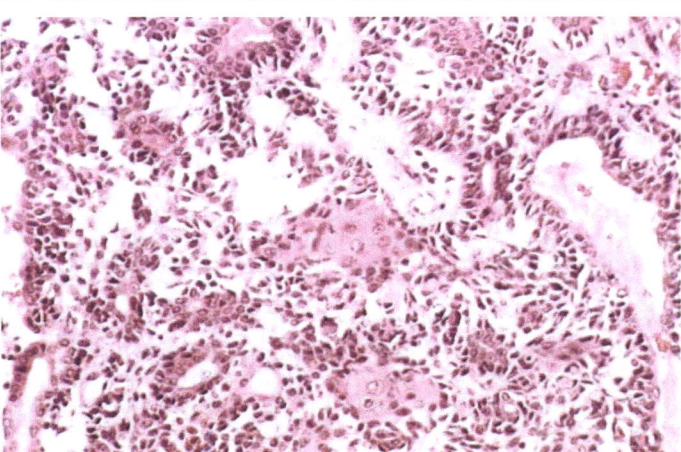

Figure 6.20 Higher power view of pleomorphic adenoma showing spindle cells in interglandular areas which appear to be in contiguity with cells lining the glands. Note also epidermoid areas. H & E (C)

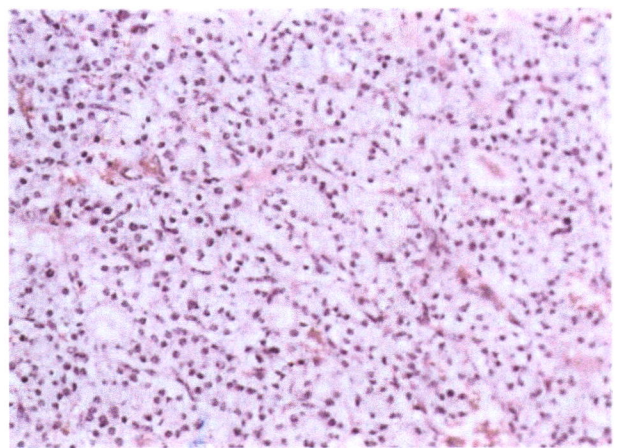

Figure 6.21 Clear cell adenocarcinoma of the nasal cavity. The tumour is composed of fairly regular cells with empty cytoplasm. H & E (C)

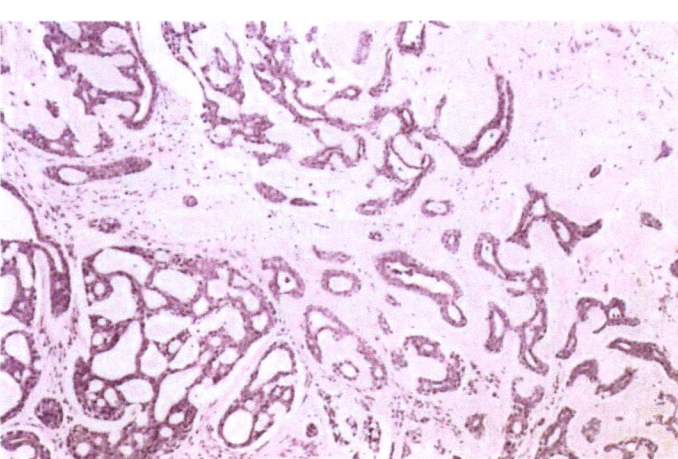

Figure 6.22 Adenoid cystic carcinoma of nasal cavity. The neoplasm shows numerous tubular areas as well as cribiform masses. H & E (B)

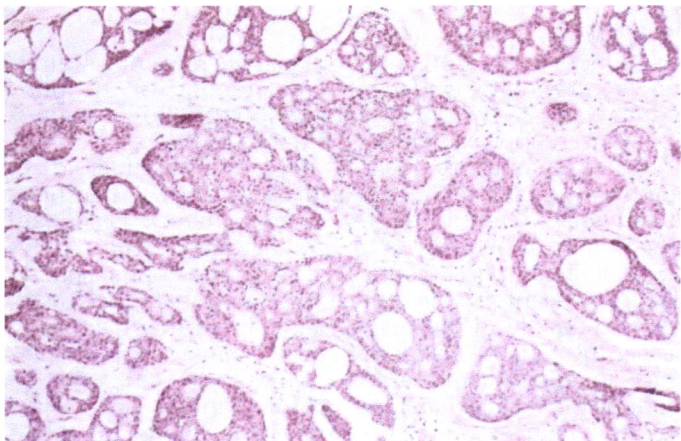

Figure 6.23 In this adenoid cystic carcinoma of the nose, cribriform areas predominate. H & E (C)

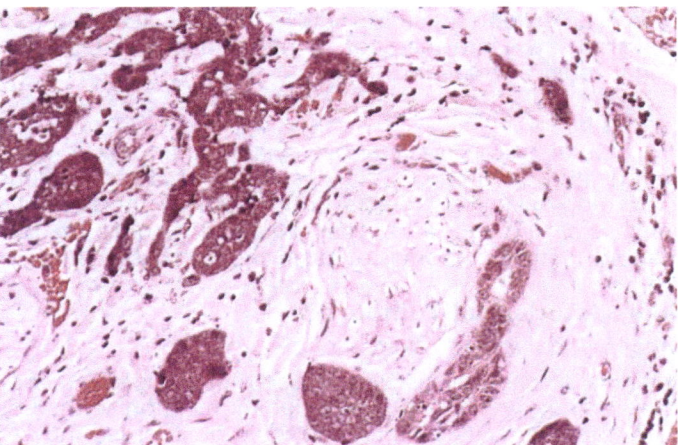

Figure 6.24 Adenoid cystic carcinoma showing perineural infiltration. H & E (C)

present in the clear cytoplasm of the tumour. A locally aggressive behaviour of this lesion with low potential for metastasis is to be expected.

In each case in which a clear cell carcinoma is seen, the possibility of a metastatic deposit from clear cell carcinoma of the kidney must be considered. The kidney tumour shows cytoplasmic lipid as well as glycogen in the tumour cells and exhibits considerable vascularity.

Adenoid cystic carcinoma

Adenoid cystic carcinoma is a malignant tumour derived from the salivary type seromucinous glands of the nose and paranasal sinuses, possibly from the myoepithelial cells of these glands.

Pathological appearances

The gross appearances of the neoplasms in the nose and sinuses are not distinctive. The nasal mass may appear polypoid. The maxillary sinus is frequently occupied by grey tumour with evidence of bony invasion.

The term 'cribriform', i.e. having numerous small holes, is descriptive of the most important feature of the variable histology of this neoplasm. It is composed of rather small regular epithelial cells with uniform nuclei staining darkly and in a homogeneous fashion. Among these cells are many holes which seem to be punched out without any definite glandular lining. These 'pseudocysts' contain amorphous material which may be eosinophilic or basophilic (Figures 6.22 and 6.23). It shows histochemical features of connective tissue mucin, such as dissolution of toluidine blue staining after incubation with hyaluronidase. In a few places, columnar epithelium may line acinar structures and the secretions found in these duct-like regions show staining reactions more characteristic of epithelial mucins.

I have not been able to separate adenoid cystic carcinomas into prognostic groups on a histological basis as has been done by others[11] and am sceptical of the possibilities of such assessment.

Spread

Local infiltration, particularly along nerve sheaths, is the most constant means of spread of this neoplasm. In fact, infiltration of the neoplasm along perineural spaces is frequently present in histological sections of the neoplasm (Figure 6.24). Lymph node involvement is infrequent. Bloodstream spread is common, however. In 174 patients with adenoid cystic carcinomas of minor salivary glands, Spiro et al.[12] reported remote spread in nearly 40%. Lungs, bones and liver are the sites of bloodstream metastasis, in that order of frequency.

Natural history

The natural history of adenoid cystic carcinoma is one of repeated recurrences after surgical excision, often continuing over many years until death of the patient. Spiro et al. indicate a 10-year cure rate of only 7% for adenoid cystic carcinomas of nasal and paranasal sinuses.

Neuroectodermal Tumours

Encephalocoele and glioma

Deposits of cerebral tissue are occasionally seen in the nose. If they are not in direct communication with the brain, they are called gliomas. It must be stressed, however, that these lesions are not actually neoplasms of glial tissue, but rather heterotopic brain tissue.

Most nasal gliomas are seen in infants soon after birth. Sixty per cent of the lesions present subcutaneously upon the bridge of the nose, which may be broadened, while 30% are situated high up within the nasal cavity and are seen as smooth pale polypoid masses. In the other 10% of cases, the lesion is both intranasal and extranasal.

Rarely, heterotopic neural tissue (glioma) may be found in the nose of adults. These are almost always found in the middle turbinate.

Nasal glioma is, in most cases, composed of astrocytes, often the plump gemistiocytic form, in a background of fibrous tissue (Figure 6.25). In a few cases, nerve cells may also be present, although their identification may be difficult because they may have shrunk to a small size. A surface covering of skin or respiratory epithelium is present, depending on the site and size of the glioma.

Encephalocoeles contain brain, meningeal tissue and sometimes even part of the ventricular system (Figure 6.26).

Meningioma

Meningiomas with a histological pattern identical to the intracranial neoplasms are sometimes encountered in the nose. The majority are derived by extension of intracranial meningiomas. Occasionally, no intracranial component is detected in a case of nasal meningioma and it must then be presumed that the lesion is primary in the nose or paranasal sinuses.

Pathological appearances

Meningiomas of the nose may present as nasal polyps. The tumours usually have a firm consistency and may be somewhat granular or fibrous on their cut surfaces.

Most intranasal meningiomas show a meningothelial (Figure 6.27) or fibroblastic pattern, in which tumour cells of epithelial or fibroblastic appearance, respectively, are arranged concentrically around small blood vessels. Both cell appearances may be present in the same meningioma. Psammoma bodies are sometimes seen.

Neurogenic tumours

Neurogenic tumours are probably all derived by proliferation of Schwann cells. There are four varieties: neurilemmoma (Figure 6.28), neurofibroma, plexiform neurofibroma and neurogenous sarcoma (malignant schwannoma). Each of these neoplasms has been identified in the nose and paranasal sinuses, the majority being neurilemmomas[13].

Malignant melanoma

Malignant melanomas, which are tumours arising from melanin-producing cells, are unusual lesions in the mucosa of the air and food passages.

Pathological appearances

The tumour may be polypoid but usually presents infiltrating features with evidence of destruction of the bony antral wall. A brownish colouration of the tumour is apparent in approximately two-thirds of the cases.

The tumours exhibit cells of polygonal (epithelioid) or spindle shape or a mixture of both kinds. The cellular shape is not related to the degree of malignancy. Malignant melanomas of the nose often contain large bizarre, polygonal or giant cells (Figure 6.29). Large eosinophilic nucleoli are present in the nuclei of about half the cases, situated mainly in the polygonal cells. In the majority of cases, the tumour cells are heavily pigmented with melanin; in some, the presence of pigment can only be identified by silver staining. Mitotic figures are always frequent in nasal and paranasal sinus malignant melanomas. Their numbers range from one in every high-power field to one in every five high-power fields. Junctional activity is an important feature of malignant melanoma of the skin but this change is unusual in the nasal variety of the tumour because, unlike the skin neoplasm, only small amounts of normal epithelium are removed with the tumour. Moreover, the epithelium is frequently ulcerated over the surface of nasal melanoma.

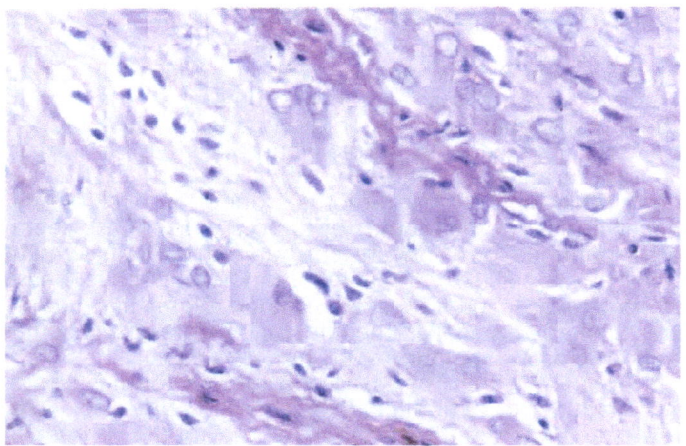

Figure 6.25 Nasal 'glioma'. The lesion is composed of gemistiocytic astrocytes and glial fibres. H & E (C)

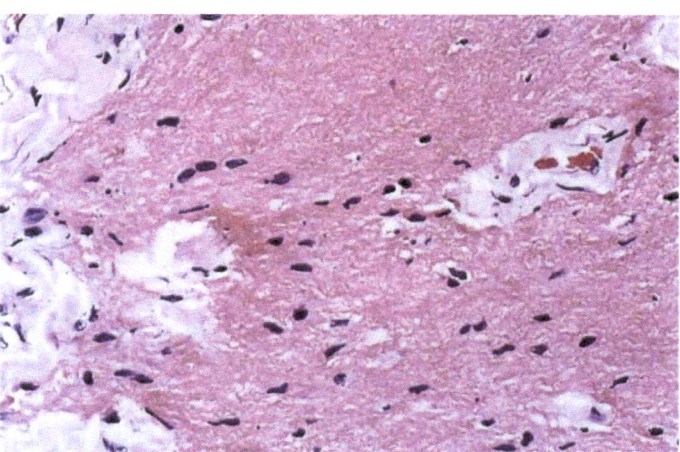

Figure 6.26 Encephalocoele of nose showing brain tissue composed of nerve cells, astocytes and glial fibres. H & E (B)

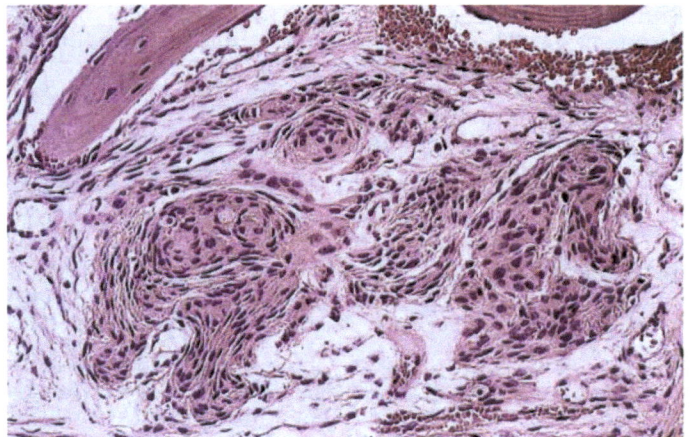

Figure 6.27 Meningothelial meningioma in the ethmoid sinus showing whorls of epithelial-like cells. H & E (B)

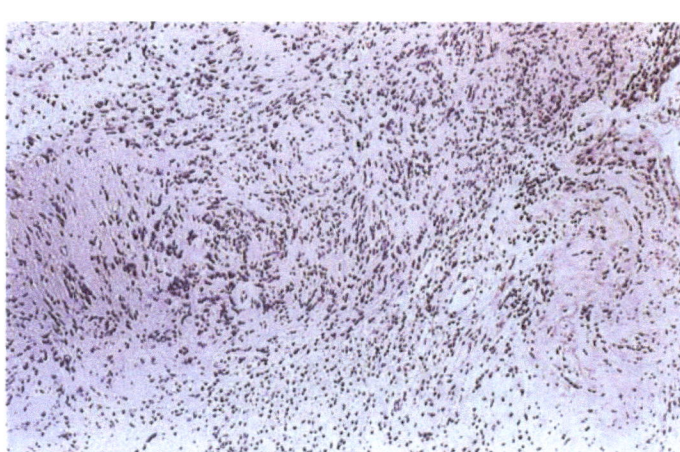

Figure 6.28 Neurilemmoma of nasal cavity showing Antoni A and B areas. H & E (A)

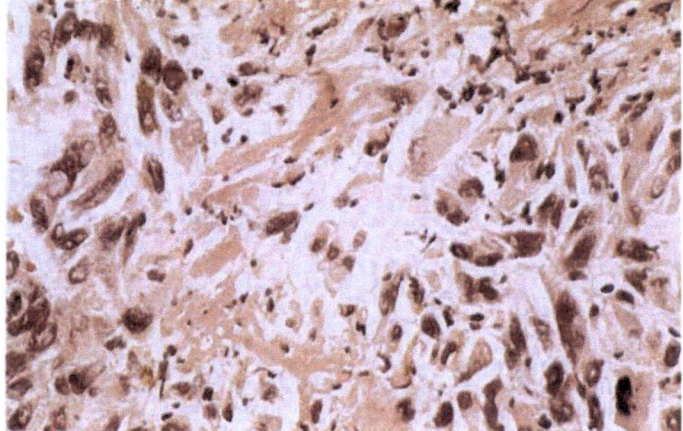

Figure 6.29 Malignant melanoma of nasal cavity showing pigmented tumour cells which are irregular with abundant cytoplasm. H & E (C)

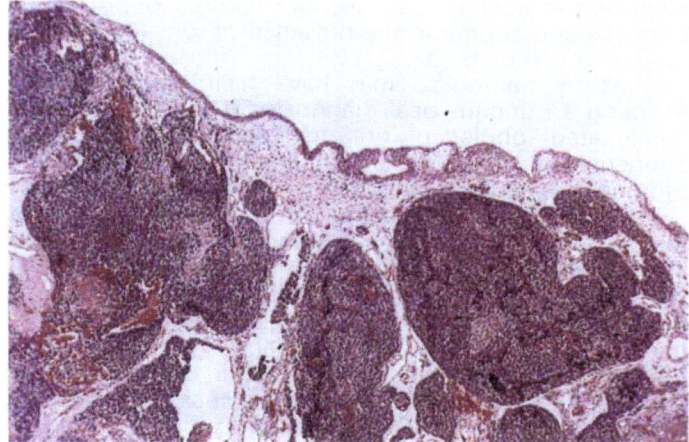

Figure 6.30 Olfactory neuroblastoma. The tumour is composed of darkly staining cells arranged in lobules of different sizes with distinct edges. H & E (A)

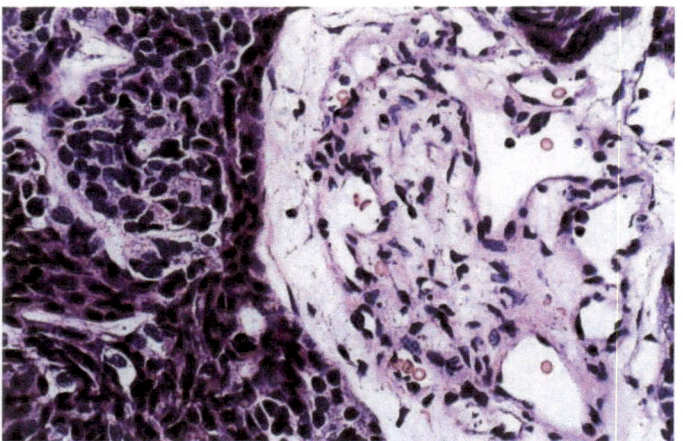

Figure 6.31 Olfactory neuroblastoma showing numerous stromal blood vessels and edge of tumour lobule composed of cells showing regular nuclei and moderate amounts of cytoplasm.   H & E (C)

Junctional activity is sometimes seen, however, in the epithelium adjacent to the main tumour mass.

The histochemical identification of the protein, S100, is an important diagnostic adjunct in malignant melanoma, since almost every case gives a positive reaction. It is particularly useful in the absence of melanin pigment when the cells are morphologically compatible with malignant melanoma.

Electron microscopy
Observation of the ultrastructure is sometimes of value in identifying a neoplasm as malignant melanoma when no pigment is present in the cells on light microscopy even after special staining. Ultrastructural examination shows ovoid bodies in the cytoplasm of the tumour cells. These bodies, known as melanosomes, which are the precursors of melanin with the cells, possess an internal structure of transversely-arranged internal striations.

Olfactory neuroblastoma
Olfactory neuroblastoma is an unusual neoplasm, arising in almost all cases from the roof of the nasal cavity where the olfactory neuroepithelium is situated.

Microscopic appearances
It is my opinion that there is but a single entity, olfactory neuroblastoma, which does have some differences from neuroblastoma arising elsewhere. The nasal neoplasm displays specific light-microscopic features for both tumour cells and stroma in the presence of which a definite diagnosis can be made.

Olfactory neuroblastomas have histological features enabling an unequivocal diagnosis. These are: (a) well-demarcated lobules of uniform tumour cells and (b) congeries of blood vessels in close apposition to the tumour lobules (Figures 6.30 and 6.31).

The nasal mucosa is expanded in all cases by tumour lobules which are somewhat round in shape and vary in size from large spheres containing many cells to small groups of some four cells. The lobules are characterized by well-defined edges. In a few cases, the neoplasm is composed mainly of wide trabeculae of tumour cells, but the presence of round bulges at their edges reveals a similar lobular configuration. In some areas, the neoplasm is formed of anastomosing files a cell or two wide. This appearance is most prominent in recurrences and advanced stages of the tumour growth. Examination of other parts of the neoplasm will usually show a more typical architecture.

Tumour cells are uniform and rather small. Nuclei are oval and finely granular with uniformly distributed chromatin, without prominent nucleoli. There is often so little cytoplasm that it is not clearly visible; when observed, it is scanty and pink staining. Mitotic figures are seen in some tumours but are never numerous. Nerve cell differentiation has been described in a few cases, and, in one case, replaced the whole neuroblast population of the tumour after irradiation therapy[14].

In about half of the tumours, round or oval empty spaces appear in the lobules of tumour cells. These seem to be punched out and are surrounded by cells which have no special structural alteration which have been referred to as pseudorosettes. Dilated gland-like structures, lined by cubical epithelium, may be present in some cases in close association with tumour cells.

In about one-third of cases, the tumour lobules show pink-staining finely fibrillar areas. These occupy a sizeable area, sometimes more than half of the lobule. It seems likely, from ultramicroscopic evidence, that such areas are neurofibrils but satisfactory identification by nerve-fibre stains, both immunochemical and with silver impregnation, is difficult to achieve.

Stromal vascularization is a diagnostically important feature of olfactory neuroblastoma. Numerous capillaries and venules, usually in conglomerates, are present in the stroma between tumour lobules and intimately associated with them. The vessels are often embedded in hyaline fibrous tissue. They may indent the lobules of tumour and may appear as vascular islands lying among tumour cells. Areas of amorphous calcification are seen in the stroma of about 15% of cases.

Olfactory neuroblastomas often stain positively by the Grimelius method for argyrophilia. Immunochemical reactions for neurone-specific enolase are positive. Epithelial (cytokeratin) markers are positive in about 50% of cases.

References

1. Woodson, G. E., Robbins, K. T. and Michaels, L. (1985). Inverted papilloma. Considerations in treatment. *Arch. Otolaryngol.*, **111**, 806–811
2. Krisch, I., Neuhold, N. and Krisch, K. (1984). Demonstration of secretory component, IgA and IgM by the peroxidase–antiperoxidase technique in inverted papillomas of the nasal cavity. *Hum. Pathol.*, **15**, 915–920
3. Robin, P. E. and Powell, D. J. (1980). Regional node involvement and distant metastases in carcinoma of the nasal cavity and paranasal sinuses. *J. Laryngol. Otol.*, **94**, 301–309
4. Ringertz, N. (1938). Pathology of malignant tumors arising in the nasal and paranasal cavities and maxilla. *Acta Otolaryngol. (Stockholm)* (Suppl.) **27**, 1–405
5. Robin, P. E., Powell, D. J. and Stassbie, J. M. (1979). Carcinoma of the nasal cavity and paranasal sinuses: incidence and presentation of different histological types. *Clin. Otolaryngol.*, **4**, 431–456
6. Heffner, D. K., Hyams, V. J., Hauck, K. W. and Lingeman, C. (1982). Low-grade adenocarcinoma of the nasal cavity and paranasal sinuses. *Cancer*, **50**, 312–322
7. Macbeth, R. (1965). Malignant disease of the paranasal sinuses. *J. Laryngol. Otol.*, **79**, 592–612
8. Acheson, E. D., Cowdell, R. H., Hadfield, E. and Macbeth, R. G. (1968). Nasal cancer in woodworkers in the furniture industry. *Br. Med. J.*, **2**, 587–596
9. Brinton, L. A., Blot, W. J., Stone, B. J. and Fraumeni, J. F. Jr. (1977). A death certificate analysis of nasal cancer among furniture workers in North Carolina. *Cancer Res.*, **37**, 3473–3474
10. Sachez-Casis, G., Devine, K. D. and Weiland, L. H. (1971). Nasal adenocarcinomas that closely simulate colonic carcinomas. *Cancer*, **28**, 714–719
11. Perzin, K. H., Gullane, P. and Clairmont, A. C. (1978). Adenoid cystic carcinomas arising in salivary glands: a correlation of histological features and clinical course. *Cancer*, **42**, 265–282
12. Spiro, R. H., Koss, L. G., Hajdu, S. I. and Strong, E. W. (1973). Tumours of minor salivary origin. A clinicopathologic study of 492 cases. *Cancer*, **31**, 117–129
13. Iwamura, S., Sugiura, S. and Nora, Y. (1972). Schwannoma of the nasal cavity. *Arch. Laryngol.*, **96**, 176–177
14. Chan, J. K. C., Lau, W. H. and Yuen, R. W. S. (1989) Ganglioneuro-blastic transformation of olfactory neuroblastoma. *Histopathology*, **14**, 425–428

Non-epithelial and Metastatic Neoplasms of the Nose and Paranasal Sinuses

7

Capillary Haemangioma of Nasal Septum

Capillary haemangioma is a common lesion which has often been designated 'pyogenic granuloma' on the basis of the active inflammatory exudate between the blood vessels. Inflammation is frequent in nasal tumours, particularly if they are polypoid, and so is unlikely to be related to the origin of this condition. I have not been able to separate a 'pyogenic' from a 'haemangiomatous' form of benign vascular lesion in this situation. The site of the tumour is most frequently the mucosa at the anterior end of the nasal septum.

Pathological appearances

Capillary haemangioma has a characteristic reddish-purple appearance with a smooth surface which may be somewhat lobulated. The spherical mass usually projects from the mucosal surface and may be polypoid.

The lesion is composed of capillary channels which are frequently arranged in small lobules. Larger vessels, often referred to as 'feeder' vessels, are situated between the capillary lobules. The capillaries are lined by endothelial cells which vary in their cytoplasmic content (Figures 7.1 and 7.2). Mitotic figures may be found among these cells but are not significant as regards recurrence. The epithelial surface of the haemangioma is frequently ulcerated and replaced by a layer of fibrin and polymorphonuclear leukocytes. A variable degree of acute and chronic inflammation is present between the blood vessels. The non-ulcerated epithelium covering the haemangioma often shows squamous metaplasia.

Haemangiosarcoma

In spite of the high degree of vascularization which is a feature of the normal nose, malignant neoplasms derived from blood vessels are rare. Bankaci et al.[1] found only 14 published cases and added one of their own. The maxillary antrum is most frequently affected. Microscopically, a spectrum of appearances can be recognized, from a well-differentiated angiosarcomatous pattern to a poorly differentiated solid pattern. It is important to ascertain that the actual endothelial cells lining blood vessels have malignant features (Figure 7.3). These cells usually (but not always) give a positive reaction in their cytoplasm for Factor VIII antigen or with the Ulex technique by the immunoperoxidase method. It is my impression from the small numbers of cases in my own experience and the literature that angiosarcoma of the nose and paranasal sinuses may have a rather better outlook after active therapy than haemangiosarcoma arising in other parts of the head and neck, including the larynx.

Haemangiopericytoma

Haemangiopericytoma is an unusual neoplasm composed of normal blood vessels surrounded by spindle-shaped or oval tumour cells.

Pathological appearances

There is no typical gross appearance. The lesions vary with regard to the degree of vascularity that is apparent on the cut surface. Microscopically, the vascularity of the neoplasm is apparent in most cases. The cells of the tumour are distinct from, and external to, the normal endothelium-lined blood vessels. The latter are either capillaries or sinusoidal channels. The cells of the haemangiopericytoma show an oval or elongated nucleus with little atypicism and indistinct cytoplasm (Figure 7.4). Mitotic rate is low. Fibrosis, diffuse or localized, is present in almost all nasal haemangiopericytomas.

Haemangiopericytomas of the nose and paranasal sinuses seem to be more benign than their counterparts elsewhere. The series of Compagno and Hyams[2] showed that, in the nose and paranasal sinuses, there was a recurrence in only 14% and metastasis in 7%.

Myogenic Neoplasms

Leiomyoma

Tumours composed of smooth muscle are rare in the nose. Fu and Perzin[3] described two cases and could find only one other in the world literature. In each of their two cases, the patients had nasal polyps and the smooth muscle tumour was found incidentally on histological examination among the polyps.

The cells of leiomyoma are spindle shaped with rounded 'cigar-shaped' ends. The cytoplasm is eosinophilic and may exhibit longitudinal striations and vacuolation due to accumulation of glycogen (Figure 7.5). Mitotic figures are rare or absent. Nuclear palisading may be present so that the neoplasm may be mistaken for a neurilemmoma. The most useful immunochemical diagnostic aid is for desmin. Leiomyoma is benign and does not usually recur after resection.

Epithelioid leiomyoma (leiomyoblastoma)

Neoplasms of smooth muscle in which the smooth muscle cells display an epithelioid shape, often with vacuolated cytoplasm, have been referred to as leiomyoblastoma. Such neoplasms have occurred mainly in the stomach but are also known at other sites. Most of these tumours are benign and are best known as epithelioid leiomyomas[4]. They are occasionally malignant, in which case the term epithelioid leiomyosarcoma may be applied. The tumours, both benign and malignant, are also often called leiomyoblastomas.

We have seen an epithelioid leiomyoma in the nose of a girl of 5 years at the Royal National Throat, Nose and Ear Hospital, London. This was a whitish pedunculated mass which was removed at lateral rhinotomy. The cytoplasm of the cells was clear and, in places, vacuolated due to glycogen (Figure 7.6). Electron microscopy of the tumour cells showed large amounts of glycogen granules, fine fibrils (actin) and pinocytic vesicles. There have been three local recurrences of the growth in the seven years since resection was carried out[5].

Leiomyosarcoma is rare in the nose and paranasal sinuses. It presents usually in the nasal cavity. It shows cells of similar appearance to leiomyoma (see above) and gives similar desmin positivity, but the cell nuclei display malignant features (Figure 7.7).

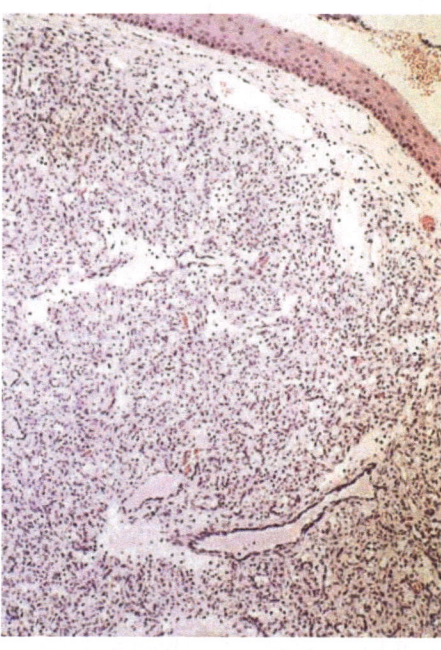

Figure 7.1 Capillary haemangioma of nasal septum showing capillaries and larger 'feeder' vessels. H & E (A)

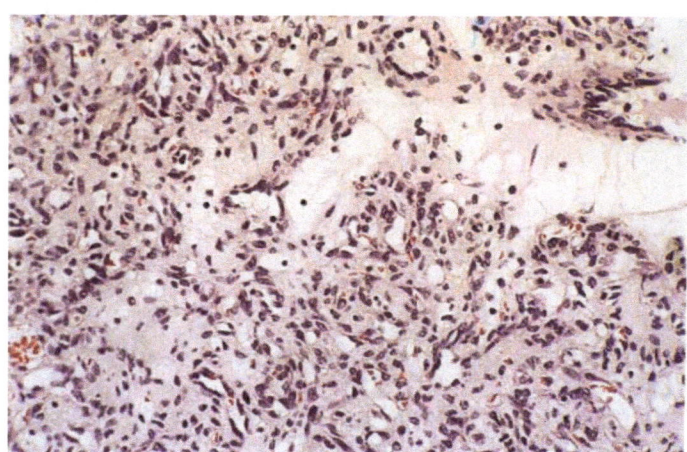

Figure 7.2 Capillary haemangioma of nasal septum showing polymorphonuclear leukocytes, plasma cells and lymphocytes infiltrating tissue between blood vessels. H & E (B)

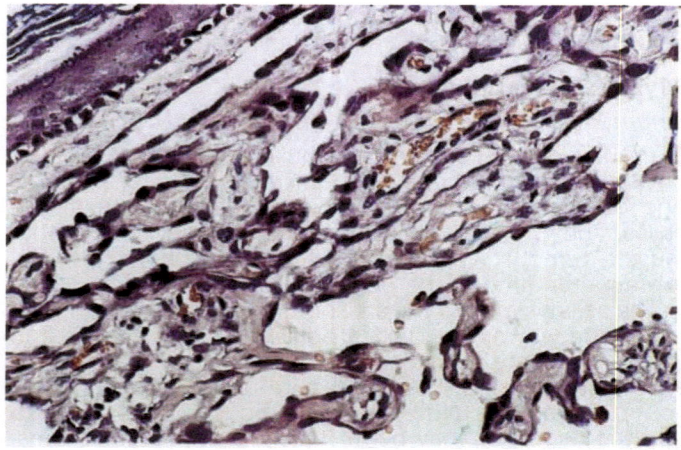

Figure 7.3 Haemangiosarcoma of nasal cavity showing a vascular tumour characterized by irregular hyperplasia of atypical endothelial cells. H & E (C)

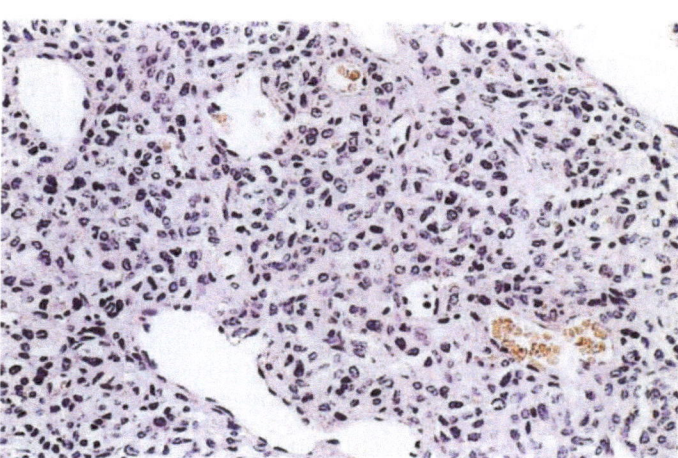

Figure 7.4 Haemangiopericytoma of nasal cavity showing neoplasm composed of oval cells situated between numerous vessels lined by normal endothelial cells. H & E (B)

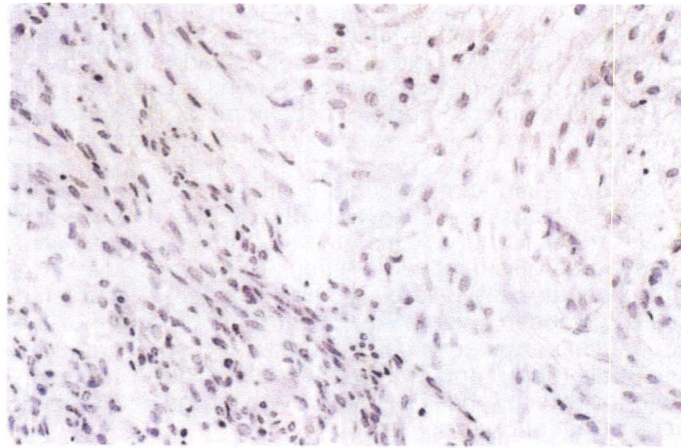

Figure 7.5 Leiomyoma of nose showing regular elongated cells with nuclei possessing rounded 'cigar-shaped' ends. H & E (B)

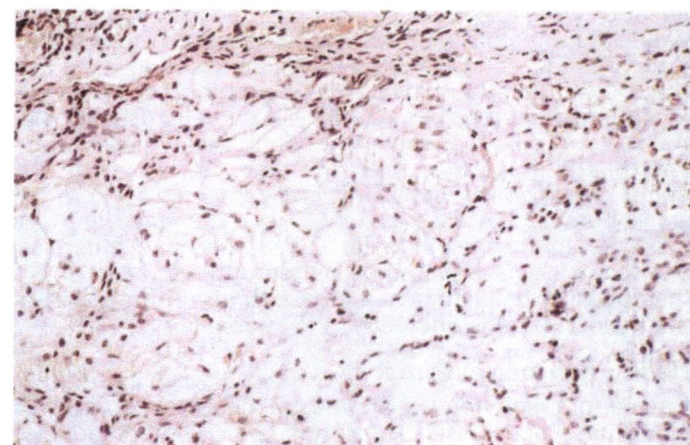

Figure 7.6 Leiomyoblastoma growing in nasal cavity of a 5-year-old girl. Vacuolated, often elongated cells beneath respiratory epithelium of nose. H & E (B)

Malignant Fibrohistiocytic Tumour
(Fibrous Histiocytoma)

In malignant fibrohistiocytic tumours (fibrous histiocytomas), the tumour cells have a decidedly atypical appearance which, according to Enzinger and Weiss[6], is a guide to the assessment of malignant potential. Perzin and Fu[7] described nine cases of fibrous histiocytoma of the nose and paranasal sinuses. Seven of these appear to have been malignant and two benign, judging by the histological descriptions and clinical courses given. Malignant-appearing as well as Touton giant cells are present in these tumours; the storiform pattern of fibroblasts is an important feature for diagnosis (Figures 7.8 and 7.9). Most of the fibrohistiocytic tumours of the nose fall into this category.

Immunochemical examination of the neoplasm is useful in identifying the neoplastic histiocytes accurately. Lysosomal enzymes, such as non-specific esterase and also α-1-antitrypsin, are usually present in the neoplastic histiocytic cells.

It may be difficult to distinguish malignant fibrous histiocytoma from other sarcomatous neoplasms, such as osteosarcoma, leiomyosarcoma or fibrosarcoma. There is a histological overlap between these neoplasms and it seems reasonable to diagnose the neoplasm according to whichever of the histological features predominates. Spindle cell carcinoma occasionally occurs in the maxillary antrum and resembles malignant fibrous histiocytoma. Immunochemical examination for epithelial antigens and electron microscopic examination for desmosomes and tonofibrils may be attempted, but, in my experience, are frequently negative in spindle cell carcinoma because of the great dedifferentiation of the neoplasm.

Myxoma

Myxoma is a benign neoplasm which is identified histologically by its infrequent small elongated or stellate cells embedded in a ground substance of mucoid material and reticulin fibres. It occurs principally in muscles and in the extremities but may also develop in the bones of the jaw, being more common in the lower than in the upper jaw. Fu and Perzin[8] described six cases of upper jaw myxoma of ages ranging from one to 52 years. I have seen three cases of upper jaw myxoma presenting in children under two years of age.

Pathological appearances

Myxomas are described grossly as being gelatinous. Microscopically, the scanty cells of the lesion show small dark nuclei with extremely thin cytoplasmic processes which merge with the reticulin fibres of the stroma to give a stellate appearance (Figure 7.10). A variable amount of collagen is present. It is sometimes abundant; in such cases, the designation of 'fibromyxoma' may be applied to the neoplasm but consideration should be given to the possibility of a fibrous tumour, such as fibromatosis. The cases of maxillary myxoma in children under two years mentioned above were all of this fibromyxomatous appearance (Figure 7.11). Blood vessels are very scanty in myxomas. The neoplasm infiltrates between the trabeculae of the maxillary bone and also produces bone resorption.

Neoplasms of Cartilage and Bone

Chondroma

Benign cartilaginous neoplasms of the nose are surprisingly infrequent although hyaline cartilage constitutes the whole anterior part of its framework.

Grossly, the lesions are firm and appear translucent. In a patient whose biopsies I have seen, the cartilaginous deposits were multiple. Microscopically, they consist of adult cartilage without nuclear atypia. It is likely that some of the cases described in the literature were chondrosarcomas rather than chondromas since some malignant features of the cartilage cells were illustrated. There is a definite propensity for recurrence after surgical excision, probably in cases where removal has been incomplete.

A chondroma of Ollier's disease may present in this situation with a histological appearance suggesting low-grade chondrosarcoma. The occurrence of such a lesion in a young person should suggest a bone scan for the presence of other chondromas of this benign condition.

Chondrosarcoma

Chondrosarcoma of the nose and paranasal sinuses is a rare condition. Fu and Perzin[9] found only 15 cases in the literature and described ten cases of their own. In five of these, the maxilla was involved by the neoplasm; in three, the sphenoid was affected. Origin from the nasal septum was described in only one of the ten cases.

Pathological appearances

Grossly, the tumours were lobulated firm grey and glistening on their cut surfaces. Microscopically, the appearances met the criteria of Lichtenstein and Jaffe[10], i.e. the tumour contained too many cells, the cells were too irregular, the nuclei stained too darkly and many were enlarged or giant cells with single, double or multiple nuclei present (Figure 7.12).

Natural history

The five-year survival of sinonasal chondrosarcoma is about 60%[9]. The tendency to recurrence of this neoplasm is said by Fu and Perzin to be related to three factors:

1. position of growth, the posteriorly located tumours having a particularly bad outlook;
2. the presence of tumour in the lines of resection after surgical excision; and
3. the degree of dedifferentiation of the growth.

Osteoma

A tumour-like lesion of lamellar bone – 'true' osteoma – is frequent in the paranasal sinuses. There is some doubt as to the neoplastic nature of this condition. The density of bone in osteoma of the sinuses is variable. Bone formation in relation to a variety of stimuli is frequent in the paranasal sinuses. It is, therefore, possible that some cases of osteoma may represent a hyperplasia of bone reacting to some unknown, or indeed known, irritant.

Grossly, osteomas are usually spherical, sometimes lobulated, hard masses of bone. Histologically, there is variation in the amount of fibrous tissue accompanying the lamellar bone. 'Ivory' osteomas usually show very little, while 'mature' osteomas show large trabeculae of mature lamellar bone, separated by moderately cellular fibrous tissue[11].

Benign fibro-osseous lesion

Fibrous dysplasia, ossifying fibroma and cementifying fibroma are said to be lesions of bone with well-defined characteristics when they are of odontogenic origin[12]. In the nose and paranasal sinuses, however, a decision as to whether a lesion is fibrous dysplasia or ossifying fibroma is more difficult and other tumours, such as benign osteoblastoma and osteoma, may also have to be considered as possible differential diagnoses. Even where some agreement is present, the criteria for the different entities show some overlap in this region. The problem is further compounded by the variable histology which is often found in different parts of the same lesion. These difficulties may be resolved to some extent by employing

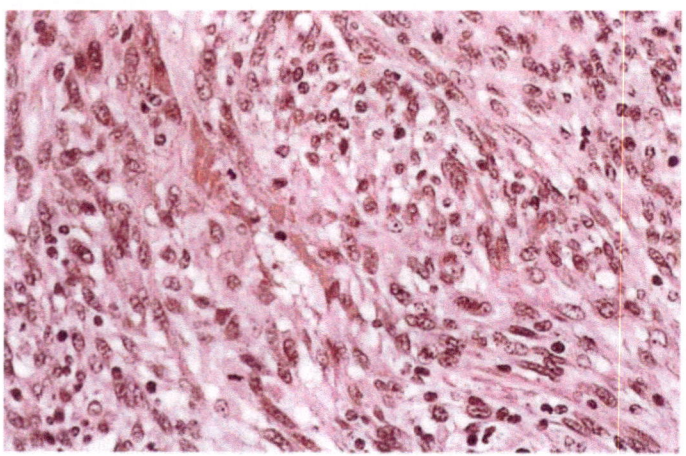

Figure 7.7 Leiomyosarcoma of nose composed of bundles of elongated atypical cells of smooth muscle appearance. H & E (C)

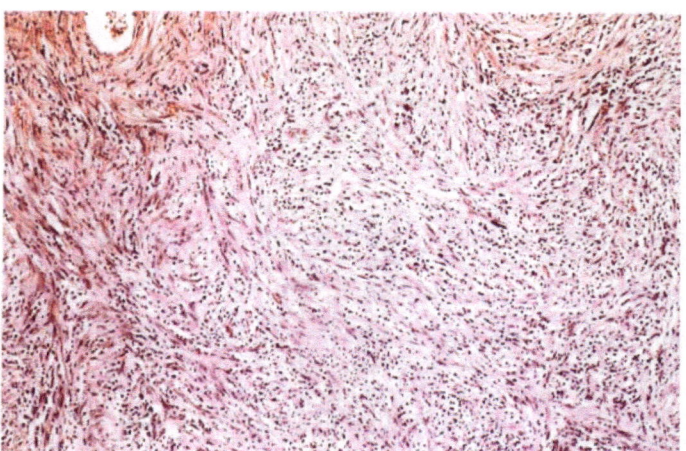

Figure 7.8 Malignant fibrous histiocytoma of nose showing fibrous tissue arranged in a storiform pattern. H & E (A)

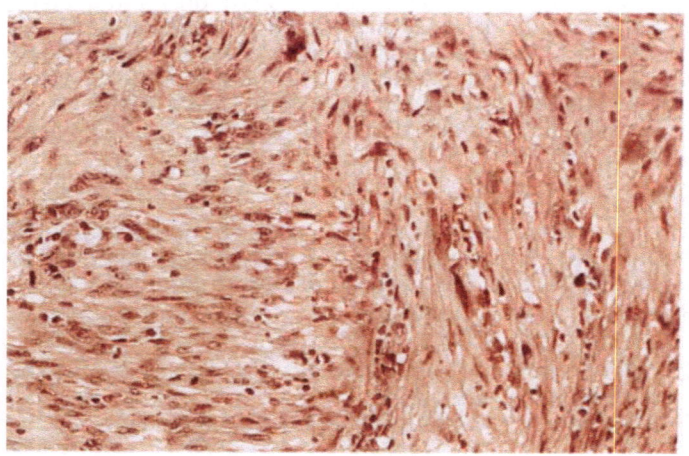

Figure 7.9 Malignant fibrous histiocytoma of nose showing histiocytes, fibroblasts and giant cells. There is some nuclear irregularity. H & E (B)

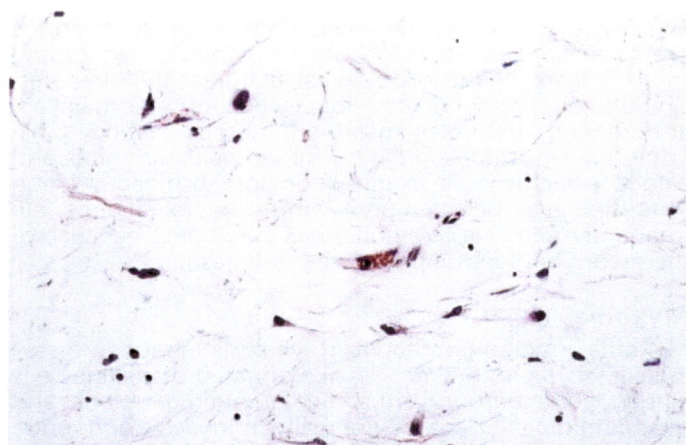

Figure 7.10 Myxoma of nose showing scanty elongated cells, some of which have a stellate appearance. H & E (B)

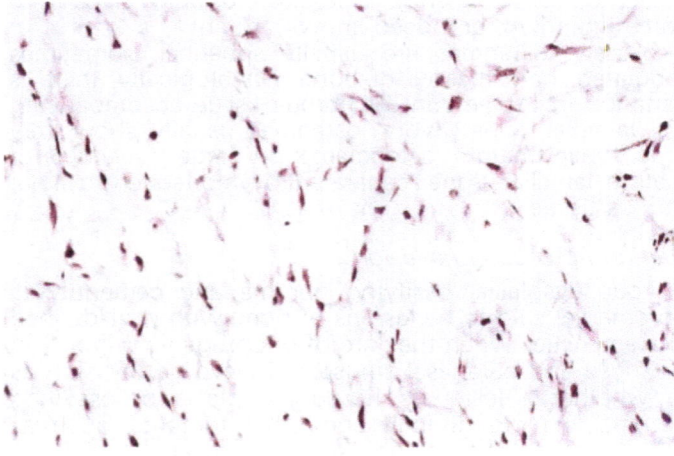

Figure 7.11 Fibrous myxoma from maxilla of 2-year-old child. Stellate cells and some fibroblasts are the component cells of this neoplasm. H & E (B)

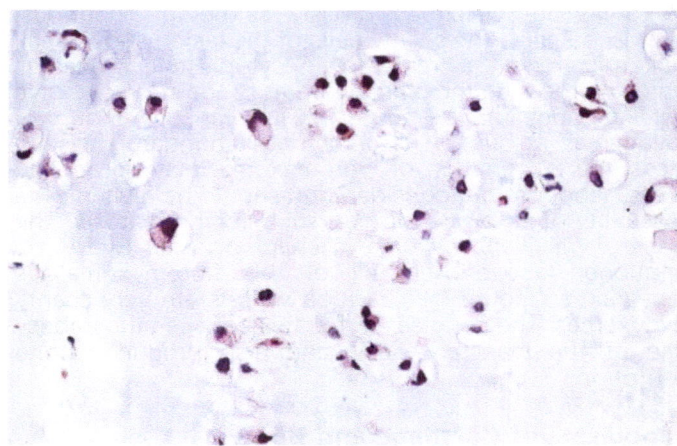

Figure 7.12 Chondrosarcoma of nose showing cartilage with chondrocytes which are more numerous, more darkly staining and larger than those of normal cartilage. H & E (C)

the umbrella term 'benign fibro-osseous lesion' for conditions in which we are not capable of giving a more specific diagnosis. Such lesions are particularly likely to be found in children, and Dehner[13] describes the features of a group of 15 cases, also using this generic term.

Pathological appearances

Biopsy of benign fibro-osseous lesions of the nose and paranasal sinuses is usually carried out by curettage, so that any differences between tumour and surrounding tissue cannot be detected.

The World Health Organization[14] defined ossifying fibroma as consisting of spindle-shaped fibroblastic cells and small islands of woven bone. The lesion is usually encapsulated and the bony trabeculae are said to be rimmed by osteoblasts. Fibrous dysplasia is defined as a non-encapsulated lesion of fibrous connective tissue containing islands of trabecular or immature non-lamellar metaplastic bone. Osteoblastic rimming is said to be absent or inconspicuous. If there are multiple bony lesions of this type and particularly in the presence of excessive skin pigmentation, the diagnosis of fibrous dysplasia is easily made. The latter features are, however, very rarely present in benign fibro-osseous lesions of the nose and paranasal sinuses. In the absence of such polyostotic features, I do not think that it is possible to decide which of the two names should be assigned to a fibro-osseous lesion in the majority of cases in this region. So a neoplasm showing a regular histological pattern of trabeculae of woven bone in a cellular fibrous stroma is best designated as benign fibro-osseous lesion. I do not ascribe any significance to the presence or absence of osteoblastic rimming (Figures 7.13 and 7.14).

Cementifying fibroma of the nose and paranasal sinuses has also been called juvenile ossifying fibroma and psammo-osteoid fibroma[15]. Margo et al.[16] have produced convincing arguments for the use of the term 'psammomatoid ossifying fibroma'. In this lesion, which occurs most commonly in the ethmoid of children and young people, small round mineralized collagenous foci are embedded in a cellular spindle cell stroma (Figures 7.15 and 7.16). This histological appearance is quite distinct from other forms of benign fibro-osseous lesion, but it should be noted that, in some cases, elongated woven bone trabeculae may also be present in the same neoplasm. The spicules are not cementum; such a tissue would hardly arise in a neoplasm as remote from dental structures as the ethmoids. Fibro-osseous lesions with similar calcified structures are seen sometimes in tumours of long bones[17]. This pattern is important to recognize in a nasal tumour, since recurrence seems to be more likely than with the other fibro-osseous lesions of this area and a more thorough excision at an early stage of the disease is required for complete cure. Lesions of this type may be mistaken for intranasal meningioma, the basophilic masses resembling psammoma bodies.

Osteosarcoma

Osteosarcoma is rare in the nose and paranasal sinuses. It is well established that osteosarcoma may develop after previous irradiation of the same bone. In one patient from our hospital, an anaplastic carcinoma of the maxillary antrum had been treated by radiotherapy 4 years before the onset of osteosarcoma of the maxillary antrum[18]. Another possible predisposing factor is Paget's disease of bone. A 58-year-old woman at our hospital showed gross Paget's disease of the skull when she presented with features of a large osteosarcoma in the nasal cavity and maxilla[18].

Pathological appearances

The gross features of osteosarcoma are those of an irregularly calcified destructive tumour. Histologically, the neoplasm is composed of sarcoma cells together with foci of malignant osteoid and/or malignant bone (Figures 7.17 and 7.18). The neoplasm is often less anaplastic than osteosarcoma of long bones and mitoses may not be numerous. Malignant cartilage is frequently present in parts of the growth and may dominate the histological appearances so that a diagnosis of chondrosarcoma rather than osteosarcoma may be preferred. The distinction is not of serious significance because chondrosarcoma of the upper jaw seems to be just as malignant locally as osteosarcoma[19], and osteosarcoma of the upper jaw, like chondrosarcoma, rarely metastasizes. Fibrosarcoma-like and myxomatous areas may also be prominent in the osteosarcoma. Some osteosarcomas of the maxilla show a marked vascularity with dilated capillary and cavernous vessels.

Extension of the neoplasm is mainly within the skull. Haematogenous metastasis is much less frequent than with osteogenic sarcoma of long bones.

Extramedullary Plasmacytoma (Malignant Lymphoma, Plasmacytic)

Extramedullary plasmacytoma is most commonly found in the upper respiratory tract, particularly the nose and paranasal sinuses.

Pathological appearances

In a small proportion of cases, plasmacytoma produces a polypoidal thickening of the mucosa. Mostly there is a grey or pink thickening of the mucosa with underlying invasion of soft tissue or bone.

Although plasma cells may be very numerous in non-neoplastic conditions, the histological recognition of the lesion as a neoplasm is usually not difficult. In chronic inflammation, plasma cells may be numerous but there is an admixture of other cells, such as lymphocytes and histiocytes. The hallmark of a plasmacytoma is the presence of large sheets of plasma cells alone, which replace tissue structures and invade locally. Fields of neoplastic plasma cells are generally very broad, being split up only by blood vessels (Figure 7.19). Sometimes the tumour cells may appear to be adherent to, or supported by, the blood vessels, and, if so, an alveolar pattern may be suggested. The actual identification of a neoplasm as one derived exclusively from plasma cells may sometimes be more difficult. The normal plasma cell has a number of specific features, all of which may be found in cells of well-differentiated plasmacytomas. The small eccentrically situated nucleus, with five to eight deeply basophilic condensations of chromatin regularly arranged around the nuclear membrane in a 'cartwheel' fashion, may be found in some plasmacytomas. A lightly stained area (the paranuclear vacuole) may also be identified near the nucleus in some tumour cells (Figure 7.20). The cytoplasm of the cells is non-granular and basophilic and the high ribonucleoprotein content of the cytoplasm may be confirmed by the Unna–Pappenheim stain, which usually produces a red (pyroninophil) reaction. Even the feature of normal plasma cells of greatest ultrastructural significance – the abundant arrays of endoplasmic reticulin – may sometimes be seen in plasmacytomas, by light microscopy, as small dilated vesicles. Russell bodies are present in extramedullary plasmacytomas in 13% of plasmacytomas of the upper respiratory tract, sometimes in large numbers. They may also be found in metastatic deposits of the plasmacytoma as well as in the primary. Some 20% of plasmacytomas are accompanied by deposits of amorphous proteinaceous material, which, in some

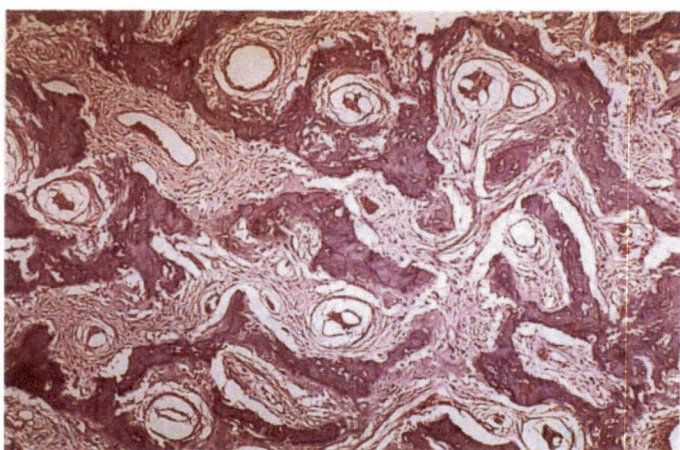

Figure 7.13 Benign fibro-osseous lesion of nose consisting of trabeculae of woven bone separated by fibrous tissue. H & E (A)

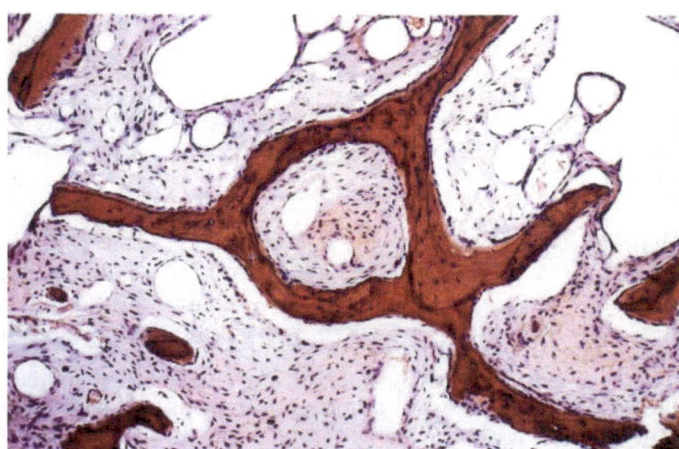

Figure 7.14 Benign fibro-osseous lesion showing trabeculae of lamellar bone separated by fibrous tissue. H & E (A)

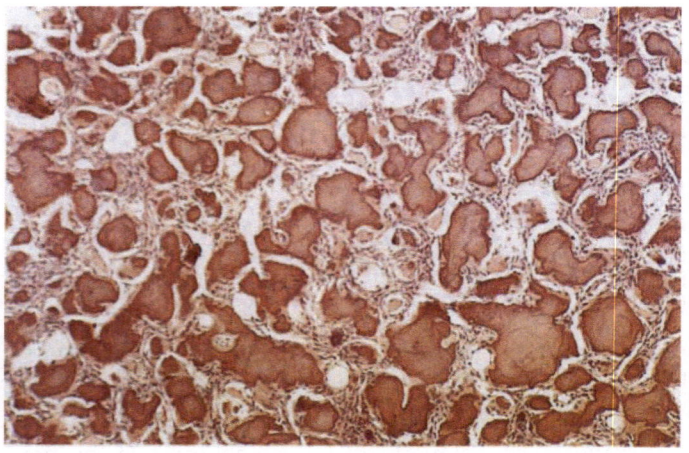

Figure 7.15 Psammomatous ossifying fibroma of ethmoid sinus showing small round bony trabeculae resembling cementum. H & E (A)

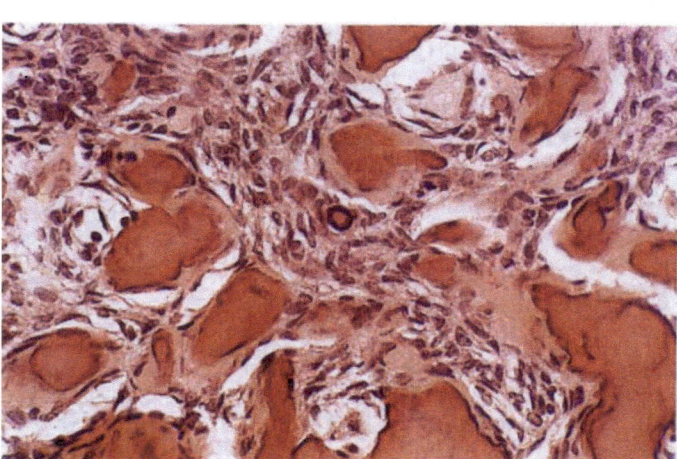

Figure 7.16 Higher power view of trabeculae of Figure 7.15. H & E (C)

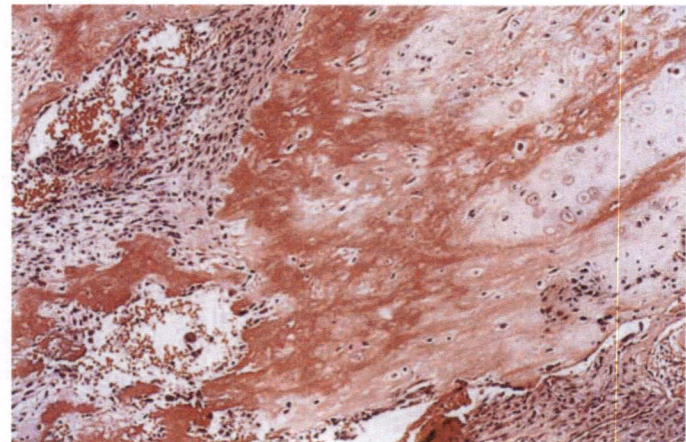

Figure 7.17 Osteosarcoma of nasal cavity showing spindle cell sarcoma in upper right together with malignant osteoid and cartilage in rest of illustration. H & E (C)

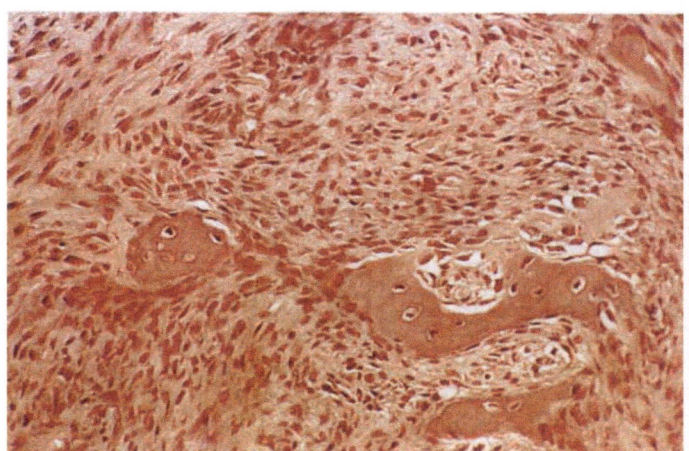

Figure 7.18 Osteosarcoma of nose showing spindle cell sarcoma and woven bone. H & E (B)

cases, is amyloid and in others immunoglobulin[20]. Amyloid in plasmacytoma tends to be deposited around blood vessels (Figure 7.21) and to show concentrically laminated masses similar to the deposits of primary amyloid of the larynx[21] (see Chapter 11).

Natural history
The most comprehensive account of the natural history of extramedullary plasmacytomas has been given by Wiltshaw[22] in her analysis both of the cases under treatment at the Royal Marsden Hospital, London, and those collected from the world literature. Nineteen per cent of all patients developed secondaries in bone but these were single, rather than multiple, and were distributed in a random fashion throughout the skeleton. Bone marrow involvement was infrequent. In 18% of all cases of extramedullary plasmacytoma collected by Wiltshaw, there was lymph node spread, but, in one-third of these, it went no further than the lymph nodes draining the primary lesion. Other sites of spread from extramedullary plasmacytoma were the skin, subcutaneous tissue, liver, lungs and pleura and the gastrointestinal tract. Among the Royal Marsden cases, Wiltshaw computed a 10-year survival rate of more than 50%. Renal failure is not a feature in the world literature (although I have personally studied tumour material from two cases with renal failure). In approximately half of all cases, further development of the plasmacytoma is to be expected, according to Wiltshaw's findings, but the pattern of spread is to local lymph nodes, random solitary bone sites and deposits in soft tissues, a pattern quite unlike that of multiple myeloma. Survivals of 15 years without recurrence after treatment by irradiation or surgery are quite common and cases are seen with long survival even after local recurrence of the tumour.

I have found, in unpublished studies, that plasmacytomas with a mean nuclear diameter of more than 6 μm tend to behave in an aggressive fashion.

Immunoglobulin secretion
Elevation of serum immunoglobulin or the presence of urinary Bence–Jones protein is seen very rarely on presentation of this neoplasm. In Wiltshaw's Royal Marsden series, about 10% of all patients subsequently developed paraproteinaemia. This was always in the advanced stage of the disease, presumably as a result of the presence of a large mass of immunoglubulin-secreting neoplasm. We have found with the immunoperoxidase staining method, used on paraffin-embedded formalin-fixed sections of extramedullary plasmacytoma, that this tumour, like multiple myeloma, may express immunoglobulin in a monotypic fashion. The heavy chain produced is usually IgG and the light chains may be either κ or λ. The finding of monoclonal immunoglobulin may be useful in deciding whether a particular collection of plasma cells in histological section is a plasmacytoma rather than an inflammatory infiltrate, and also in identifying an undiagnosed tumour as a plasmacytoma, but the method frequently presents unexplained difficulties in the study of this neoplasm, even in the best immunohistochemical laboratories.

Metastatic carcinoma
Metastasis via the bloodstream to the nose and sinuses is sometimes observed. It should be suspected by the pathologist in biopsies of neoplasms that do not resemble the usual pattern of primary growths in the sinonasal tract. The most frequent source of metastatic carcinoma to the nose and sinuses is renal cell carcinoma[23]. Carcinomas of the lung and breast and, even more rarely, of the gastrointestinal tract, have also been sources of metastatic neoplasm.

Grossly, metastatic renal carcinoma is pale yellow in colour. Microscopically, the large clearly-defined pale vacuolated cells with a vascular stroma are characteristic (Figures 7.22 and 7.23). Useful histochemical aids in making the diagnosis are stains for the presence of lipid and glycogen in the tumour cells. These substances are also seen well as cytoplasmic inclusions with the electron microscope, and the presence of fine microvilli emanating from tumour cells is also helpful in identifying the renal origin of the tumour cells (Figure 7.24).

References

1. Bankaci, M., Myers, E. N., Barnes, L. and DuBois, P. (1979). Angiosarcoma of maxillary sinus: literature review and case report. *Head Neck Surg.*, **1**, 274–280
2. Compagno, J. and Hyams, V. J. (1976). Hemangiopericytoma-like intranasal tumors: a clinicopathological study of 23 cases. *Am. J. Clin. Pathol.*, **66**, 672–683
3. Fu, Y. S. and Perzin, K. H. (1975). Nonepithelial tumors of the nasal cavity, paranasal sinuses, and nasopharynx: a clinicopathologic study. IV. Smooth muscle tumors (leiomyoma, leiomyosarcoma). *Cancer*, **35**, 1300–1308
4. Enzinger, F. M. and Weiss, S. W. (1988). *Soft Tissue Tumours.* 2nd Edn. (St Louis: CV Mosby)
5. Papavasiliou, A. and Michaels, L. (1981). Unusual leiomyoma of the nose (leiomyoblastoma): Report of a case. *J. Laryngol. Otol.*, **95**, 1281–1286
6. Weiss, S. W. and Enzinger, F. M. (1978). Malignant fibrous histiocytoma. An analysis of 200 cases. *Cancer*, **41**, 2250–2266
7. Perzin, K. H. and Fu, Y. S. (1980). Non-epithelial tumors of the nasal cavity, paranasal sinuses and nasopharynx: a clinicopathologic study. XI. Fibrous histiocytomas. *Cancer*, **45**, 2616–2626
8. Fu, Y. S. and Perzin, K. H. (1977). Non-epithelial tumors of the nasal cavity, paranasal sinuses and nasopharyx: a clinicopathologic study. VII. Myxomas. *Cancer*, **39**, 195–203
9. Fu, Y. S. and Perzin, K. H. (1974). Non-epithelial tumors of the nasal cavity, paranasal sinuses and nasopharynx: a clinicopathologic study. III. Cartilaginous tumors (chondroma, chondrosarcoma). *Cancer*, **34**, 453–463
10. Lichtenstein, L. and Jaffe, H. L. (1943). Chondrosarcoma of bone. *Am. J. Pathol.*, **19**, 553–589
11. Fu, Y. S. and Perzin, K. H. (1974). Non-epithelial tumors of the nasal cavity, paranasal sinuses, and nasopharynx: a clinicopathologic study. II. Osseous and fibro-osseous lesions, including osteoma, fibrous dysplasia, ossifying fibroma, osteoblastoma, giant cell tumor, and osteosarcoma. *Cancer*, **33**, 1289–1305
12. Pindborg, J. J. and Kramer, I. R. H. (1971). *Histological Typing of Odontogenic Tumours, Jaw Cysts and Allied Lesions. International Histological Classification of Tumours. No. 5.* (Geneva: World Health Organization)
13. Dehner, L. P. (1973). Tumors of the mandible and maxilla in children. I. Clinicopathologic study of 46 histologically benign lesions. *Cancer*, **31**, 364–384
14. Shanmugaratnam, K. (1978). *Histological Typing of Upper Respiratory Tract Tumours. International Histological Classification of Tumours, No. 19.* (Geneva: World Health Organization)
15. Damjanovm, I. Maenza, R. M., Snyder, G. G., Ruiz, J. W. and Toomay, J. M. (1978). Juvenile ossifying fibroma. An ultrastructural study. *Cancer*, **42**, 2668–2674
16. Margo, C. E., Ragsdale, B. D., Perman, K. I., Zimmerman, L. E. and Sweet, D. E. (1985). Psammomatoid (juvenile) ossifying fibroma of the orbit. *Ophthalmology*, **92**, 150–159
17. Friedman, N. B. and Goldman, R. L. (1969). Cementoma of long bones; extragnathic odontogenic tumor. *Clin. Orthop.*, **67**, 243–248
18. Windle-Taylor, P. C. (1977). Osteosarcoma of the upper jaw. *J. Maxillofac. Surg.*, **5**, 62–68
19. Garrington, G. E., Scofield, H. H., Cornyn, J. and Hooker, S. P. (1967). Osteosarcoma of the jaws. Analysis of 56 cases. *Cancer*, **20**, 377–391
20. Wright, D. H. and Isaacson, P. G. (1985). *Biopsy Pathology of the Lymphoreticular System.* (London: Chapman and Hall)
21. Michaels, L. and Hyams, V. J. (1979). Amyloid in localized deposits and plasmacytoma of the respiratory tract. *J. Pathol.*, **128**, 29–38
22. Wiltshaw, E. (1976). The natural history of extramedullary plasmacytoma and its relation to solitary myeloma of bone and myelomatosis. *Medicine*, **55**, 217–238
23. Miyamoto, R. and Helmus, C. (1973). Hypernephroma metastatic to the head and neck. *Laryngoscope*, **83**, 898–905

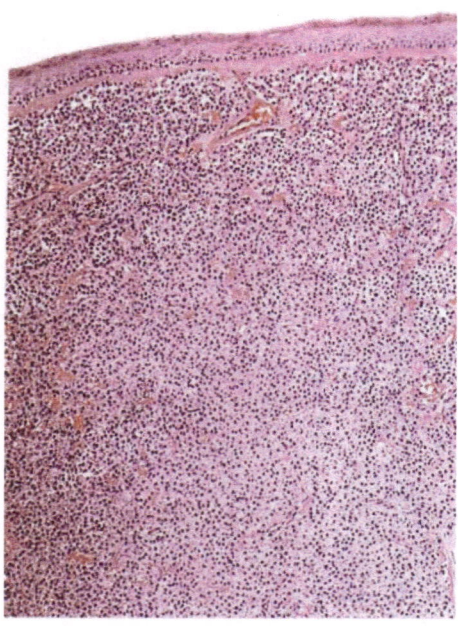

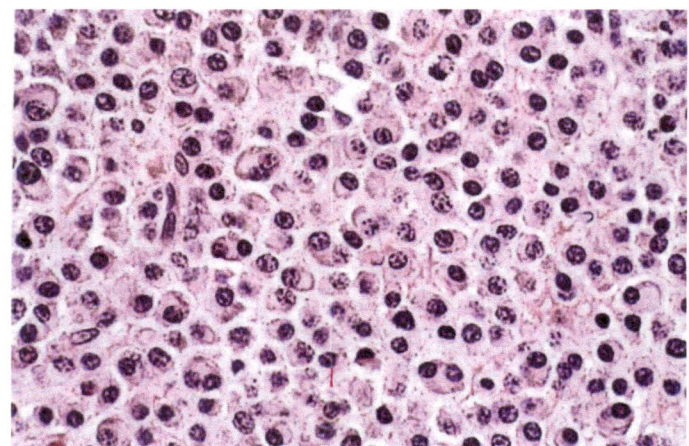

Figure 7.19 Plasmacytoma of nasal cavity showing large sheets composed of plasma cells only. H & E (A)

Figure 7.20 Plasmacytoma of nasal cavity composed of atypical plasma cells. H & E (C)

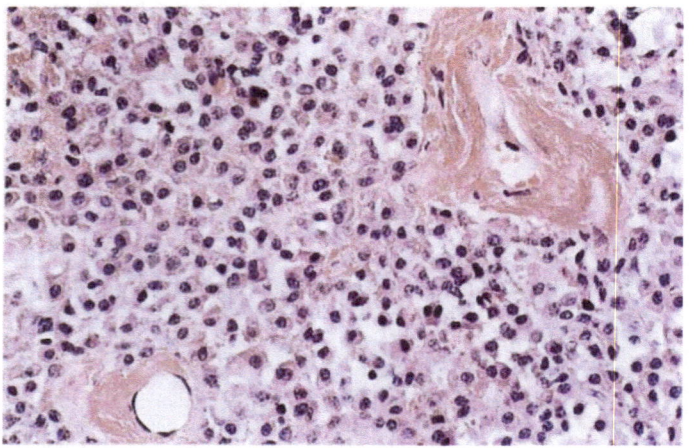

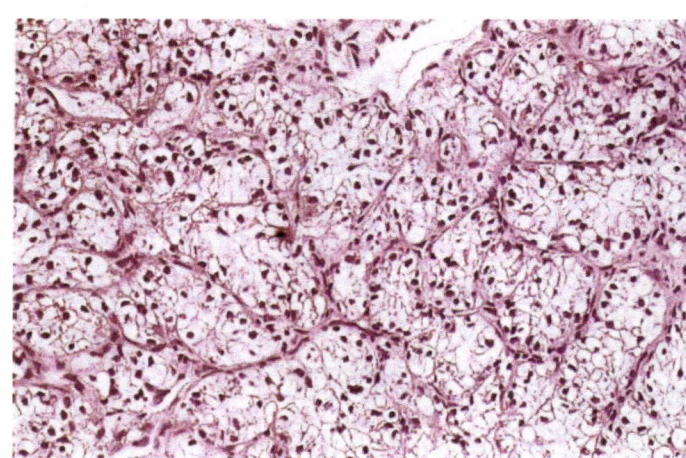

Figure 7.21 Plasmacytoma of nose showing perivascular amyoid. H & E (B)

Figure 7.22 Metastasis of clear cell carcinoma of kidney to paranasal sinus. Vacuolated clear cells in clusters with numerous blood vessels. H & E (B)

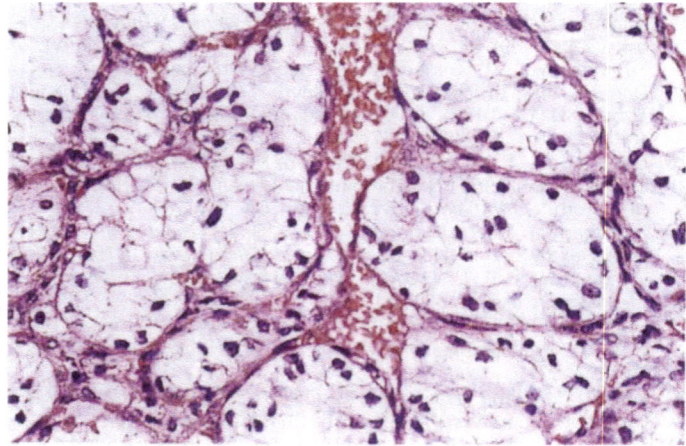

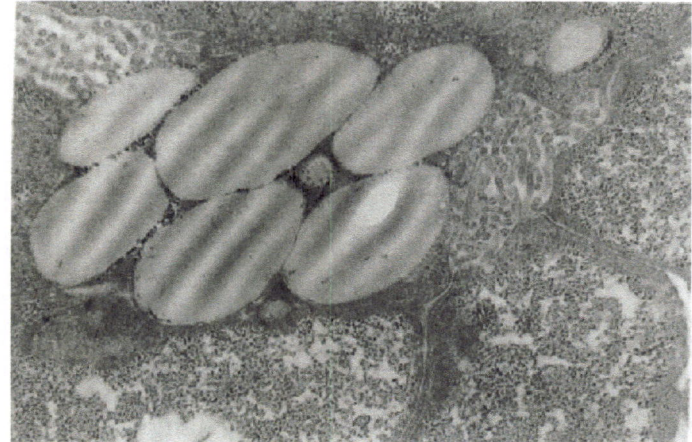

Figure 7.23 Higher power of tumour seen in Figure 7.22. H & E (C)

Figure 7.24 Electron micrograph of metastatic deposit of clear cell carcinoma of kidney to nasal bone. There are deposits of glycogen granules and large lipid-containing globules. Collections of microvilli are also present. × 18 000

Nasopharynx

8

Anatomy

The nasopharynx (nasal part of the pharynx) lies behind the nose, with which its lining and cavities are continuous. It has an arbitrarily fixed lower level at the posterior edge of the soft palate. The bony superior and posterior walls make a concavity composed of the body of the sphenoid above and the atlas and axis cervical vertebrae below. The mucosa and submucosa of the nasopharynx are separated from these bony structures by the retropharyngeal space, a layer of very loose connective tissue.

The Eustachian tube on each side opens into the nasopharynx, where it is bounded by an elevation which is produced by the medial end of the cartilage of the tube. The latter is shaped like a shepherd's crook (or an inverted 'J') so that the tubal elevation (torus) has a similar shape, the long limb being posterior. The mucosa of the posterior wall of the nasopharynx shows an irregular bulging, caused by the presence of lymphoid tissue in the mucosa, which is known as the pharyngeal tonsil.

Histology

At birth, the nasopharynx is lined by respiratory epithelium similar to that of the nose. However, later in childhood and in the adult, most of the surface epithelium has become replaced by stratified squamous epithelium[1]. Crypts lined by modified squamous epithelium of identical appearance to those found in the palatine tonsil (see Chapter 9) may also be seen in the nasopharynx. Seromucinous glands, both serous and mucous, are also present in the submucosa of the nasopharynx. The lymphoid tissue of the nasopharyngeal tonsil is subepithelial and composed of diffusely scattered lymphocytes and secondary lymphoid follicles with germinal centres. Lymphoid cells have a particularly close relationship with the epithelium. Among the lymphocytes beneath the eipthelium, both of the surface and of the crypts and gland ducts, plasma cells are found in abundance and this is their main location in the nasopharyngeal lymphoid tissue.

Adenoids

The term 'adenoids' is applied to an enlargement of the nasopharyngeal tonsil which occurs in the majority of children between the ages of 3 and 7 years. Grossly, adenoids show corrugated surfaces and pale grey fleshy cut surfaces. Microscopically, the surface epithelium is of either stratified squamous or respiratory columnar varieties. The lymphoid follicles of the pharyngeal tonsil are enlarged and more numerous than normal. Their germinal centres are swollen and contain many tingible body macrophages (Figures 8.1 and 8.2).

Hairy Polyp (Teratoid Tumour)

A striking lesion of the nasopharynx, which arises during development but is so far not satisfactorily explained, is the hairy polyp or teratoid tumour. This lesion would seem to come under the designation of a choristoma, i.e. a formation of non-neoplastic tissue, which does not normally arise in that situation. Hairy polyps arise from the lateral wall of the nasopharynx or from the nasopharyngeal surface of the soft palate. They are frequently pedunculated and may be up to 6 cm in diameter.

The polyp is covered by skin with both hair follicles and sebaceous glands. More deeply, adipose tissue, smooth and striated muscle, cartilage and bone may be found (Figure 8.3)[2]. Neoplastic tissue is never seen and the lesion does not recur after removal.

Nasopharyngeal Carcinoma

Classification

In a classification proposed by the World Health Organization[3], there were three histological types of nasopharyngeal carcinoma:

1. Squamous cell carcinoma (keratinizing squamous cell carcinoma;
2. Non-keratinizing squamous cell carcinoma;
3. Undifferentiated carcinoma.

There is evidence, however, from light and electron microscopic studies of surgical biopsies[4] and from autopsy material in a Chinese population[5] that these three forms do not represent sharp categories: they appear to merge into each other, each being a variety of epidermoid carcinoma with a greater or lesser degree of squamous differentiation.

Epidemiology and aetiology

Nasopharyngeal carcinoma is infrequent in Europe and North America but much more frequent among Mongoloid populations living in or derived from Southern China; groups with an intermediate incidence occur in the North African littoral and in East Africa. A close relationship between nasopharyngeal carcinoma and Epstein–Barr virus is now extensively documented.

Microscopic appearances

Most nasopharyngeal carcinomas present an undifferentiated pattern. Undifferentiated carcinoma cells often show branching trabeculae or seemingly isolated masses. In some biopsies, the tumour is composed of cells that lie loosely in connective tissue without any tendency to form groups. In others, the tumour cells adopt a spindle shape similar to spindle cell carcinoma. Between the tumour cells, the stroma may be fibrous or show numerous lymphocytes and plasma cells. Downgrowths of undifferentiated carcinoma from overlying squamous cell epithelium are frequently present (Figures 8.4 and 8.5).

The cytology of undifferentiated carcinoma presents distinctive features. Nuclei have well-defined membranes but nuclear chromatin is scanty. One or two nucleoli of eosinophilic appearance are prominent in most nuclei. The cytoplasm, on the other hand, is poorly defined, often presenting a syncytial appearance where a number of cells appear to merge together (Figure 8.6). The foregoing pattern is so characteristic of carcinoma of the nasopharynx that, when it is seen in a biopsy of a cervical lymph node, as is frequently the case, even without

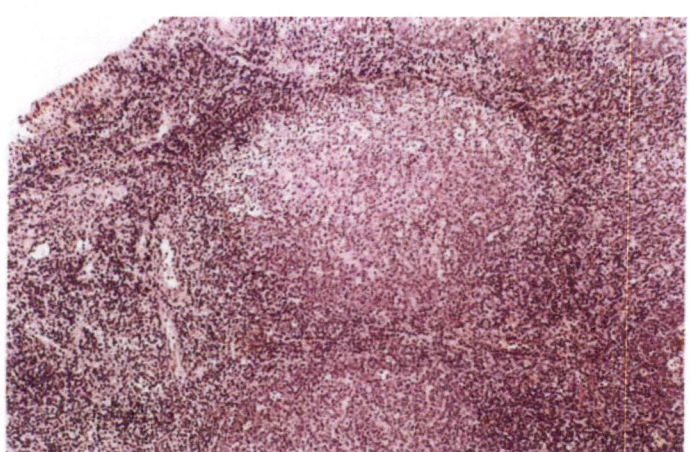

Figure 8.1 Adenoid of nasopharynx showing an epithelial covering of respiratory type. There is a large lymphoid follicle with a lymphocytic cap on the epithelial side and a swollen germinal centre containing tingible body macrophages. H & E (B)

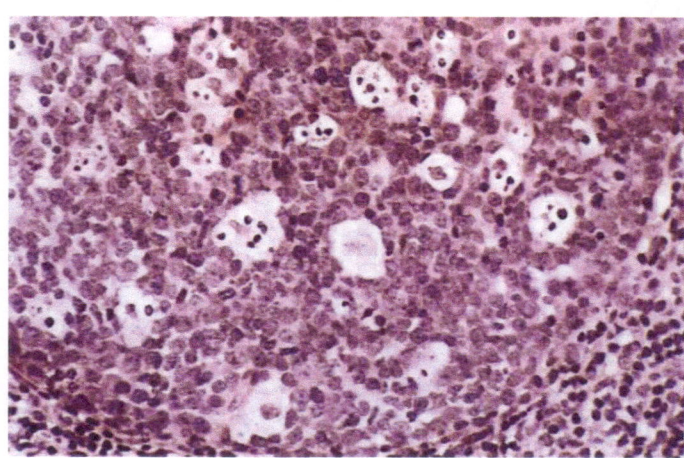

Figure 8.2 Higher power of germinal centre of adenoid showing tingible body macrophages. H & E (C)

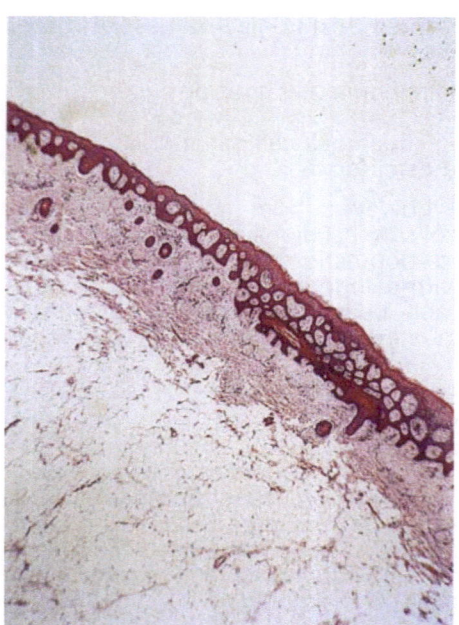

Figure 8.3 Covering of hairy polyp of nasopharynx showing hair follicles, one of which is horizontally aligned. H & E (A)

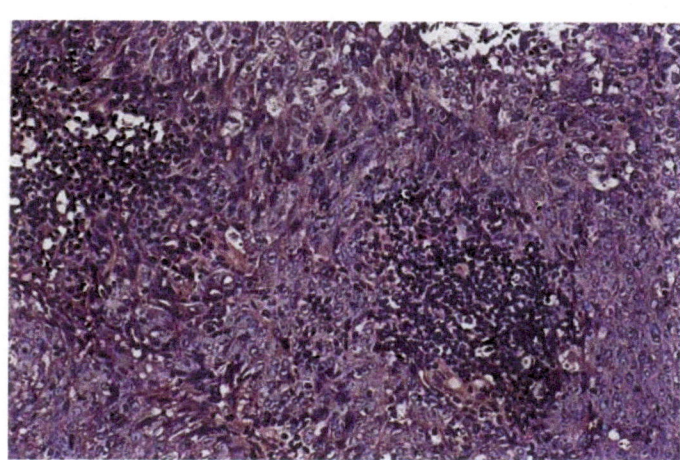

Figure 8.4 Undifferentiated carcinoma of the nasopharynx showing trabeculae of growth arising from basal layers of covering malignant epithelium (above). H & E (B)

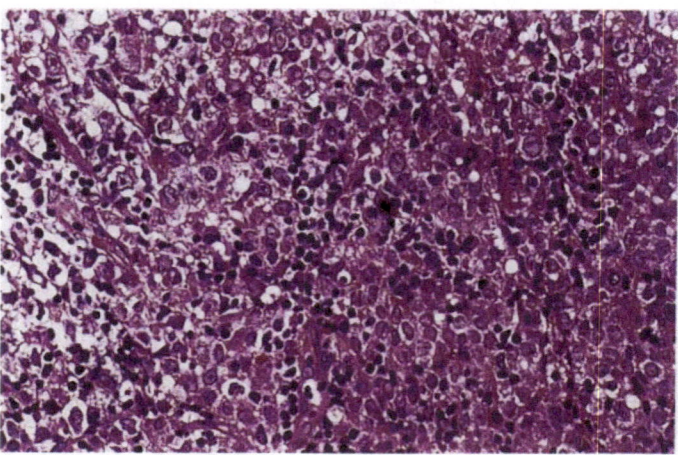

Figure 8.5 Undifferentiated carcinoma of nasopharynx. The cytoplasm of the cells appears to merge to give a syncytial pattern. Note lymphocytes and plasma cells around groups of carcinoma cells and infiltrating among them. H & E (C)

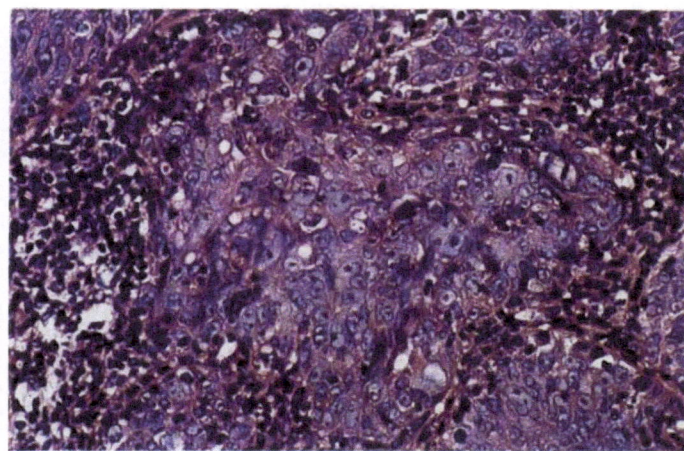

Figure 8.6 In this example of undifferentiated carcinoma of nasopharynx, groups of carcinoma cells are surrounded by lymphocytes. H & E (C)

symptoms or signs of nasopharyngeal disease, an occult nasopharyngeal primary should be suspected.

Staining of tumour cells for keratin antigen gives a positive result while that for leukocyte common antigen gives a negative result[6].

Spread

At postmortem, in most cases, invasion of the basi-occiput and posterior part of the body of the sphenoid with erosion of the bone is revealed. Cervical lymph node involvement in nasopharyngeal carcinoma is common. Metastases to remote organs, mainly liver, lungs and bones, in that order of frequency, were found in most cases at autopsy in Teoh's material[5].

Angiofibroma (Juvenile Nasopharyngeal Angiofibroma)

Angiofibroma, or juvenile nasopharyngeal angiofibroma, is a fibrous and vascular tumour-like swelling of the nasopharynx which occurs only in young males between 10 and 25 years of age.

Pathological appearances

When received in the laboratory, the resected tumour shows a lobular surface and is grey or pinkish grey depending on the degree of its vascularity. If the vascularity is marked, the cut surface will have a spongy appearance. In some cases, the vessels near the surface of the tumour are so dilated that they appear as cysts with a smooth lining (Figure 8.7).

Angiofibroma has a characteristic structure of blood vessels set in a stroma of fibroblasts and collagen. Blood vessels are thick walled in the deeper parts of the tumour. Here some vessels show gaps in their muscle and elastic layers. More superficially, all vessels are thin walled with few or no muscle fibres. The capillary vessels are often extremely thin and elongated. In some parts of angiofibroma, pink-staining deposit is found around the periphery of the vessel walls. The stroma is composed of collagen fibres and fibroblastic stromal cells. The former may be excessive in amount at the expense of the latter. Stromal cells have vesicular nuclei which may be atypical in appearance. Mitotic figures are absent among these cells, however, the sole mitotic activity in angiofibromas occurring among the heaped up vascular endothelial cells. The stromal cells may be multinucleate (Figures 8.8 to 8.11).

The overlying epithelium of the tumour is either respiratory or stratified squamous in type.

Treatment and natural history

Treatment of angiofibroma is by surgical excision via the nose, palate or maxillary sinus. Radiotherapy is no longer used. Recurrence of tumour after treatment is frequent. Embolization of the tumour via the common carotid artery using Silastic beads or Gelfoam particles has been undertaken recently in an attempt to reduce its vascularity at surgery.

There is no solid evidence for the spontaneous involution of nasopharyngeal angiofibromas. The lesion seems to maintain its growth unless treated vigorously. Cases are rarely seen nowadays which reach the proportions of that removed by maxillectomy in 1841, the specimen of which was described by Myrhe and Michaels[7] (Figure 8.12). However, malignant change does not occur.

Rhabdomyosarcoma

Malignant tumours of the skeletal muscle are the commonest form of sarcoma in the head and neck. Most cases are of the embryonal type. The nasopharynx is the second most frequent situation within the head and neck, the orbit being the most frequent. The average age at presentation is about 7 years.

Pathological appearances

The tumour is often composed of multiple grape-like polypoid masses. This gross feature gives rise to the designation of sarcoma botyroides (which is histologically identical to the embryonic form). Most of the nasopharyngeal neoplasms in this latter category consist of loosely arranged primitive cells. In some, there is a condensation of tumour cells immediately beneath the epithelium, the deeper cells being more loosely arranged. The superficially condensed cell layer is often referred to as the cambial layer by analogy with plant tissue.

The cells of embryonal rhabdomyosarcoma are round or elongated and the nuclei are usually hyperchromatic, irregularly shaped and showing numerous mitotic figures. The cytoplasm in many areas shows vacuolation which, on special staining with periodic acid–Schiff reagent (with and without prior treatment by diastase), is revealed to be glycogen (Figure 8.13). Cross-striations are not usually observed, although they may sometimes be found in a few tumour cells that are thin and elongated. Detection of cross-striations when they are present is usually easy in routinely stained sections; the examination of such sections in polarized light for the alternating light and dark stripes is sometimes useful, as is the staining of sections with phosphotungstic acid haematoxylin. Large round cells with abundant eosinophilic cytoplasm containing pink-staining masses but without cross-striations are much more frequent than cross-striations, however (Figure 8.14). An alveolar pattern may sometimes be adopted in parts of the tumour (Figure 8.15).

Immunochemical markers are useful in the histological diagnosis of embryonal rhabdomyosarcoma. Antibodies to fast myosin and skeletal muscle actin are said to be more diagnostic for poorly differentiated rhabdomyosarcomas than those to myoglobin, which is, in general, only present in cytoplasm-rich well-differentiated tumour cells[8]. We have found the presence of desmin to be a valuable marker for this neoplasm. Transmission electron microscopy is also of value, when the specific feature revealed is the presence of alternating thick (myosin) and thin (actin) filaments. The neoplasm spreads deeply into the skull and often reaches the meninges[9]. Lymph node metastases are occasionally seen. Distant metastasis is common, particularly to the lungs and bones.

Treatment

A drastic improvement has occurred in recent years with the introduction of triple therapy – surgery, radiotherapy and chemotherapy – for embryonal rhabdomyosarcoma.

Chordoma

Chordoma is a neoplasm which is derived from the primitive notochord. The largest proportion of chordomas occur in the sacrococcygeal region, with a rather smaller number in the cranio-occipital region, and it is members of this latter group that involve the nasopharynx. A third group of chordomas occur along the vertebral column, most frequently in the cervical region.

Pathological appearances

At postmortem, chordoma has been described as producing a mass in the spheno-occipital region posterior to the pituitary, optic nerves and carotid vessels. There is infiltration through the body of the sphenoid into the nasopharynx[10]. The tumour shows a well-demarcated edge often with a fibrous capsule. It may be lobulated. The cut surface is usually pale grey and mucoid with a rather softer, more mucoid texture than that presented by cartilage.

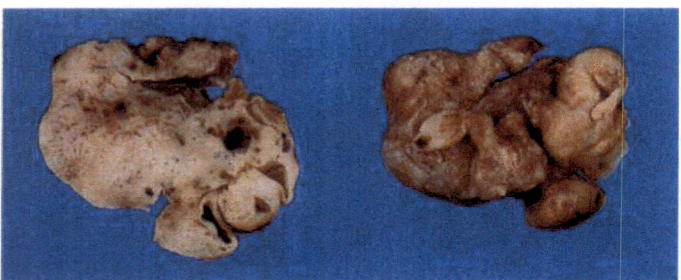

Figure 8.7 Gross specimen of angiofibroma. The cut surface is shown on the left and the outer surface on the right. Cysts with smooth linings are present within prominent swellings of the tumour. These are distended blood vessels and blood is seen in the cut surfaces of some of them

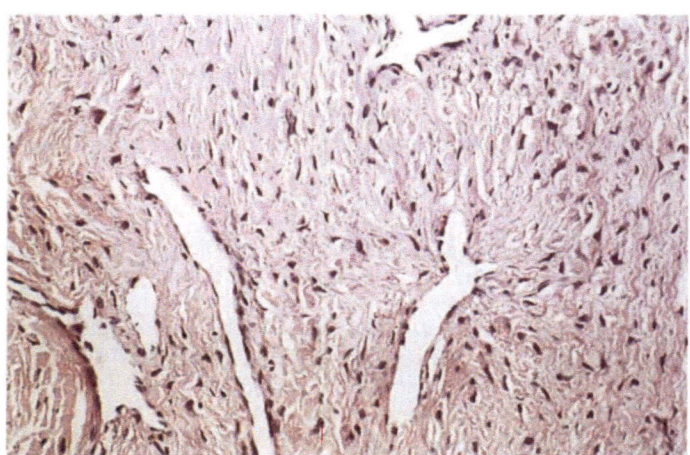

Figure 8.8 Nasopharyngeal angiofibroma showing thin-walled blood vessels and fibroblastic stromal cells. H & E (B)

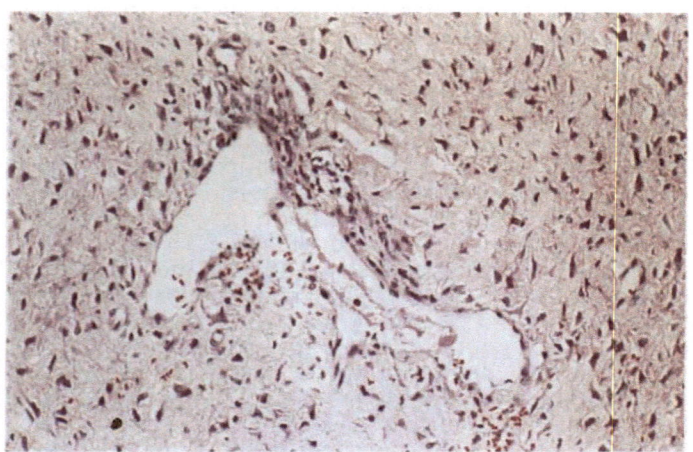

Figure 8.9 Vessel in nasopharyngeal angiofibroma showing thickening in part of its wall. H & E (B)

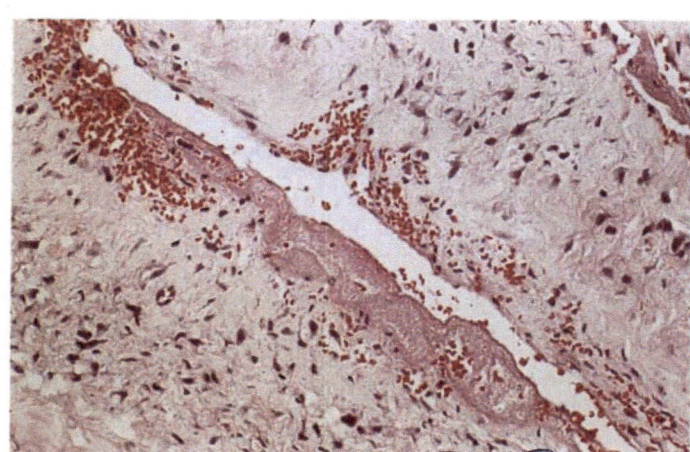

Figure 8.10 Fibrin thrombus on wall of vessel in angiofibroma. H & E (B)

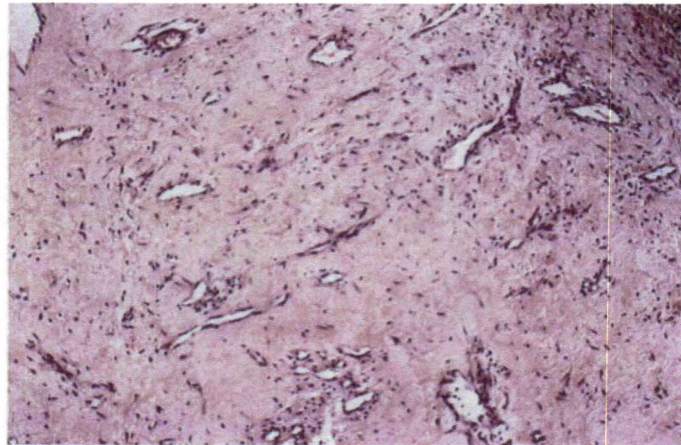

Figure 8.11 Nasopharyngeal angiofibroma showing marked collagenous infiltration of stroma. H & E (A)

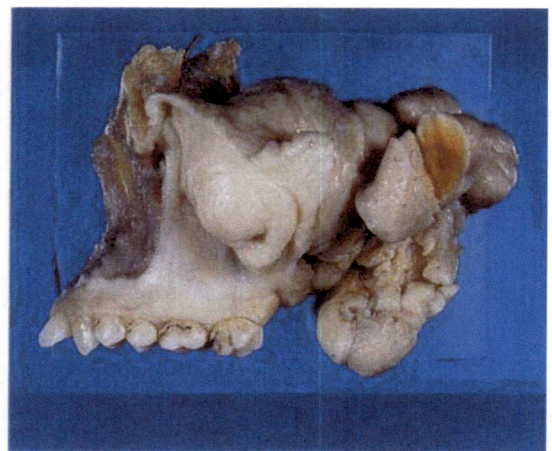

Figure 8.12 Advanced nasopharyngeal angiofibroma showing extension of nasopharyngeal growth lateral to maxilla. From a specimen of maxillectomy performed by Liston in 1841 at University College Hospital and preserved as museum specimen

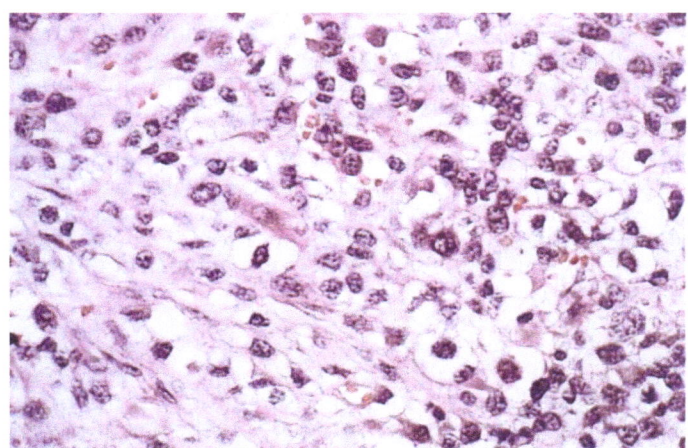

Figure 8.13 Embryonal rhabdosarcoma showing round and spindle-shaped cells, many of which are vacuolated due to accumulation of glycogen in the cytoplasm. There are also cells with eosinophilic cytoplasm. H & E (C)

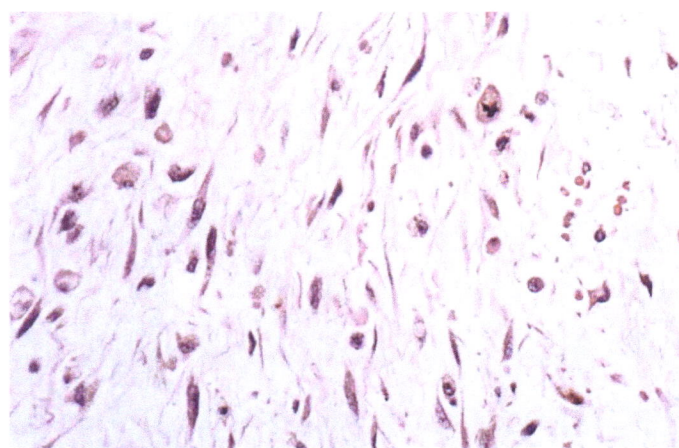

Figure 8.14 Embryonal rhabdomysarcoma showing predominance of spindle-shaped cells. H & E (C)

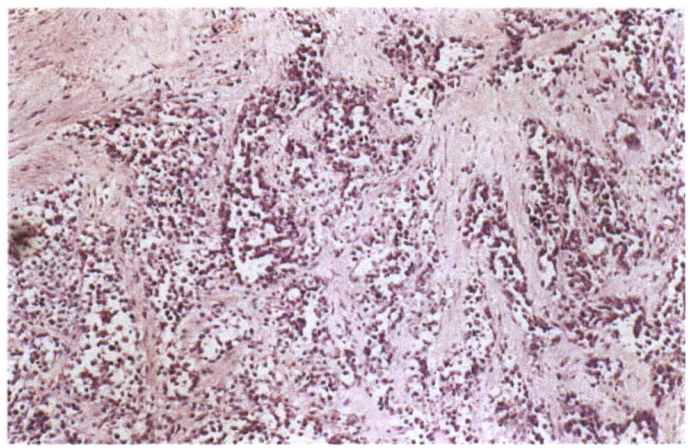

Figure 8.15 Alveolar rhabdosarcoma showing non-cohesive cells arranged in an alveolar pattern. H & E (C)

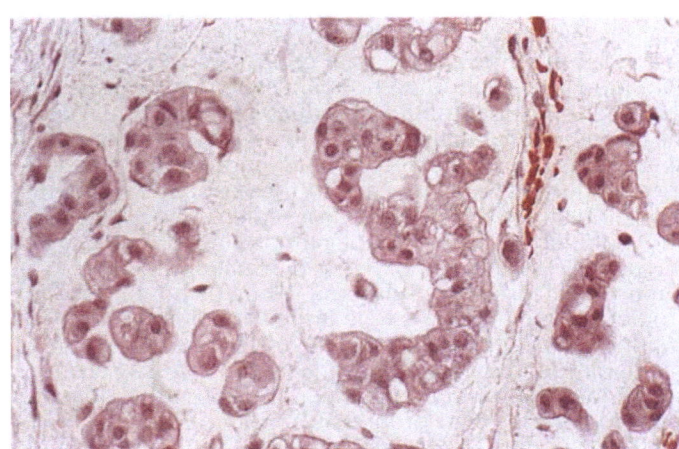

Figure 8.16 Chordoma presenting in nasopharynx with epithelioid tumour cells many of which are distended with a vacuolar material. The cells are suspended within a mucoid ground substance. H & E (C)

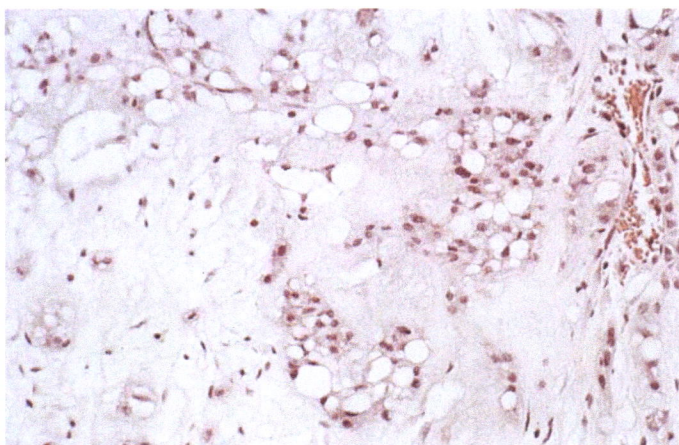

Figure 8.17 Another example of chordoma showing more prominent vacuolar distension of tumour cells. H & E (C)

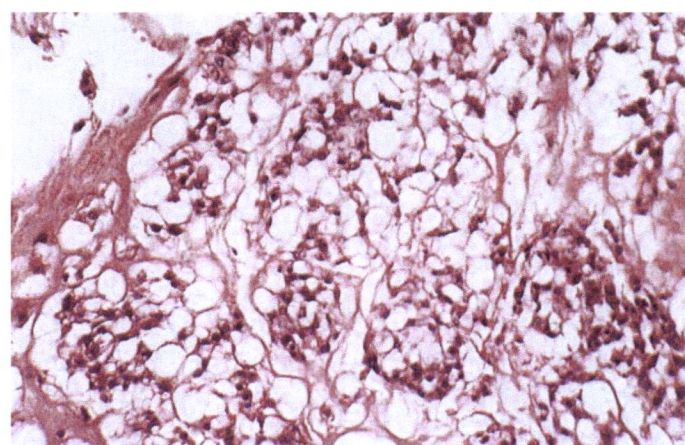

Figure 8.18 In this example of chordoma, most of the material is composed of the distended cells with little representation of the ground substance. H & E (C)

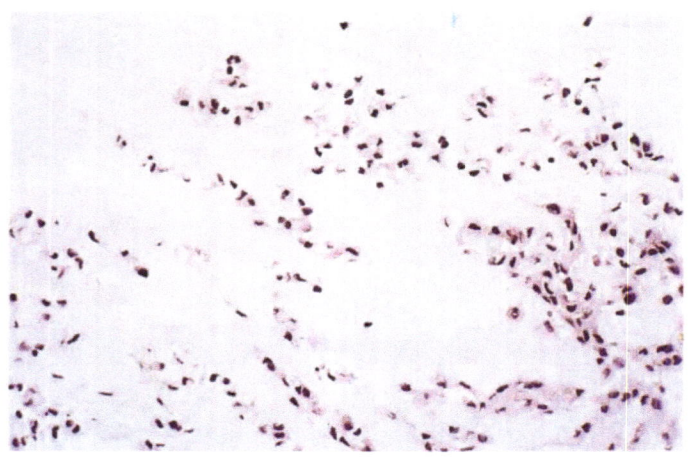

Figure 8.19 Chondroid chordoma. The small, often separate, tumour cells in a basophilic ground substance create an impression of a cartilaginous tumour. H & E (C)

The histology of this tumour is very variable. However, three constant features may be recognized: the formation of large lobules or alveoli of tumour; strands of tumour cells; 'physaliferous' (bubble) cells. The lobules of growth may be enveloped by a fibrous capsule. In many places this is absent, however, and growth is seen in direct contact with surrounding normal tissue. The capsule may also intersect the tumour to produce fibrous septa. Within the tumour, a characteristic growth pattern is the formation of strands of tumour cells within a mucoid ground substance (Figure 8.16). The cells in these strands frequently show indistinct boundaries. Physaliferous cells possess fine bubbles in their cytoplasm produced by droplets (Figures 8.17 and 8.18). They can usually be found in some parts of every chordoma. The fusion of the fine droplets of mucus to a single large vacuole gives the cell a 'signet-ring' appearance. Nuclei of chordoma cells show a variable degree of pleomorphism and mitoses are few. Sometimes there is much nuclear atypia but this does not seem to be related to prognosis.

Stains for mucus are usually positive in the ground substance and the cytoplasm often contains glycogen. Immunochemical markers for cytokeratins and S100 protein are positive.

Chondroid chordoma

Chordomas seen in the base of skull (but not in the sacrococcygeal variety) have been observed in about one-third of cases to possess a chondroid appearance. In these areas, the cellularity is high, the nuclei large and many of the cells are multinucleate. The ground substance surrounding these cells takes on a bluish staining so that the appearances are closely similar to those of chondrosarcoma, although more typical chordoma may be identified in adjacent parts of the section[11]. The separation of this chondroid group is important because patients with chondroid chordoma have a much longer survival time than those with typical chordoma (Figure 8.19).

Spread

In most cases, the spread of the tumour is into the bony tissue of the base of the skull, outwards to the nasopharynx and inwards to the brain. Metastasis is rare.

References

1. Ali, M. Y. (1965). Histology of the human nasopharyngeal mucosa. *J. Anat.*, **99**, 657–672
2. Chaudry, A. P., Lore, J. M. Jr., Fisher, J. E. and Gambrino, A. G. (1978). So-called hairy polyps or teratoid tumors of the nasopharynx. *Arch. Otolaryngol.*, **104**, 517–525
3. Shanmugaratnam, K. (1978). *Histological Typing of Upper Respiratory Tract Tumours. International Histological Classification of Tumours, no. 19.* (Geneva: World Health Organization)
4. Michaels, L. and Hyams, V. J. (1977). Undifferentiated carcinoma of the nasopharynx. A light and electron microscopical study. *Clin. Otolaryngol.*, **2**, 105–114
5. Teoh, T. B. (1957). Epidermoid carcinoma of the nasopharynx among Chinese: a study of 31 necropsies. *J. Pathol. Bact.*, **73**, 451–465
6. Gusterson, B. A., Mitchell, D. P., Warburton, M. J. and Carter, R. C. (1983). Epithelial markers in the diagnosis of nasopharyngeal carcinoma. *J. Clin. Pathol.*, **36**, 628–631
7. Myrhe, M. and Michaels, L. (1987). Nasopharyngeal carcinoma treated in 1841 by maxillectomy. *J. Otolaryngol.*, **16**, 390–392
8. Roholl, P. J., de Jong, A. S. and Ramaekers, F. C. (1985). Review. Applications of markers in the diagnosis of soft tissue tumours. *Histopathology*, **9**, 1019–1035
9. Tefft, M., Fernandez, C., Donaldson, M., Newton, W. and Moon, T. E. (1978). Incidence of meningeal involvement by rhabdomyosarcoma of the head and neck in children. A report of the Intergroup Rhabdomyosarcoma Study (IRS). *Cancer*, **42**, 232–258
10. Dahlin, D. C. (1981). *Bone Tumors*, 3rd Edn. (Springfield Ill.: Charles C. Thomas)
11. Heffelfinger, M. J., Dahlin, D. C., McCarty, C. S. and Beabout, J. W. (1973). Chordomas and cartilaginous tumors at the skull base. *Cancer*, **32**, 410–420

Palatine Tonsil and Oropharynx

9

Normal Histology

The palatine tonsil is composed of lymphoid tissue within which are channels lined by squamous epithelium – crypts – that open onto the surface (Figure 9.1). It is part of a ring of lymphoid tissue in the oral cavity and nasopharynx – Waldeyer's ring – which includes also the lingual tonsil at the base of the tongue and the pharyngeal tonsil or adenoid in the nasopharynx. There are about 20 crypts reaching the deepest part of the structure. Submucosal glands lie in the peripheral part.

Epithelium

The epithelium of the tonsillar surface is non-keratinizing stratified squamous, similar to that covering the mucosa of the rest of the oral cavity. In the crypts, however, although continuous with the surface, the squamous epithelium has a more prominent component of basal cells and is infiltrated by lymphocytes and plasma cells (Figure 9.2). Particularly in children, the crypt epithelium conveys such an impression of activity that neoplasia may be suggested by those unfamiliar with this normal feature (Figure 9.3). Beneath the epithelium, the tonsil is formed mainly by lymphoid follicles which are surrounded by loosely distributed lymphoid tissue. Each follicle consists of a germinal centre and a lymphocytic cap which becomes thicker towards the crypt (Figure 9.4). The germinal centre is composed of precursors of lymphocytes: centrocytes (cleaved cells), which have indented nuclei and indistinct cytoplasm, and centroblasts (large non-cleaved cells), which show nucleoli near the nuclear membrane and a thin rim of basophilic cytoplasm. There are also macrophages often containing numerous particles of phagocytosed material (tingible body macrophages) and dendritic reticulum cells. The lymphocytic cap is composed entirely of B lymphocytes. T lymphocytes – mainly helper cells – are located in the perifollicular tissue.

The function of the tonsil is the supply of B cells which produce specific immunoglobulin following antigenic stimulation through the crypts.

Cartilage and bone

Islands of bone and cartilage are found in about a fifth of all tonsils (Figure 9.5). Bone is said to occur only in the presence of cartilage but the latter may occur without bone. These tissues are present in older individuals but otherwise have no known significance.

Inflammatory Diseases

Tonsillitis

Attacks of tonsillitis are among the commonest of all infections. Children are the most frequent sufferers but adults are not spared.

Gross appearances

The pathological changes characteristic of tonsillitis are difficult to define. The tonsils are rarely removed at the time of an acute attack and there is some uncertainty about the significance of the changes found between attacks. The tonsils may be of equal or unequal size. The relative sizes are no reflection of the degree of pathological change in one or the other. The external (crypt orifice) surface may show crypts distended by white foci, greyish casts or even calcified casts of the crypt (tonsilloliths). Cut surface may show cysts filled with white debris or grey cast material. Fibrosis is rare. The majority of surgically removed tonsils show no gross abnormalities.

Microscopic appearances

The specific feature of inflammatory change in the tonsil is the presence of neutrophils under the crypt epithelium, which may form small abscesses and may extend through the epithelium to the lumen. The overlying squamous epithelium may be thinned or even ulcerated. In areas of resolved inflammation, the crypt epithelium may show a papillary arrangement in which numerous small swellings of squamous epithelium associated with plasma cells and lymphocytes project into the lumen (Figure 9.6). Lymph follicles are swollen by enlargement of germinal centres which contain many tingible body macrophages. As a result of focal compression of the lumen of crypts by abscess formation or enlarged lymph follicles, there may be a damming up of crypt products, leading to swelling of the crypt proximal to the obstruction with, eventually, the formation of a cyst lined by squamous epithelium and filled with squamous debris. In a few cases, the stagnant material becomes calcified, resulting in a tonsilolith.

Another feature of crypt lumina in most surgically excised tonsils is the presence of colonies of *Actinomyces israeli* (Figure 9.7) which are microaerophilic and, therefore, flourish well under the conditions existing in the crypt. It is doubtful how much they contribute to the inflammation of the tonsil. Fibrosis is sometimes seen in tonsils.

Infectious mononucleosis

Infectious mononucleosis is an infection caused by the Epstein–Barr virus. Changes are mainly in the mononuclear cells of the blood and in the lymph nodes, and an antibody against sheep red cells is present in the blood. Complete recovery from the infection is the rule. In a few cases, the tonsils become markedly enlarged during the course of the infection and may even impede swallowing and breathing. In such cases, the patient recovers completely after tonsillectomy. Microscopic appearances are those of massive replacement of crypt epithelium and follicles by lymphoid cells of blast-cell appearance (Figures 9.8 and 9.9). In a few places, the remains of keratinous cysts formed from crypt epithelium are present. An occasional surviving follicle may also be seen. Areas of necrosis are frequent. Some lymphoid cells may even invade the walls of small arteries. The histological pattern would be highly suggestive of a lymphoma but for the proven condition of infectious mononucleosis. Immunohistochemical studies on the sections of tonsillar tissue show both λ and κ light chains (i.e. immunoglobulin polyclonality) in the proliferated cells. Such an investigation is necessary in

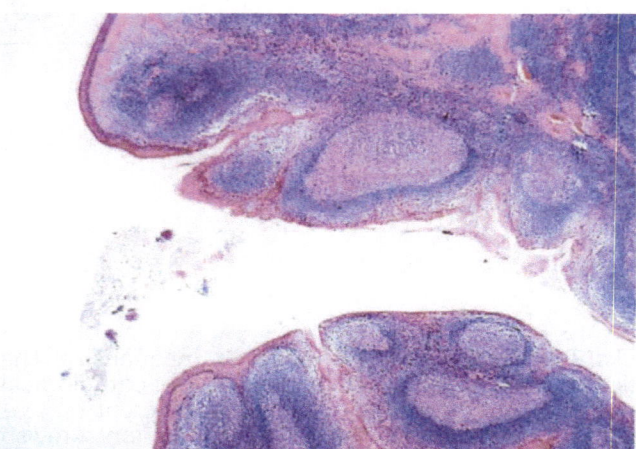

Figure 9.1 Opening of crypt of palatine tonsil onto the surface. The crypt is lined by stratified squamous epithelium which is thinner than that lining the mucosal surface. Note lymphoid follicles beneath the crypt epithelium.   H & E (A)

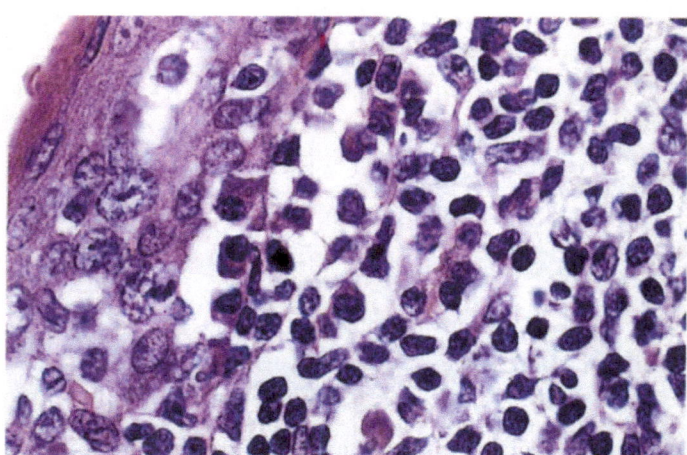

Figure 9.2 Lining of crypt of tonsil showing close association of basal cells with adjacent lymphoid cells composed mainly of plasma cells and lymphocytes.   H & E (C)

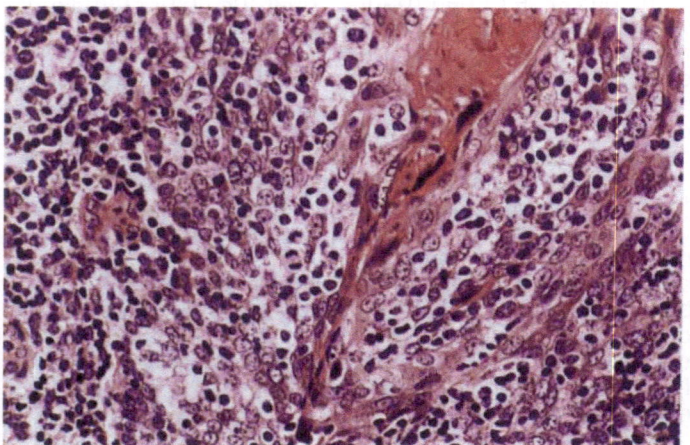

Figure 9.3 Deeper part of crypt epithelium from normal tonsil. Showers of epithelial cells extend from keratinized stratified squamous epithelium towards underlying lymphoid follicles.   H & E (C)

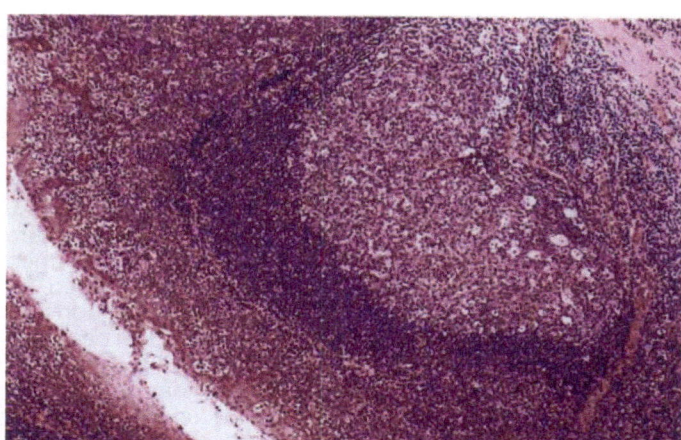

Figure 9.4 Lymphoid follicle near lining of crypt of tonsil. Note lymphocytic cap of follicle which is thickest towards the crypt. H & E (B)

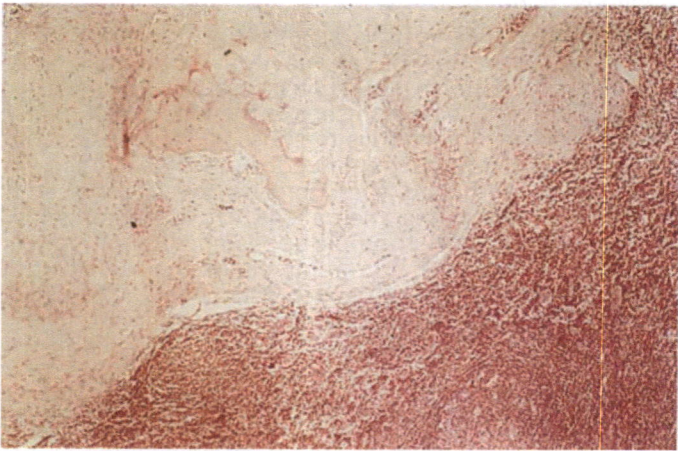

Figure 9.5 Normal cartilage with a small piece of bone which has been deposited in the tonsillar lymphoid tissue.   H & E (B)

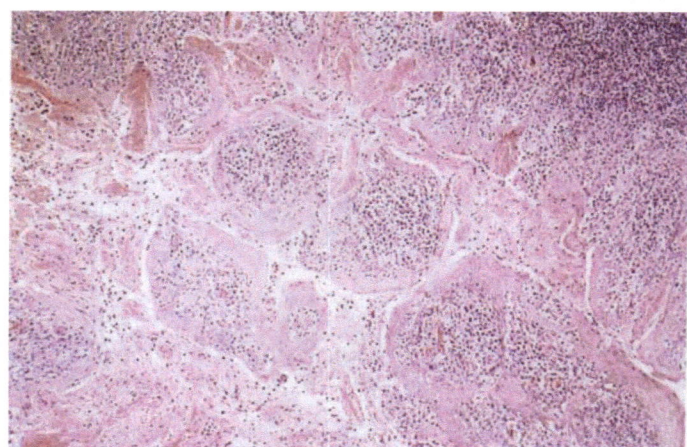

Figure 9.6 Crypt of tonsil showing papillary formation of lymphoid cells with a covering of squamous epithelium.   H & E (B)

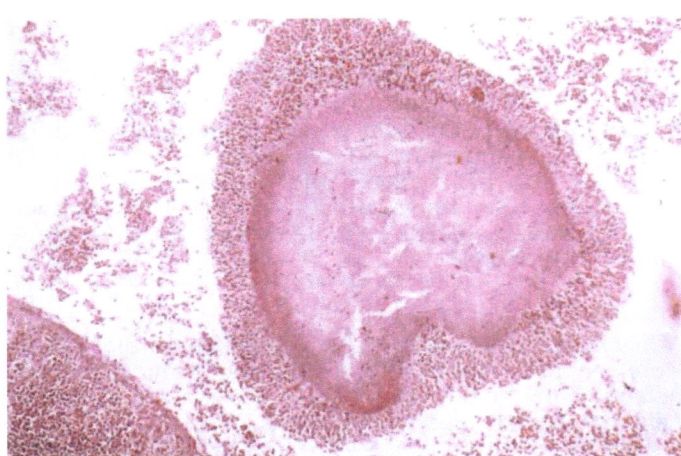

Figure 9.7 Actinomyces and numerous pus cells in crypt of tonsil H & E (B)

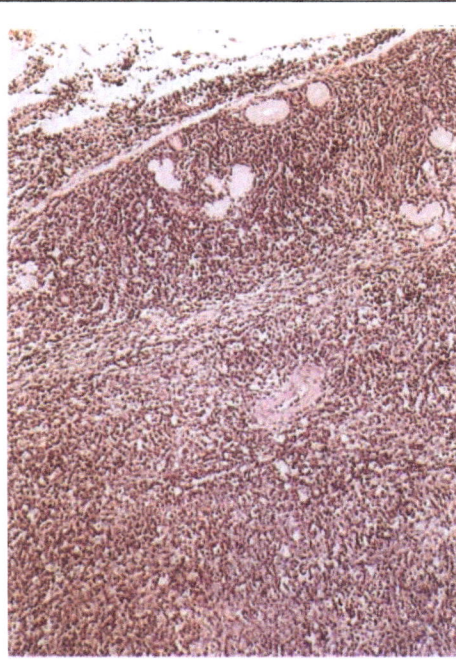

Figure 9.8 Hyperplasia of tonsillar lymphoid tissue in infectious mononucleosis with infiltration of region of mucous glands. H & E (B)

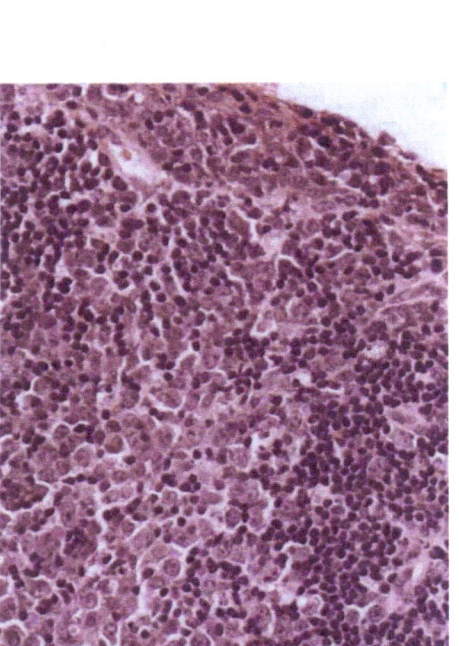

Figure 9.9 Infectious mononucleosis showing infiltration of atypical lymphoid cells with infiltration of epithelium of crypt. H & E (C)

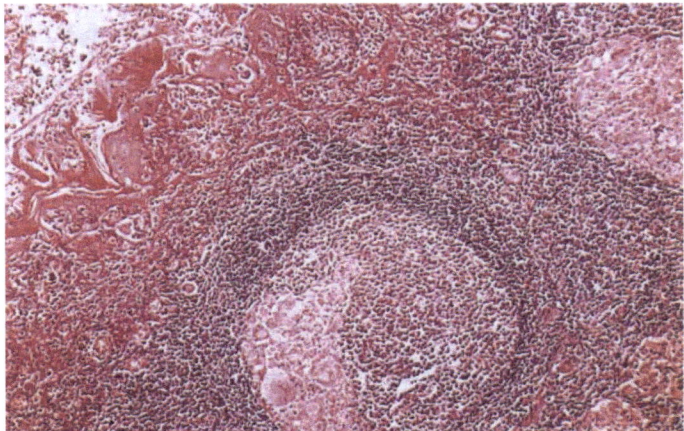

Figure 9.10 Granulomatous infiltration of lymphoid tissue of tonsil. The granulomas are composed of epithelioid cells with an occasional giant cell. H & E (B)

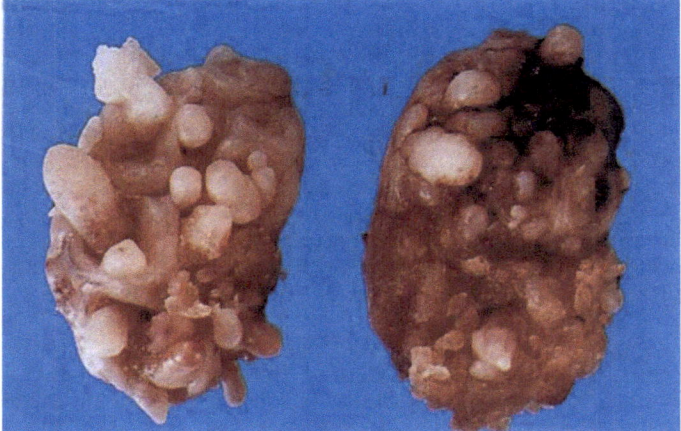

Figure 9.11 Multiple squamous papillomas growing from the surface of both tonsils.

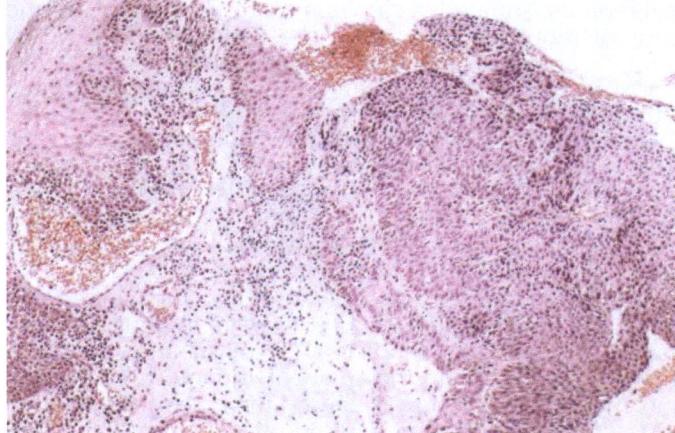

Figure 9.12 Poorly differentiated squamous cell carcinoma of tonsil showing ribbons of malignant epithelial cells arising from dysplastic epithelium of tonsil. H & E (B)

doubtful cases to exclude the monoclonal immuno-globulin secretion of malignant lymphoma.

Diphtheria

Diphtheria is an acute mucosal inflammation of the tonsils and adjacent soft palate produced by *Corynebacterium diphtheriae*. The organism is present in large numbers in the surface inflammatory exudate, and exotoxin produced by it enters the bloodstream and has a specific damaging effect on the myocardium.

The gross appearance of the tonsillar inflammation is that of a dull greyish yellow layer – the false membrane – which covers the surface of the tonsil and a variable amount of surrounding tissue. This membrane separates off with difficulty. The membrane may extend or may, indeed, be confined to the laryngeal or the nasopharyngeal mucosae. Microscopically, the false membrane contains fibrin and neutrophils with, in the early stages, large numbers of diphtheria bacilli. The squamous epithelium of the tonsil forms part of the membrane.

Granulomas

Tuberculosis of the tonsil was once a common disease but has now been almost entirely eradicated. Non-caseating tuberculoid granulomas are occasionally seen in the tonsils. These are usually small and scattered evenly in the tonsillar lymphoid tissue (Figure 9.10). A few of these cases may show evidence of sarcoidosis on further investigation. The others do not and usually remain unexplained.

Neoplasms

Squamous cell papilloma

Squamous cell papilloma commonly arises on the surface of the palatine tonsil and adjacent oral epithelium. It has the appearance typical of an everted squamous papilloma seen elsewhere in the upper air and food passages, showing branching fronds and, microscopically, first-, second- and third-order branching of the papillae from a central stalk. The papillary processes show a connective core and a covering of squamous epithelium. Occasionally, numerous papillomas are present on each tonsil (Figure 9.11). Malignant change does not occur.

Squamous cell carcinoma

This neoplasm is said to be second in frequency to laryngeal carcinoma among malignant neoplasms of the upper air and food passages, although, in some geographical regions, squamous carcinoma of the tongue, lips and floor of mouth is probably more common. Both heavy smoking and excessive alcohol intake are important aetiological factors[1]. Common clinical features are sore throat, a throat lump, haemoptysis and deafness.

Gross appearances are those of a tumour usually situated in the upper pole of one tonsil. In advanced cases, there is involvement of the retromolar trigone, fauces, tongue and soft palate. The more highly keratinizing growths are exophytic. The less differentiated ones are often ulcerated.

The microscopic structure of most cases is of epidermoid malignancy with moderate degrees of keratinous differentiation (Figures 9.12 and 9.13). Dysplasia and carcinoma in situ are common in the adjacent squamous epithelium and may extend as far as the epithelium of the tongue and soft palate. In a small proportion of tonsillar carcinomas, the neoplasm is completely undifferentiated and closely resembles undifferentiated carcinoma of the nasopharynx (see Chapter 8). Such neoplasms grow rapidly. They metastasize more readily and are more sensitive to radiotherapy than the better differentiated squamous carcinomas.

Lymph node involvement is present in 65% of patients at the time of diagnosis[1]. The commonest lymph node group to be affected is said to be the subdigastric, at the angle of the mandible, but lower and even contralateral ones may also be involved. Bloodstream metastasis is quite common. In many cases, the cervical lymph node metastases may precede the clinical presentation of the primary in the tonsil.

Malignant melanoma

Primary malignant melanomas are rare in the oral cavity. More common is the development of metastatic malignant melanoma in one or both tonsils in cases of disseminated melanomatosis (Figures 9.14 and 9.15).

Salivary gland neoplasms

Neoplasms may arise from the seromucinous glands situated near the palatine tonsil. These include pleomorphic adenoma, mucoepidermoid carcinoma and adenocystic carcinoma. The histological appearances of these neoplasms are similar to those of tumours arising in the seromucinous glands of the nose (see Chapter 6).

The commonest neoplasms of the parapharyngeal space are salivary gland tumours, most frequently pleomorphic adenomas. These neoplasms may arise from the parotid gland, when they are situated lateral to the superior constrictor muscle, or from glands of the pharyngeal mucosa, when they are placed medial to the superior constrictor[2].

Synovial sarcoma

This malignant neoplasm has occasionally arisen primarily in the tonsil (Figure 9.16).

Malignant lymphoma

Malignant neoplasms derived from cells of the reticulo-endothelial system are common in the tonsils and other parts of the upper air and food passages. The tonsil is the commonest site of primary malignant lymphoma in the upper air and food passages.

Non-Hodgkin's lymphoma

The classification of non-Hodgkin's lymphomas has achieved considerable uniformity in Europe following the work of Lennert[3] and the publications of Wright and Isaacson[4] and of Stansfeld[5]. The classification in the latter two works follows the Kiel system of Karl Lennert which will form the framework of the following presentation of non-Hodgkin's lymphomas.

In the tonsil, lymphoma invades the lymphoid tissue and replaces crypts to produce a solid pinkish-yellow homogeneous neoplasm which conforms to the outline of original tonsil. An occasional keratin cyst may be visible on the cut surface (Figure 9.17). Histologically, traces of the crypt structure may be observed. Residual crypts may be markedly compressed and elongated by the lymphomatous neoplasm (Figure 9.18). In a few places, compression of crypts has produced retention of keratin production proximal to obstruction (Figure 9.19).

Malignant lymphoma, lymphocytic: Lymphocytic lymphomas are usually composed of B cells, occasionally of T cells. The normal lymphoid tissue is replaced by small lymphocytes which also invade the crypt epithelium.

Malignant lymphoma, lymphoplasmacytoid (lymphoblastic immunocytoma): In this type, substantial numbers of lymphocytes are differentiated towards plasma cells, forming also half-way cells, 'plasmacytoid' cells (Figure 9.20). Such changes are recognized by the presence

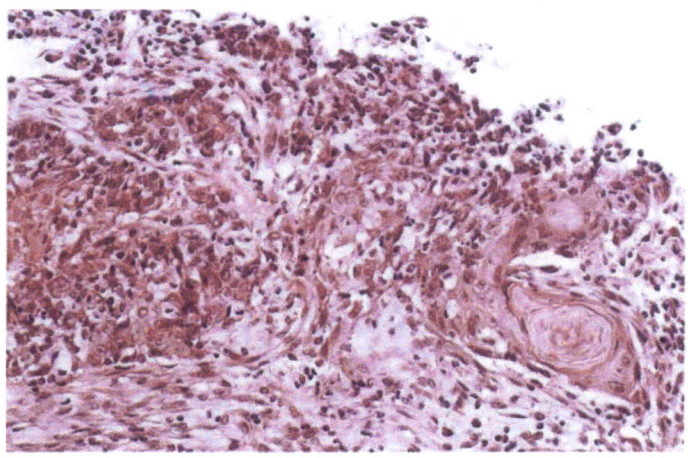

Figure 9.13 Moderately differentiated squamous carcinoma of tonsil showing keratinizing squamous carcinoma invading from the surface epithelium.   H & E (C)

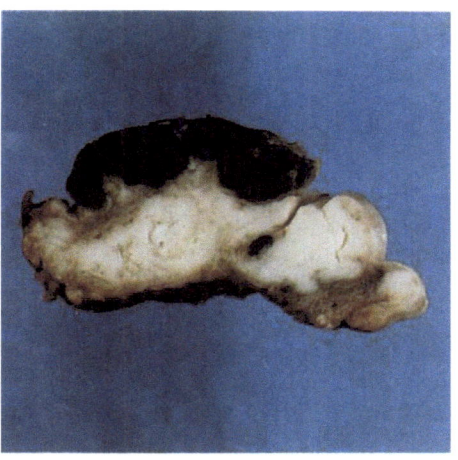

Figure 9.14 Metastatic malignant melanoma of tonsil

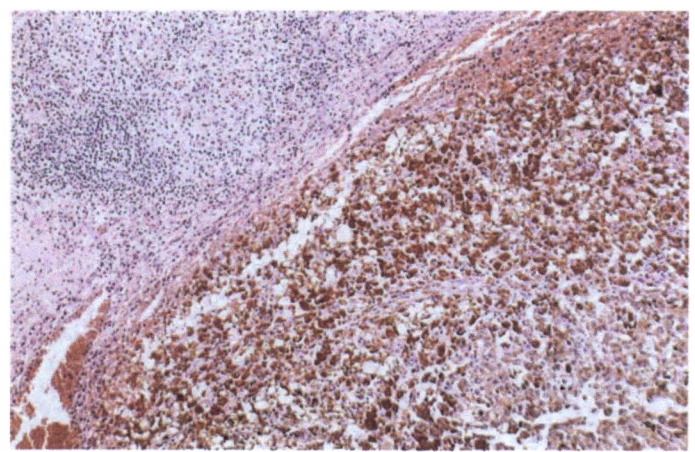

Figure 9.15 Metastatic malignant melanoma of tonsil showing pigmented malignant cells. An epithelioid granuloma is also present. This has been produced by local BCG inoculation in an attempt to restrict the growth of the neoplasm.   H & E (B)

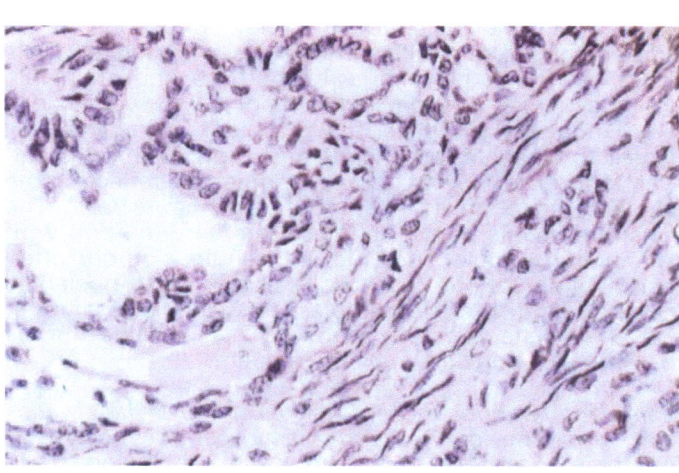

Figure 9.16 Synovial sarcoma of tonsil showing biphasic pattern of gland-like structures and mesenchymal cells.   H & E (C)

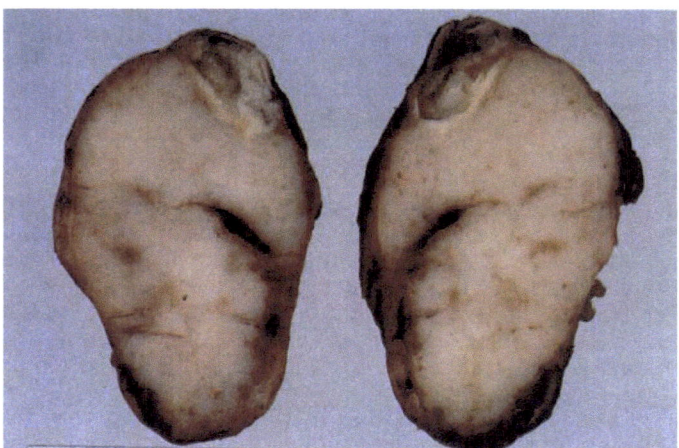

Figure 9.17 Malignant lymphoma of the palatine tonsil. The tonsil is replaced by homogeneous lymphomatous tissue. Note elongated dark cyst which is a retention cyst formed from a crypt

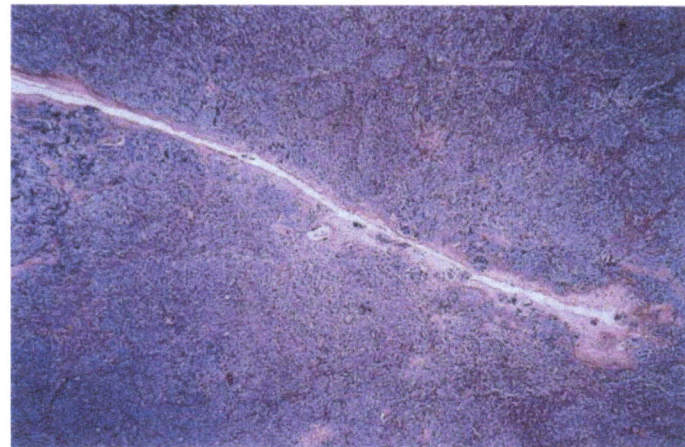

Figure 9.18 Compressed and elongated crypt surrounded by malignant lymphoma.   H & E (A)

of intracytoplasmic or intranuclear periodic acid–Schiff staining immunoglobulin inclusions. Immunohistochemical studies usually show IgM cytoplasmic immunoglobulin in a 'monoclonal' pattern, i.e. demonstration of only that immunoglobulin. The commonest form of lymphoplasmacytoid lymphoma is that of a widespread neoplasm involving lymph nodes, spleen and extranodal tissue, including Waldeyer's ring. In some cases the IgM secreted by the tumour cells leads to a paraproteinaemia and even to symptoms due to the hyperviscosity of the blood, a condition known as Waldenstrom's macroglobulinaemia. The lymphoma which occasionally occurs in certain autoimmune conditions, Hashimoto's thyroiditis and Sjogren's syndrome of salivary glands, is of this type.

Malignant lymphoma, plasmacytic: A synonym for this neoplasm is extramedullary plasmacytoma. The nose and paranasal sinuses are the commonest sites for plasmacytic lymphoma in this region and an account of it is given in Chapter 7.

Malignant lymphoma, centrocytic: The cells in this neoplasm are derived from centrocytes, the small cells normally found in the follicle centre. They correspond to the cleaved cells of the Lukes and Collins terminology[4]. This condition usually presents as lymph node and/or splenic swellings, but extranodal involvement may be very extensive. Under the microscope, the tumour may sometimes appear to emanate from surviving lymphoid follicles and even to form somewhat nodular aggregates, reflecting the follicle centre origin of the tumour cells (Figure 9.21). The constituent cells of the neoplasm are very uniform with pale-staining nuclei showing an irregular contour often seen as indentations ('cleaved' cells). A small nucleolus may be identified. The cytoplasm is variable in amount and always stains faintly (Figure 9.22). Hyaline fibrous thickening of capillary walls is frequent.

Malignant lymphoma, centroblastic–centrocytic: Malignant lymphoma of the centroblastic–centrocytic type is the commonest form of lymphoma in lymph nodes and the extranodal areas of the head and neck. The two cell forms involved in this neoplasm are the B-lymphocyte precursors which are abundant in normal germinal centres. Centrocytic–centroblastic lymphomas frequently show a follicular pattern which may be clearer on reticulin staining of the sections. Most of the tumour cells are small centrocytes (see above). Centroblasts are an important diagnostic component of the tumour although they may be quite scanty. They have large round pale-staining nuclei with one to three nucleoli which are often, but not always, situated near the nuclear membrane. The cytoplasm is scanty and basophilic (Figure 9.23). The neoplasm may show broad bands of fibrosis.

Malignant lymphoma, centroblastic: The already mentioned forms of non-Hodgkin's lymphoma are each examples of low-grade lymphoma which are composed of moderately differentiated cells and show a rather low degree of invasiveness. In this and the following forms – the high-grade non-Hodgkin's lymphomas – the cells are of blast type and invasive activity of the tumour is marked (Figure 9.24). Centroblastic lymphoma may be primary or it may arise by an acceleration of a lower-grade lymphoma, often centroblastic–centrocytic.

Malignant lymphoma, lymphoblastic: The lymphoblasts referred to in the designation of this neoplasm are primitive lymphoid precursors and do not correspond to a cell with a recognizable counterpart in normal postnatal life. A B-type, a T-type and a U-type (unclassified) are recognized. The latter corresponds in many cases to the tumorous phase of acute lymphoblastic leukaemia and shows immunohistochemical reactions for the antigens of that condition. Invasion outside the tonsil is active in this condition (Figure 9.25). Lymphoblasts may often be seen to form a single- 'Indian'-file formation around the walls of small blood vessels (Figure 9.26).

Many of the cases of the B type of lymphoblastic lymphoma correspond to Burkitt's lymphoma. This tumour of children, particularly of the male sex, occurs frequently in certain African territories and all cases are associated with Epstein–Barr virus infection of the tumour cells. Neoplasms of similar histological appearance have been reported sporadically in other parts of the world; these are not associated with an Epstein–Barr virus infection. Most patients present with tumours of the jaws. The ovaries, salivary glands, thyroid and other sites are also frequently involved. Lymph nodes are rarely affected (Figure 9.27).

Malignant lymphoma, immunoblastic: This highly malignant form of lymphoma is composed of transformed lymphocytes, usually of B cell type. The tumour cells have round or oval nuclei with a single prominent central nucleolus and a well-defined pyroninophilic cytoplasm (Figure 9.28). Immunoperoxidase studies show a strong positivity of the cells for immunoglobulin on a monoclonal basis. This neoplasm may be regarded as a high-grade (very malignant) form of lymphoplasmacytoid lymphoma and indeed it may arise as a complication of the latter.

T cell lymphoma: A variety of T cell lymphomas are recognized but their place in the Kiel classification has not been clearly established. They are usually skin tumours; the slowly developing mycosis fungoides belongs to this group. A group of T cell lymphomas affecting the nose is emerging as a distinct entity[6] (Figure 9.29). Mention should be made at this juncture of lymphoepithelioid T cell lymphoma, often known as Lennert's lymphoma. This was, at first, thought to be a form of Hodgkin's disease, but Reed–Sternberg cells have usually been absent or scanty and the lymphoma is now classified as non-Hodgkin's, possibly of T cell type. Lymph nodes are mainly affected but Lennert found tonsillar involvement at the outset in a quarter of the cases.

'True' histiocytic lymphoma: These are neoplasms of the monocytic-macrophage system and are said to be rare if immunological and cytochemical markers are used to specify fully the nature of the cells. They are often found to be T cell lymphomas after such categorization. The cells of this tumour resemble histiocytes and may often demonstrate lysosomal enzymes, such as α-1-antitrypsin.

Hodgkin's disease

In the upper air and food passages, Hodgkin's disease occurs only in Waldeyer's ring. Todd and Michaels[7] reviewed 16 cases in that situation from the files of the Royal Marsden and the Royal National Throat, Nose and Ear Hospitals, London. It now seems possible that the four cases in this series presenting as isolated neoplasms of Waldeyer's ring were, in fact, a form of lymphomas known as lymphoepithelioid T cell type (see above). True Hodgkin's disease occurring in Waldeyer's ring alone is now thought to be extremely rare (Professor P. Isaacson, personal communication). The course of the disease in Hodgkin's involving Waldeyer's ring did not seem to differ from that of cases of Hodgkin's disease in general. Involvement of Waldeyer's ring, thus, does not seem to be of any special significance in the natural history of the disease.

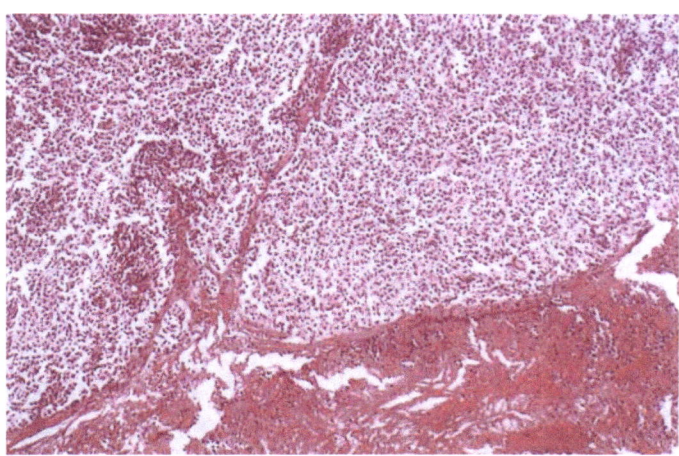

Figure 9.19 Keratin cyst in tonsil produced by compression and obstruction of a crypt caused by malignant lymphoma. H & E (B)

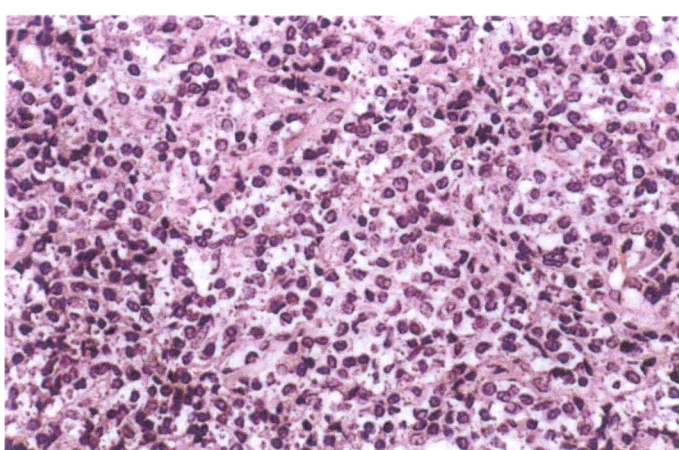

Figure 9.20 Malignant lymphoma, lymphoplasmacytoid, of tonsil. The neoplasm is composed of lymphocytes and cells differentiated towards plasma cells. H & E (C)

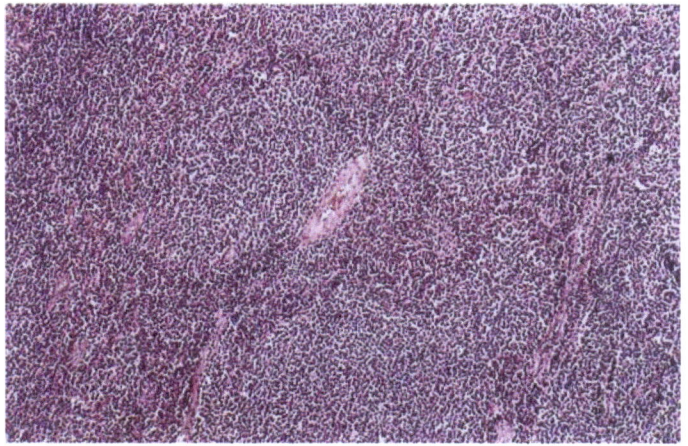

Figure 9.21 Follicular lymphoma of tonsil in which nodular aggregates are formed. The lymphoma type is centrocytic, i.e. of follicular centre origin. H & E (C)

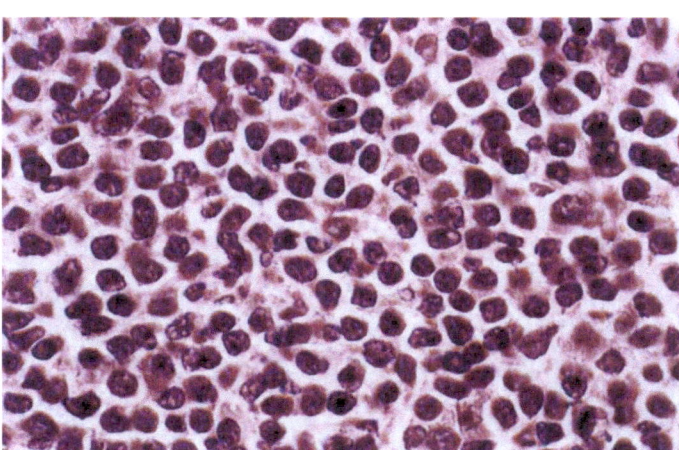

Figure 9.22 Centrocytic cell proliferation in centrocytic centroblastic lymphoma of tonsil. The centrocytes are uniform with pale-staining nuclei showing an irregular contour and are often 'cleaved'. The cytoplasm stains faintly. H & E (D)

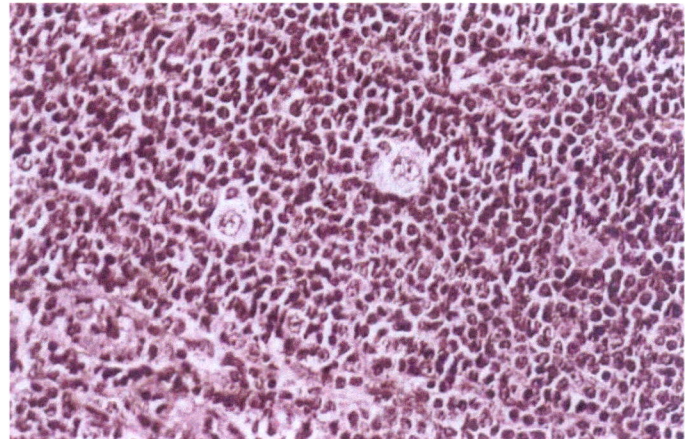

Figure 9.23 Centroblastic centrocytic lymphoma of the tonsil. Scanty centroblasts are seen among large numbers of centrocytes. H & E (C)

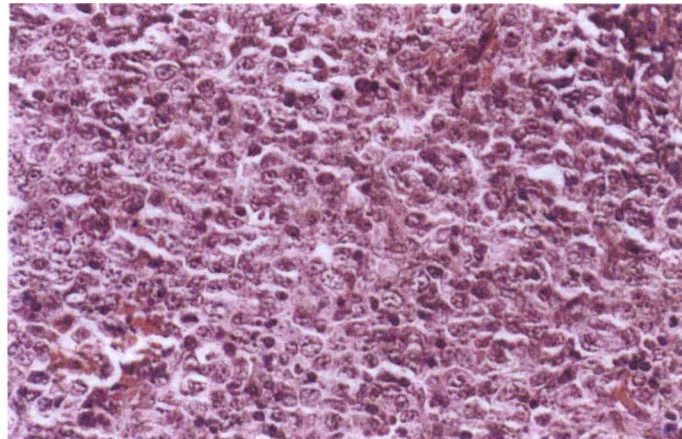

Figure 9.24 Centroblastic lymphoma of tonsil. The tumour is composed of centroblasts alone. H & E (C)

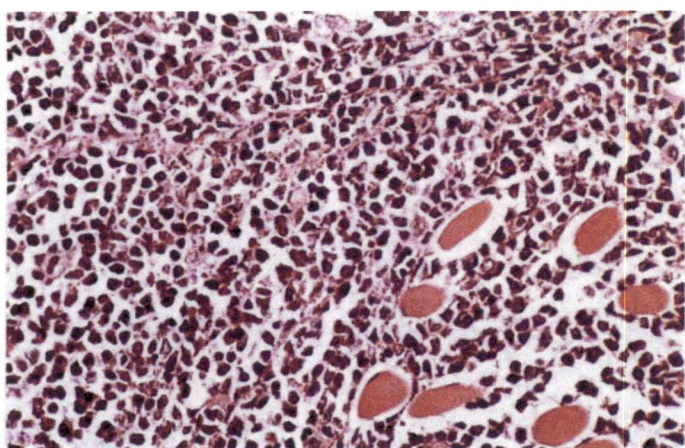

Figure 9.25 Lymphoblastic lymphoma of tonsil. The tumour cells are malignant lymphoid precursors and are invading skeletal muscle tissue adjacent to the tonsil.   H & E (C)

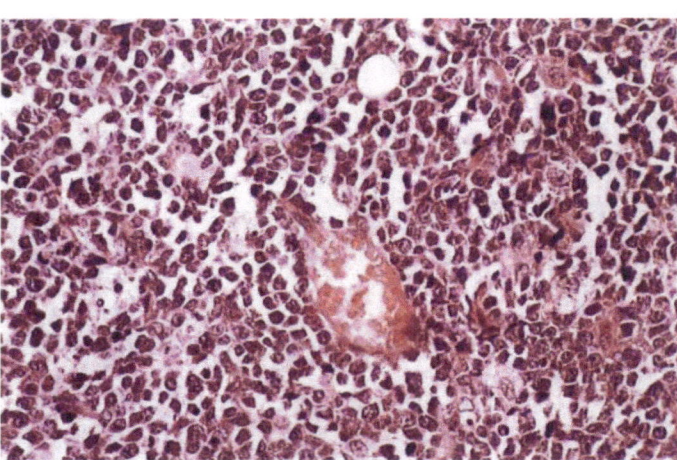

Figure 9.26 Lymphoblastic lymphoma showing 'Indian-file' pattern of lymphoma cells around small blood vessel.   H & E (C)

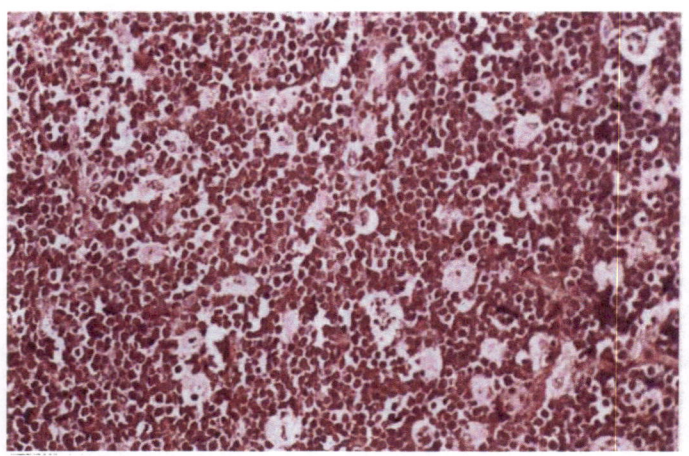

Figure 9.27 Lymphoblastic lymphoma of Burkitt's type in epiglottic region of 10-year-old child. Note foamy macrophages among primitive lyphoid cells ('starry sky' appearance).   H & E (B)

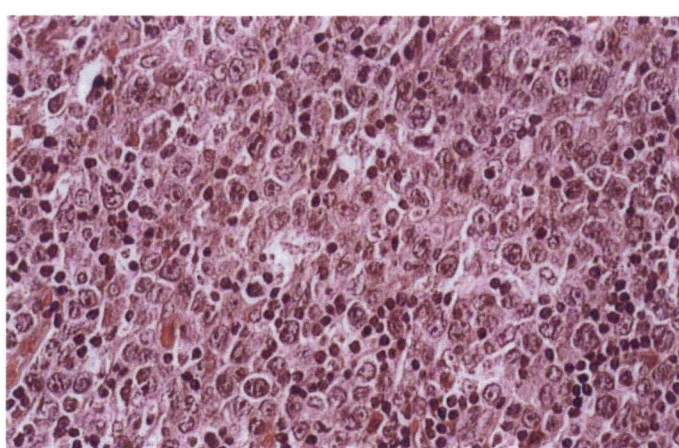

Figure 9.28 Immunoblastic lymphoma of tonsil. The tumour cells have round or oval nuclei with well-defined pyroninophilic cytoplasm. H & E (C)

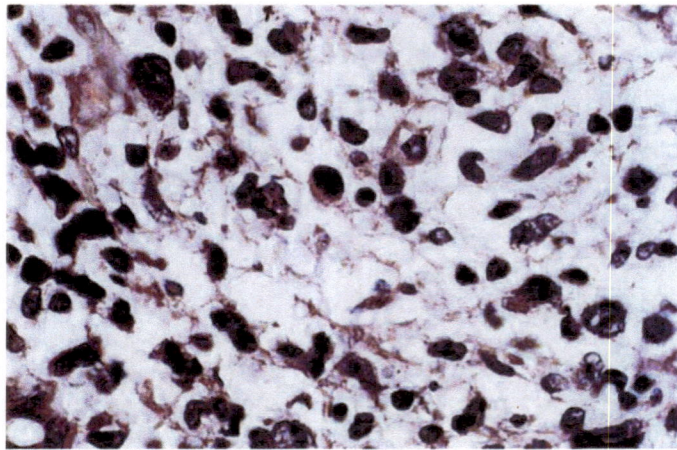

Figure 9.29 T cell lymphoma of nose.   H & E (C)

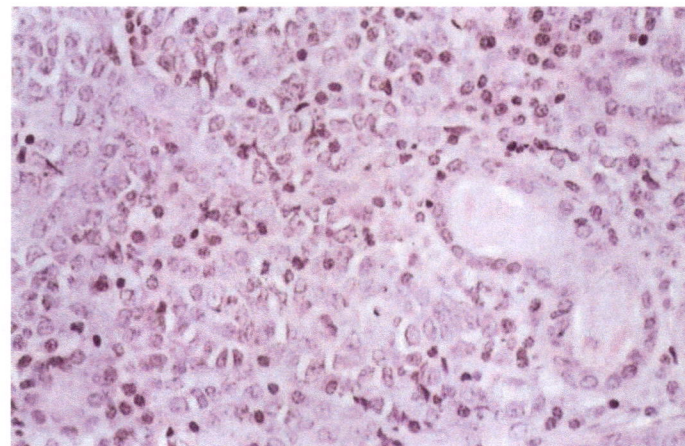

Figure 9.30 Granulocytic sarcoma occurring in inferior turbinate. The tumour cells are primitive with an occasional cell cf an appearance suggestive of a myelocyte.   H & E (C)

Granulocytic sarcoma (chloroma): Granulocytic sarcoma is a variant of acute myeloid leukaemia which is characterized by the formation of a green deposit of an invasive and destructive nature. The deposits are composed of immature cells of the granulocytic series, with myeloblasts frequently predominating so that the lesions may be mistaken for a lymphoma. The presence of myelocytes helps to alert the pathologist to the correct diagnosis and the use of special stains, such as chloracetate esterase, will confirm the myeloid nature of the deposit (Figure 9.30).

References

1. Ogrady, M., Doyle, P. J. and Flores, A. D. (1985). Cancer of the tonsil. *J. Otolaryngol.*, **14**, 221–225
2. Warrington, G., Emery, P. J., Gregory, M. M. and Harrison, D. F. N. (1981). Pleomorphic salivary gland adenomas of the parapharyngeal space. Review of nine cases. *J. Laryngol. Otol.*, **95**, 205–218
3. Lennert, K. (1981). *Histopathology of Non-Hodgkin's Lymphomas (Based on the Kiel Classification). In Collaboration with H. Stein.* (Berlin, Heidelberg, New York: Springer)
4. Wright, D. H. and Isaacson, P. G. (1983). *Biopsy Pathology of the Lymphoreticular System.* (London: Chapman and Hall)
5. Stansfeld, A. G. (ed.) (1985). *Lymph Node Biopsy Interpretation.* (Edinburgh: Churchill Livingstone)
6. Chan, J. K., Ng, C. S., Lau, W. H. and Lo, S. T. (1987). Most nasal/nasopharyngeal lymphomas are peripheral T-cell neoplasms. *Am. J. Surg. Pathol.* **11**, 418–429
7. Todd, G. B. and Michaels, L. (1974). Hodgkin's disease involving Waldeyer's lymphoid ring. *Cancer*, **34**, 1769–1778

Anatomy

Mainly for purposes of classification of neoplasms, the larynx has been divided into three regions: supraglottis, glottis and subglottis. The supraglottis is that region above the true vocal cords, including the epiglottis, the false cords, the ventricles and the saccules. The glottis comprises the vocal cords, the vocal processes of the arytenoids, and the anterior and posterior commissures. The subglottis is that region of the larynx below the true vocal cords down to the level of the lower border of the cricoid cartilage, below which the trachea commences.

Cartilages and elastic membranes

The complexity of laryngeal anatomy is the result of the curious relationships that exist among the five laryngeal cartilages. A useful approach to depicting these relationships has been made by Paff[1] and is reproduced in Figure 10.1. In this figure, the cartilages of the larynx are built up in their final relationship to each other. Diagram 1 shows the unembellished thyroid cartilage, the largest single cartilage in the laryngeal framework. In this diagram, the thyroid cartilage is seen from behind. Below the anterior notch, a square area is depicted where the handle of the spoon-shaped epiglottis is attached (Diagrams 2 and 3). The two false cords are inserted anteriorly at the pointed area and the true vocal cords are inserted into the two small oval areas below these.

In Diagram 4, the cricoid lamina (situated at the back of the ring-shaped cricoid cartilage) is depicted from behind. The two lower facets are for articulation with the inferior cornua of the thyroid cartilage (as in Diagram 5). The two upper facets are for articulation with the arytenoid cartilages. These are shown separately from behind in Diagram 6, with the minute corniculate cartilage joined to the apex of each arytenoid. In Diagram 7, the arytenoids are shown in position on top of the cricoid lamina, forming the cricoarytenoid joints. The arytenoids are thus in the posterior wall of the larynx. The hyoid bone is also related to the larynx by connection through ligaments and muscles. It is not shown in the diagram, but would be represented as a horseshoe-shaped structure, closed in front of the epiglottis and open behind.

Only the apical portion of the arytenoid and its lateral muscular process are shown in the posterior view. What is not shown is a short anterior projection from each arytenoid – the vocal process – which gives origin to the elastic tissue of the true vocal cord on each side. Beneath the mucosa of the larynx, superficial to the cartilage, an elastic membrane is present. (A similar structure is present in the trachea and bronchi.) The quadrangular membrane (the name given to the elastic membrane in the upper part of the larynx) is shown in Diagram 8, stretching from the corniculate cartilage to the epiglottis above, and from the muscular process of the arytenoid to the lower part of the epiglottis below. The upper part represents the framework of the aryepiglottic fold. The recess between the lateral surface of the quadrangular membrane medially and the medial side of the thyroid cartilage lamina laterally on each side is occupied by the piriform fossa – a pouch

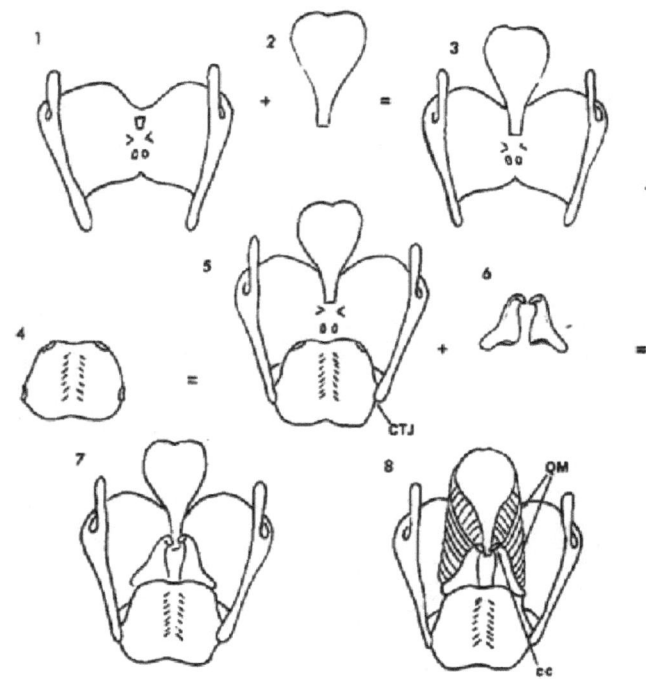

Figure 10.1 The cartilaginous framework of the larynx. In this series of diagrams, the cartilages of the larynx are built up into their actual relationships with each other. Diagram 1 shows the shape of the thyroid cartilage from behind. Diagram 2 shows the epiglottic cartilage, placed in position in Diagram 3. Diagram 4 shows the cricoid lamina from behind; the ring of the cricoid is not seen. Diagram 5 shows the position of the lamina in relation to the thyroid cartilage. The arytenoids are seen in Diagram 6 and are placed in position in Diagram 7. In Diagram 8, the elastic quadrangular membrane (QM) is in place. The vertically hatched part of this represents the aryepiglottic folds. cc: position of insertion of cuneiform cartilage at apex of arytenoid; CTJ: cricothyroid joint. From Reference 1 with permission of the publishers

of hypopharyngeal mucosa that serves for the passage of food and drink, on each side of the larynx. The quadrangular membrane ends inferiorly in the false cords. Beneath the false cords, there is a gap in the elastic lamina of the larynx, which makes way for the ventricle of the larynx and its upward extension, the saccule. The core of the true vocal cord on each side is an elastic layer – the vocal ligament – which extends from the vocal process forwards to be inserted in the back of the thyroid cartilage (the pointed area in Figure 10.1, Diagrams 1, 3 and 5). From this elastic tissue of the true vocal cord, the lower laryngeal elastic membrane – the conus elasticus or cricothyroid membrane – extends downwards to be attached into the upper surface of the cricoid ring. Thus, the upper part of the subglottic larynx, i.e. the part of the larynx below the true vocal cords but above the cricoid ring, is bounded anteriorly by the conus elasticus.

Gross Examination of the Larynx in the Histopathology Laboratory

I have found in experience of surgically excised larynges that the most suitable method for gross examination is horizontal slicing at 0.4 cm thickness, using a delicatessen-type slicing machine. With such a machine, a complete gross picture of the tumour in situ in the larynx can be obtained, and very satisfactory histological studies may also be carried out in the material so sliced[2]. The following normal structures may be identified in the tissue slices: epiglottis, laminae of the thyroid and cricoid cartilages, corniculate and cuneiform cartilages, false vocal cords, ventricles and saccules, true vocal cords, arytenoid cartilages, inferior cornua of the thyroid cartilage, cricoarytenoid joints, cricothyroid membrane and arch of the cricoid cartilage. An example of a laryngeal slice at the level of the true vocal cords is given in Figure 10.2. Any small structure that is not displayed on the surface of a block for microscopy may be included within a paraffin block and can be subsequently displayed in histological section by cutting down on to the required area during microtomy. Portions of hypopharynx that are removed with the larynx can be studied in the horizontal sections, and the method described is also suitable for examining hypopharyngeal carcinoma that has been treated by pharyngolaryngectomy. In addition to the normal structures mentioned above, the intrinsic laryngeal muscles may be conveniently displayed and sampled for histological examination by this method.

Normal Histology

Epiglottis

The pear-shaped epiglottic cartilage contains elastic tissue and does not undergo ossification. The elastic cartilage is perforated in the lower two-thirds by numerous foramina, which are associated with seromucinous glands that open through the posterior epithelial surface. The mucosa lining the anterior epiglottic surface is stratified squamous epithelium in continuity with that of the posterior surface of the tongue (vallecula) and surrounding hypopharynx. The posterior (or laryngeal) epiglottis is covered by a similar stratified squamous epithelium in its upper half, but, lower down, this changes into the ciliated pseudostratified columnar type characteristic of most of the internal laryngeal lining. The submucosa of the lingual epiglottic surface is comparatively loose areolar tissue, compared with the dense compact connective tissue of the posterior epiglottic surface (Figure 10.3).

False cords

The false and true cords of the larynx are two pairs of mucous folds situated above and below (respectively) an invagination of the laryngeal mucosa known as the ventricle. The epithelium of the false cords is of the respiratory type. However, squamous metaplasia is common. The submucosa is characterized by a large number of seromucinous glands embedded in a fibro-areolar stroma (Figure 10.4). Metaplasia of the connective tissue of the false cord to elastic cartilage was seen in 12% of males and 17% of females by Hill et al.[3]. This new formation of cartilage may encroach on the laryngeal lumen and give rise to symptoms of respiratory obstruction.

True vocal cords

The true cords are composed of elastic tissue covered by mucosa, and extend from the angle of the thyroid cartilage anteriorly to the vocal process of the arytenoid cartilage posteriorly. The epithelium of the true vocal cord is of stratified squamous variety from early in development.

This epithelium continues for a variable distance on to the floor of the ventricle and downwards towards the subglottis. The deep margin of the epithelium lining the ventricular floor (horizontal portion) is smooth, but the airway part of the vocal cord shows rete ridges. Melanocytes are found among the squamous epithelial cells in some Caucasians and Negroes[4]. The lamina propria of the true vocal cord is bounded, on its deep aspect, by the vocal ligament and, at its upper and lower extents, by respiratory mucosa. It contains no seromucinous glands (Figure 10.5). This vocal cord lamina propria is said to be deficient in lymphatic drainage and forms a space (Reinke's space). The vocal ligament (which is continuous below with the conus elasticus) is a nodular thickening composed of elastic tissue to which the vocalis portion of the thyroarytenoid muscle is tethered (Figure 10.6). The region of the vocal ligament may contain nodules of elastic cartilage.

Anterior and posterior commissures

A poorly demarcated area at the junction of the vocal cords anteriorly, the anterior commissure, is a region where the mucosa is not folded into vocal cords, but where it is in close proximity to the thyroid cartilage at the angle region. The core of the anterior commissure is fibrous tissue containing blood vessels and lymphatics. The epithelium in this region is respiratory in type (Figure 10.7). The interarytenoid area of the glottis is sometimes known as the posterior commissure. The epithelium here is also respiratory in type (Figure 10.8).

Ventricle and saccule

The ventricle and saccule are the proximal and distal parts (respectively) of an out-pouching of the laryngeal mucosa between the true and false cords. The saccule, which is of variable length, is an upward extension of the ventricle, derived from its anterior part. A similar lining consisting of respiratory epithelium with numerous glands is present in both the ventricle and the saccule (Figure 10.9). Squamous metaplasia is unusual.

Laryngeal joints

Both the cricoarytenoid and the cricothyroid joints are diarthrodial – that is, they contain a joint cavity. The articular surfaces are smooth and composed of a layer of cartilage, the thickness of which depends on the degree of ossification of the underlying arytenoid, cricoid and thyroid cartilages. The synovial membranes are lined by flattened synovial cells, beneath which there is a connective-tissue layer. Synovial membrane is confined to a recess which surrounds the articular cartilaginous surface but does not cover it. A tongue of synovium is regularly seen springing from the lateral recess of the cricoarytenoid joint (Figure 10.10).

Subglottis

Histological sections of the larynx in the subglottic region are characterized by the solid cartilaginous lamina of the cricoid behind, and, in the lower part of the subglottis, the ring is completed by the cricoid arch anteriorly. In the upper part of the subglottis, between the lower border of the thyroid cartilage and the cricoid arch, the cricothyroid membrane is seen – a thick elastic lamina which is perforated by blood vessels and lymphatic channels. At least one lymph node is usually found near the outer surface of the cricothyroid membrane.

Hyaline cartilage

The thyroid, cricoid and arytenoid cartilages are hyaline in nature. The apex (body) of the arytenoid has been

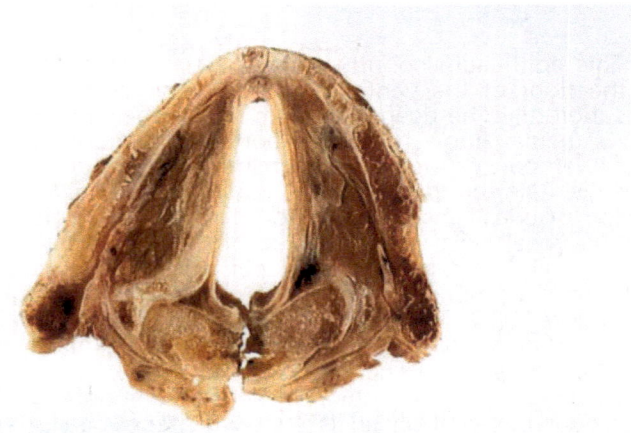

Figure 10.2 Transverse slice of normal larynx prepared on a motorized slicing machine. Note true vocal cords lateral to which is a block of muscle on each side. The anterior part of this muscle is represented by the transversely aligned fibres of the thyroarytenoid muscle; the posterior part is represented by the coarser vertically aligned lateral cricoarytenoid muscle. The cricoid lamina is seen posteriorly. It has been bisected to open up the larynx. Note the cricoarytenoid joint on the right side

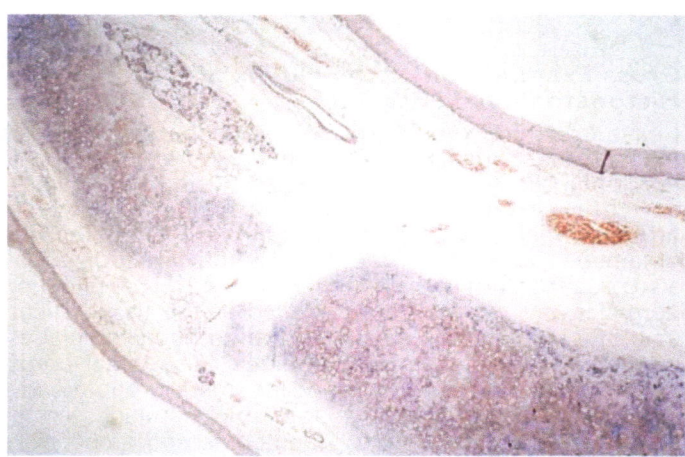

Figure 10.3 Transverse section of epiglottis showing anterior epithelium, above right, posterior epithelium, below left, and foramen in epiglottic elastic cartilage. The posterior submucosa is thinner than the anterior. H & E (A)

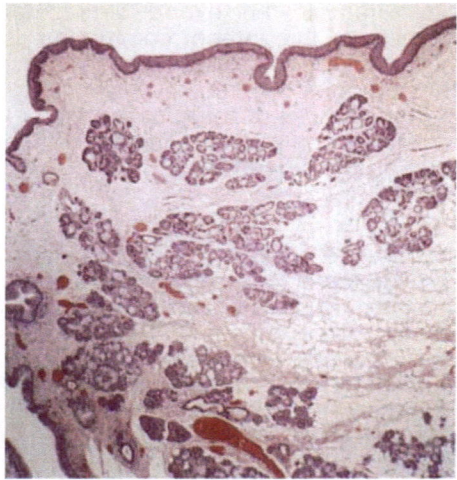

Figure 10.4 False cord. The ventricle is seen at the top left. Note large amounts of seromucinous glands and adipose tissue. The surface epithelium, but not that of the ventricle, has undergone squamous metaplasia. H & E (A)

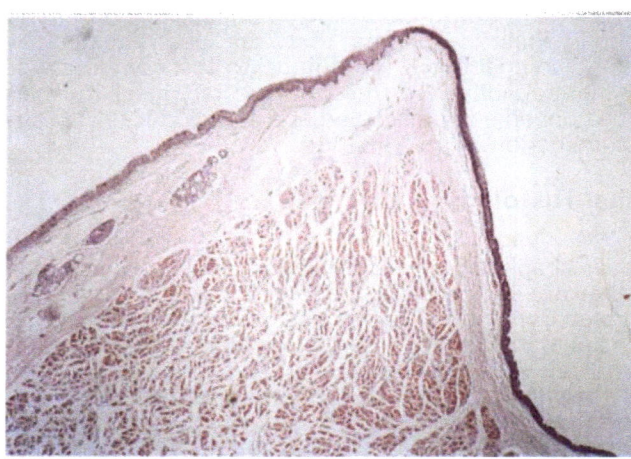

Figure 10.5 Vertical section of true vocal cord. The lining of the ventricle is passing horizontally above. It consists of stratified squamous epithelium without rete ridges medially and pseudostratified columnar epithelium laterally. The external surface of the cord is covered by stratified squamous epithelium with rete ridges. It merges with columnar epithelium inferiorly. Reinke's space lies between the mucosa of the vocal cord and the vocal ligament which lies superficial to the vocalis skeletal muscle, a superficial extension of the thyroarytenoid muscle. H & E (A)

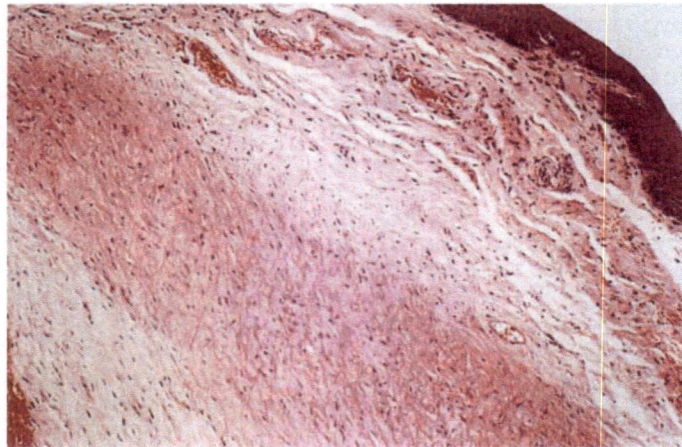

Figure 10.6 Superficial part of vocal cord showing epithelium, Reinke's space and vocal ligament. The epithelium is dysplastic in this specimen. H & E (B)

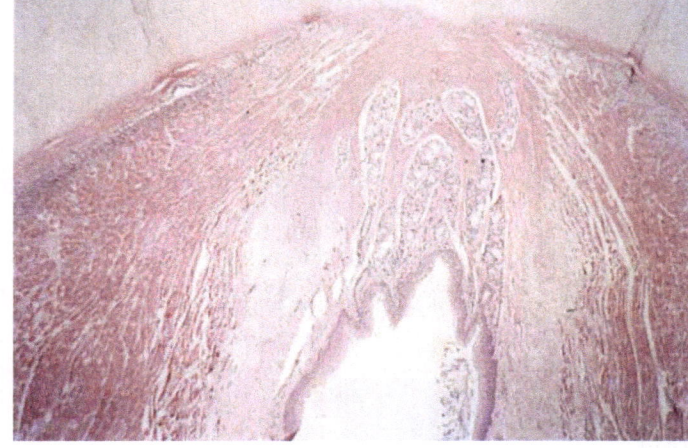

Figure 10.7 Anterior commissure. The epithelium has undergone squamous metaplasia. The space between it and the overlying thyroid cartilage is occupied largely by seromucous glands. H & E (A)

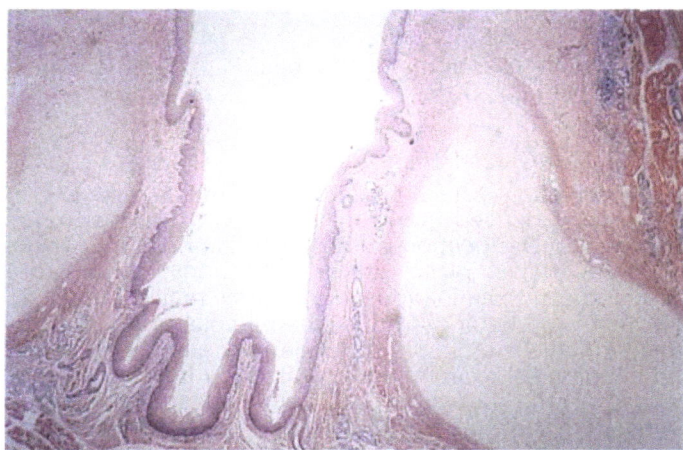

Figure 10.8 Posterior commissure showing epithelium, here metaplastic to stratified squamous, occupying the region between the two cartilaginous vocal processes of the arytenoids. H & E (A)

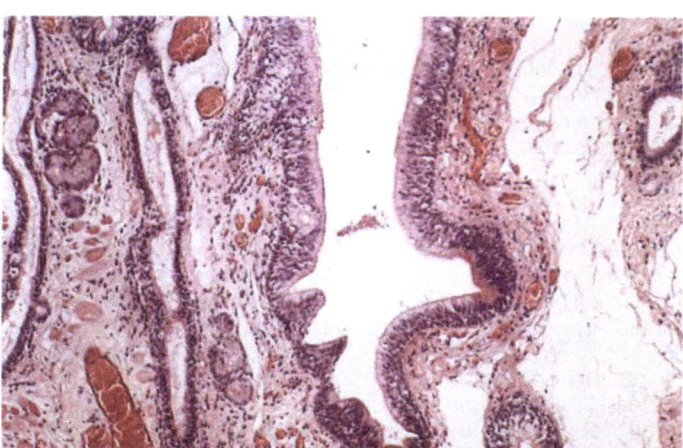

Figure 10.9 Saccule showing folded epithelial surface and underlying seromucinous glands. H & E (B)

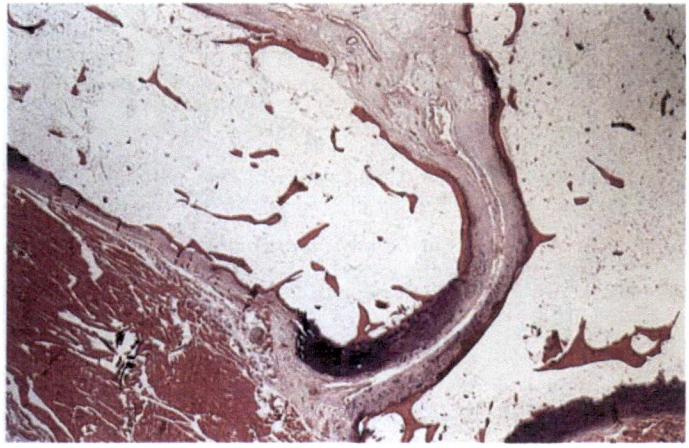

Figure 10.10 Normal cricoarytenoid joint. The articular ends of both the arytenoid (right) and cricoid (left) are covered by hyaline cartilage. A triangular tongue of synovium is arising from the joint at its lower pole. H & E (A)

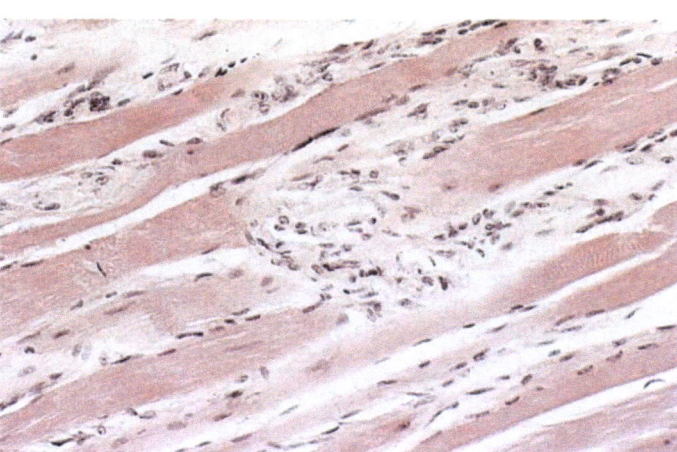

Figure 10.11 Posterior cricoarytenoid muscle showing loss of transverse striations and atrophy of muscle fibres in some areas with increase in sarcolemmal nuclei. H & E (B)

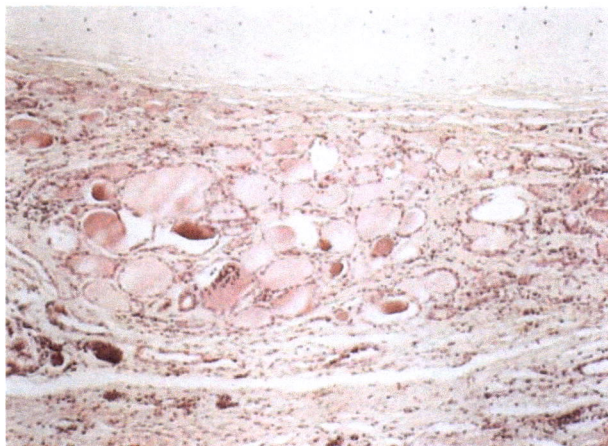

Figure 10.12 Thyroid heterotopia showing thyroid gland follicles internal to cricoid cartilage which lies across the upper part of figure. H & E (B)

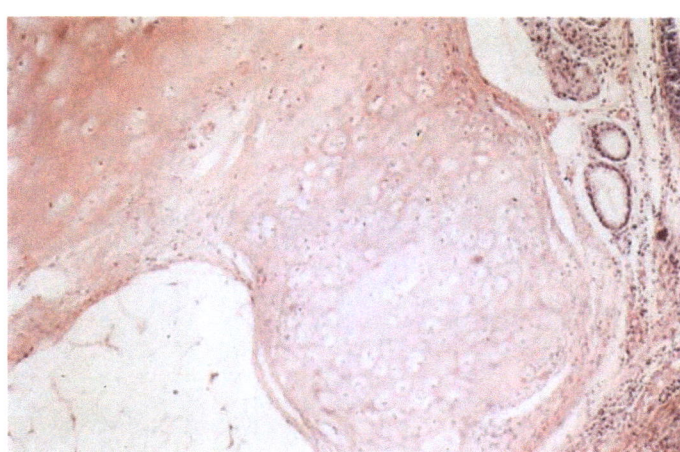

Figure 10.13 Tracheopathia osteochondroplastica. There is an ingrowth of cartilage from the tracheal ring into the tracheal mucosa. H & E (A)

stated to be elastic cartilage; the epiglottis, corniculate and cuneiform cartilages are definitely so. Hyaline cartilage undergoes ossification with developing age; elastic cartilage does not.

Laryngeal muscles

The laryngeal muscles show the features of normal skeletal muscles. On routine staining, we have found, however, that the posterior cricoarytenoid muscles constantly show abnormal features; the transverse arytenoid, thyroarytenoid, cricoarytenoid and lateral cricoarytenoid muscles do not[5]. The abnormalities comprise focal deposits of coarse brown pigment granules (lipofuscin) situated in the sarcoplasm near the sarcolemma, rows of up to 30 small deeply staining nuclei near the sarcolemma, and a loss of transverse striation (Figure 10.11).

Heterotopia

Thyroid tissue within the larynx

It is well known that thyroid gland tissue may be found along the pathway of embryological descent of the thyroid gland from the tongue downwards. Thyroid tissue may also be found within the subglottic larynx and upper trachea. The usual position for such aberrant thyroid gland is between the lower border of the cricoid cartilage and the upper rings of the trachea just beneath the mucosa[6]. In laryngectomy specimens removed from carcinoma, it is common to find islands of thyroid gland tissue within the fibrous capsule of the larynx and trachea, just outside the cricothyroid membrane. Occasionally, thyroid tissue is internal to the cartilage of the larynx and trachea, often extending over a broad area of the subglottis. The thyroid tissue in these cases is usually not recognized grossly, but is a chance finding on routine examination of the larynx specimen. The follicles of the thyroid are small and regular in such cases, with well-formed colloid, and are in proximity to seromucinous glands of the laryngeal mucosa (Figure 10.12).

Tracheopathia osteochondroplastica

In tracheopathia osteochondroplastica, multiple ingrowths of cartilage derived from the cartilages of tracheal rings are present. Ossification of these cartilaginous ingrowths frequently takes place. At bronchoscopy or at gross pathological examination, the lesion may present as irregular protuberances under the mucosa of the trachea and bronchi. The cricoid cartilage may also be involved. On histological examination, cartilage or lamellar bone is seen under the epithelium within and beneath the mucosa. Depending on the plane of the section, the aberrant cartilage or bone may be seen as a protrusion of the main cartilage towards the lumen (Figure 10.13) or an isolated mass of mucosal tissue. The condition would seem to produce no harmful effects[7].

References

1. Paff, A. G. E. (1973). Anatomy of the Head and Neck. (Philadelphia: Saunders)
2. Michaels, L. and Gregor, R. T. (1980). Examination of the larynx in the histopathology laboratory. J. Clin. Pathol., 33, 705–710
3. Hill, M. J., Taylor, C. L. and Scott, G. B. D. (1980). Chondromatous metaplasia in the human larynx. Histopathology, 4, 205–214
4. Goldman, J. L., Lawson, W., Zak, F. G. and Roffman, J. D. (1972). The presence of melanocytes in the human larynx. Laryngoscope, 82, 824–835
5. Guindi, G. M., Michaels, L., Bannister, R. and Gibson, W. (1981). Pathology of the intrinsic muscles of the larynx. Clin. Otolaryngol., 6, 101–109
6. Willis, R. A. (1962). The Borderland of Embryology and Pathology, 2nd Edn. (London: Butterworth)
7. Ashley, D. J. B. (1970) Bony metaplasia in trachea and bronchi. J. Pathol., 103, 186–188

Infections and Non-infective Inflammatory Conditions of the Larynx

11

Infections

Although the larynx is subject to infections caused by a wide variety of organisms, none of them presents in clinical practice with any frequency.

Acute inflammation

Acute inflammation may take a variety of forms in the larynx. There are four groups, each with a characteristic aetiological basis and pathological appearance, into which most cases would seem to fit:

1. Acute epiglottitis. This is usually caused by bacteria, in the majority of cases *Haemophilus influenzae*;
2. Acute laryngotracheobronchitis. This inflammatory lesion is probably caused by viruses, and the glottis and subglottic regions are particularly affected;
3. Allergic laryngitis;
4. Diphtheritic laryngitis.

The majority of patients are children in whom, because of the narrowness of the airway, the obstruction is serious and sometimes fatal.

Acute epiglottitis

The clinical features of this serious childhood infection are those of sore throat and pain on swallowing. The voice is relatively unaffected and there is little cough. The condition progresses rapidly to shock, leading to severe respiratory obstruction in 1–24 h. The clinical diagnosis is confirmed by observation of the fiery-red swollen epiglottis above the tongue. Acute epiglottitis also affects adults more frequently than has been generally realized.

The causative agent of acute epiglottitis in children is *Haemophilus influenzae*, type B. In adults, a broader spectrum of organisms, especially pyogenic cocci, has been associated with the condition.

Pathological appearances: At autopsy, not only does the epiglottis show signs of acute inflammation, but the adjacent tongue and pharyngeal structures are also swollen. An accentuation of the normal posterior concavity of the epiglottis is seen in some cases. The aryepiglottic folds are swollen and the laryngeal inlet is greatly narrowed (Figure 11.1).

In all cases, histological sections taken across the whole thickness of the epiglottis show an acute inflammatory exudate with neutrophils, red cells and fibrin infiltrating the anterior part of the epiglottis deep to the squamous epithelium (Figure 11.2). The inflammatory exudate extends widely in the pre-epiglottic space, but never penetrates the epiglottic cartilage posteriorly. There is a lymphocytic exudate in the posterior epiglottic mucosa, sometimes with germinal centres (Figure 11.3). Sections taken from the posterior part of the larynx, hypopharynx, supraglottic larynx, including aryepiglottic folds, and vocal cord region show acute inflammatory exudate similar in intensity to the anterior epiglottic region affecting the vallecula, hypopharynx and aryepiglottic fold region. The exudate is also present in the deep tissues of the larynx, extending downwards deep to the thyrohyoid, thyro-arytenoid and interarytenoid muscles, but the false and true cord mucosae do not show this change, exhibiting only a similar lymphocytic exudate to that seen in the posterior epiglottis.

It is clear from the above description that acute epiglottitis does not originate as a laryngeal disorder, but as an acute inflammatory condition affecting the oropharynx and hypopharynx.

Acute laryngotracheobronchitis

The majority of patients with this disease are less than 3 years of age, and some cases occur in the first year of life. The onset of the condition is more gradual than that of acute epiglottitis. When fully developed, there is a croupy cough with inspiratory and expiratory stridor. A viral aetiology for this condition has been emphasized but the evidence is far from conclusive.

Pathological appearances: The mortality from acute laryngotracheobronchitis has been very low for many years. Thus, to obtain a description of the pathological appearances, it is necessary to refer to accounts given before the antibiotic era[1]. They are characterized by neutrophil exudate in the subglottis, accompanied by mucus and fibrin, with degeneration of epithelial cells. A gummy rope-like exudate and crusting of necrotic epithelium are observed grossly. These changes take place mainly at the subglottic level in the larynx. There is a sparing of the seromucinous glands until late in the disease (unlike diphtheritic laryngitis, in which a specific necrosis of glands takes place with sparing of the surrounding tissue). The process extends downwards as tracheitis, bronchitis and bronchiolitis associated with similar rope-like secretions and dried crusts.

Diphtheritic laryngitis

The mucosal inflammation of diphtheria may spread to, or may be confined to, the larynx. In these cases, the epiglottis, false cords and true cords are covered by a false membrane, a dull greyish-yellow thickened layer which may extend down into the trachea.

Microscopically, the false membrane is composed of fibrin and neutrophils with, in the early stages, large numbers of diphtheria bacilli. On the deeper aspects, the laryngeal epithelium is included with the membrane. Where this epithelium is respiratory columnar in type, the membrane peels easily off the basement membrane (it may indeed by coughed up), but, in the squamous-epithelium-lined vocal cords, the false membrane separates off with difficulty and airway obstruction may result. The submucosal seromucinous glands underlying the diphtheritic membrane often show necrosis; in other forms of acute laryngitis, this is said not to happen[1].

Chronic bacterial infections and related conditions

Tuberculosis

Tuberculosis of the larynx is almost always associated with tuberculosis of the lungs which has now become unusual[2]. Hoarseness and painful dysphagia are usually complained of. The laryngoscopic appearances are those of a localized lesion, usually mimicking laryngeal carcinoma.

Pathological appearances
The commonest sites for the infection in the larynx are the true vocal cords, followed by the false cords. The lesions are often nodular, sometimes ulcerated. Microscopic examination may show the fully developed appearance of tuberculosis. The epithelium may be intact or ulcerated. Pseudo-epitheliomatous hyperplasia is common (Figure 11.4). Variable areas of mucosa are occupied by inflammatory tissue consisting of epithelioid cells, lymphocytes and Langhans' giant cells. Caseous necrosis is present to a variable degree. If the epithelium is ulcerated, acute inflammatory changes may be present (Figures 11.5 and 11.6). Special stains may reveal acid-fast bacilli in some cases, but very often these are not seen.

The clinical diagnosis of tuberculous laryngitis is usually made as a result of the pathologist's suggestion from his examinations of the endoscopic biopsy material. Since the histological appearances may be indefinite, the pathologist should adopt a high index of suspicion with regard to tuberculosis, especially in the presence of giant cells of any type, granulomatous lesions or unusual necrotic changes. The important step is to alert the clinician to the possibility of tuberculosis so that radiological examination of the chest and bacteriological examination of the sputum may be carried out.

Leprosy
Leprosy is an infective disease of the skin, mucosa of upper respiratory tract and peripheral nervous system, caused by *Mycobacterium leprae*. A spectrum of the disease exists between lepromatous leprosy, in which numerous mycobacteria are present, and tuberculoid leprosy, with few organisms. The difference between these forms is based on the immunological relationship of the host to the organism, the lepromatous form representing a state of low cell-mediated immunity and the tuberculoid a high one. Leprosy frequently attacks the larynx as well as the nose. Laryngeal involvement is seen only in the lepromatous, not the tuberculoid, form of the disease.

Microscopic appearances: The laryngeal lepromatous lesion consists, in its active stage, of a mucosal thickening containing macrophages, many of which appear as large foam cells (Virchow cells) (Figure 11.7). The latter contain the acid-fast bacilli of *Mycobacterium leprae* in large numbers. The organisms also appear in round basophilic structures known as globi, which are degenerated macrophages.

Syphilis
The introduction of penicillin to treat syphilis has eliminated laryngeal syphilis in advanced countries. Tertiary syphilis was once frequently manifested in the larynx by gummata, granulomatous foci which commenced as nodules, but which broke down eventually to form ulcers. They were often very deep, even penetrating the laryngeal cartilage. The ulcers eventually healed to produce scars, which underwent severe contraction, distorting the structure of the larynx and sometimes producing severe stenosis. Microscopically, the centre of the gumma shows coagulation necrosis. This is surrounded by an inflammatory exudate composed of plasma cells, lymphocytes, epithelioid cells and fibroblasts with variable numbers of giant cells. There is usually marked obliterative endarteritis.

Non-infective Inflammatory Conditions

Vocal cord polyp and other exudative processes of Reinke's space
Reinke's space is a potential space of the true vocal cord (see Chapter 10). It has been suggested that, because it does not possess an adequate lymph drainage, blood products may accumulate in Reinke's space without resolution and give rise to tissue reactions; together, the blood products and their tissue reactions in Reinke's space constitute the vocal cord polyp and some other lesions of the true vocal cord. Among the factors that have been invoked to explain these lesions in many of the affected patients are: the trauma of vocal cord abuse, cigarette smoking and other airborne irritants, nasal disease and hypothyroidism.

Clinical and gross appearances
Laryngologists observing the vocal cord at microlaryngoscopy insist that there are specific clinical forms of this process[3]. In Reinke's oedema the whole of both vocal cords is diffusely involved in the process. Vocal cord nodules are sessile swellings which are said to be present at the junction of the anterior and middle thirds of the true vocal cord. They are often bilateral, being present in the same position on both cords. The vocal cord polyp grows from the anterior two-thirds of a single cord taking the form of a pale spherical smooth grape-like structure up to 2 cm in diameter. In some forms of vocal cord polyp, bright red blood may be observed on the surface or within the polyps.

Microscopic appearances
The histological appearances of these lesions show combinations of the following features:

1. Blood, blood products and tissue ⎫ These two
2. Connective tissue cellular reaction ⎬ features are
   ⎭ present in
   all cases.

3. In a small number of cases squamous epithelial changes may also be present.

Fibrin is the main blood product which has exuded into the space in most of these lesions. This is observed as hyaline pink-staining amorphous material, sometimes with threads, which is usually extravascular (Figures 11.8 and 11.9). It often surrounds blood vessels. The fibrin is frequently accompanied, in haematoxylin and eosin preparations, by a blue-staining amorphous mucoid material, probably formed by sulphated glycosaminoglycans. Occasionally, fibrin may be seen within blood vessels as part of thrombus (Figures 11.10 and 11.11). Frank haemorrhage is also often present in these lesions (Figure 11.12). That this represents a real part of the tissue change and is not an artefact resulting from the surgery may be confirmed by the frequent presence of haemosiderin which usually accompanies the haemorrhage (Figure 11.13).

Variable, often extensive, degrees of connective tissue proliferation always contribute to the subepithelial swelling of vocal cord polyp or the other related lesions. Fibroblasts are always abundant (Figure 11.13). Frequently, they are small and stellate, and vocal cord polyps with a predominance of such cells have been described as 'myxoid' (Figure 11.14). Blood vessels – arteries, veins and capillaries – are often very prominent, particularly in the presence of fresh haemorrhage. Thrombosis may be seen within some of them (Figures 11.10 and 11.11). Cysts lined by flat cells sometimes develop among the connective tissue cells. The appearances of the exudate and connective tissue reaction in the vocal cord lesions secondary to myxoedema are identical to those described above (Figure 11.15).

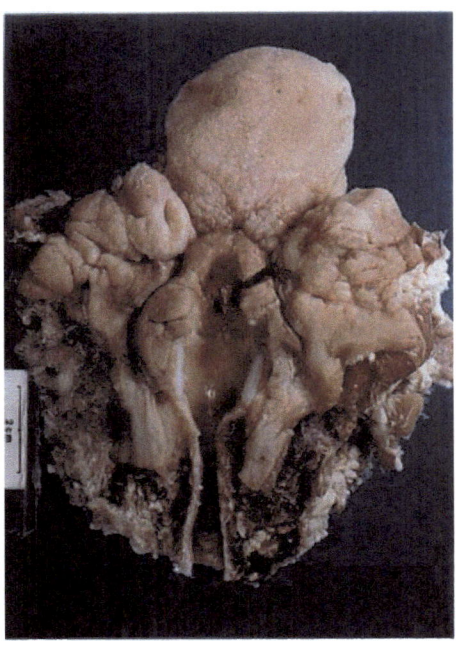

Figure 11.1 Acute epiglottitis in a child (necropsy specimen). Note marked oedema of rim of epiglottis, aryepiglottic folds and posterior pharyngeal wall. A wedge of tissue has been removed from the right side of the epiglottis for histological section

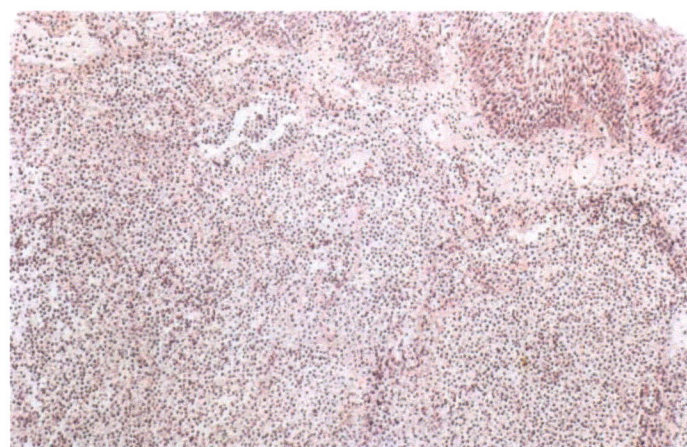

Figure 11.2 Deep part of squamous epithelium and mucosa of anterior surface of epiglottis in a case of acute epiglottitis. There is a dense accumulation of neutrophils beneath the epithelium. H & E (B)

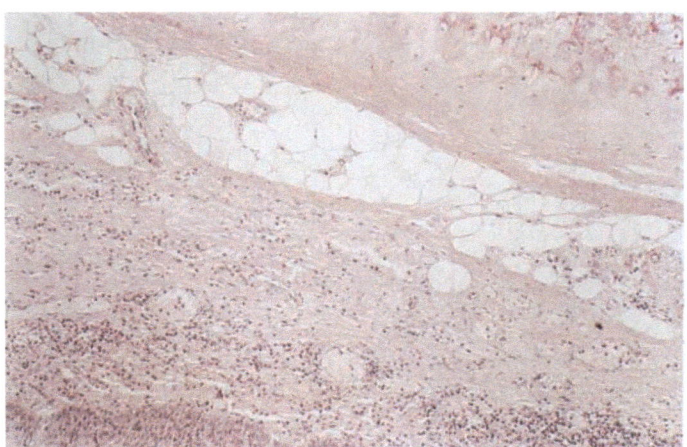

Figure 11.3 Posterior mucosa, submucosa and part of the epiglottic cartilage in a case of acute epiglottitis. Lymphocytes are present under the epithelium. H & E (B)

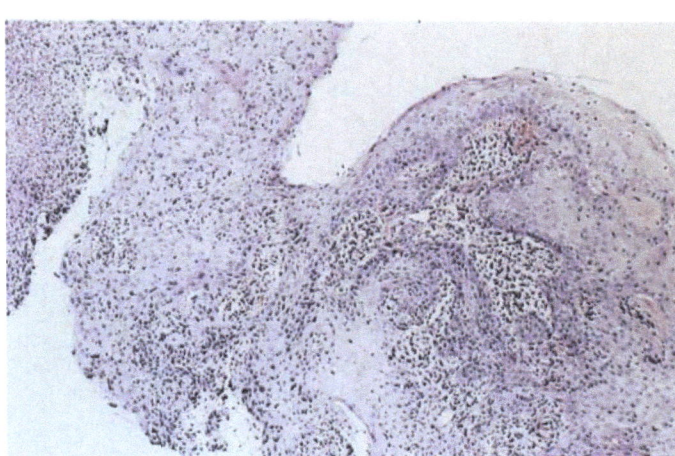

Figure 11.4 Pseudoepitheliomatous hyperplasia of vocal cord epithelium in tuberculosis of vocal cord. H & E (B)

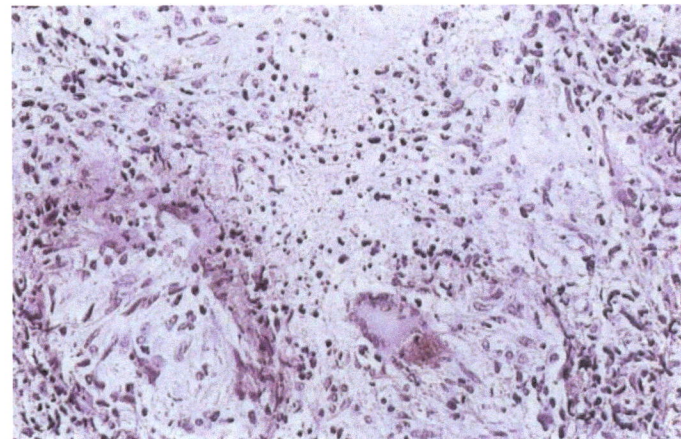

Figure 11.5 Tuberculosis of vocal cord showing epithelioid cells, a Langhans' giant cell and caseous necrosis. H & E (B)

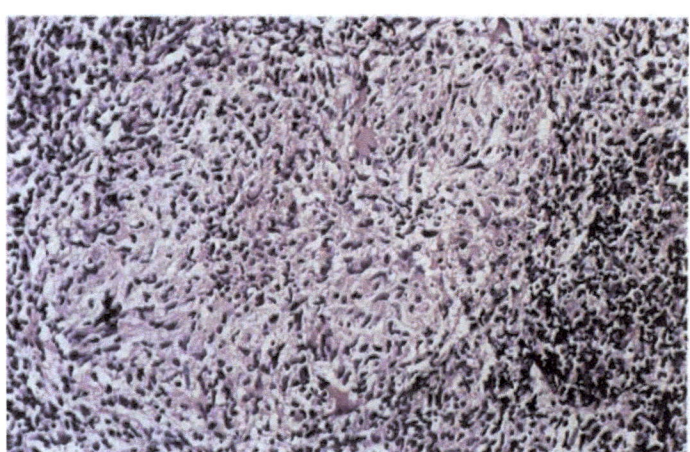

Figure 11.6 Tuberculosis of vocal cord showing epithelioid cells. H & E (B)

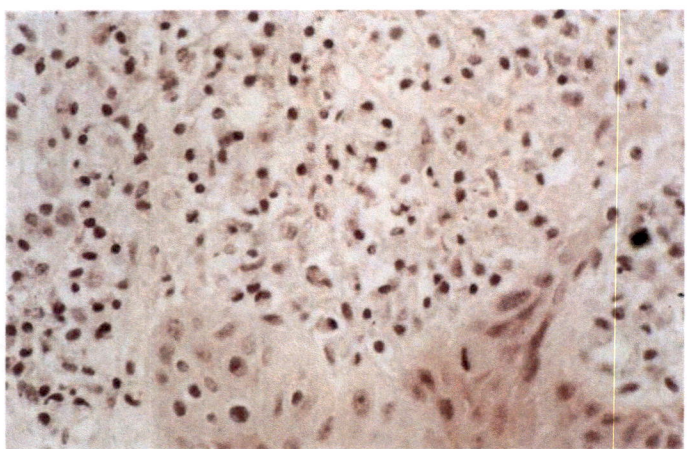

Figure 11.7 Lepromatous leprosy involving the supraglottic mucosa. Beneath the epithelium (above) there is an inflammatory infiltrate composed of foamy histiocytes and lymphocytes.   H & E (C)

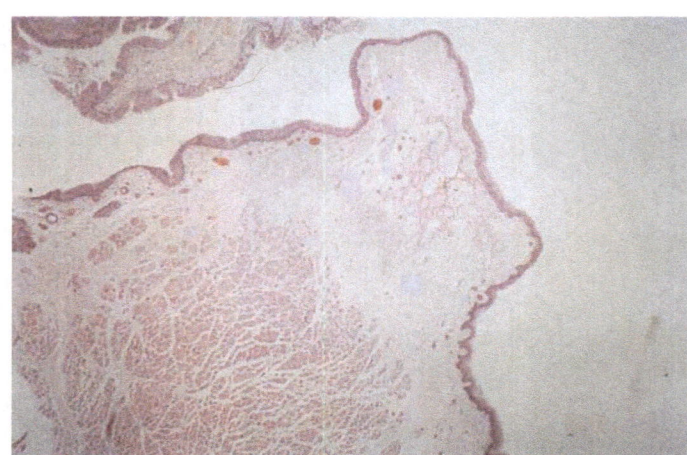

Figure 11.8 Section of vocal cord showing widening of Reinke's space by fibrin constituting a small vocal cord nodule.   H & E (A)

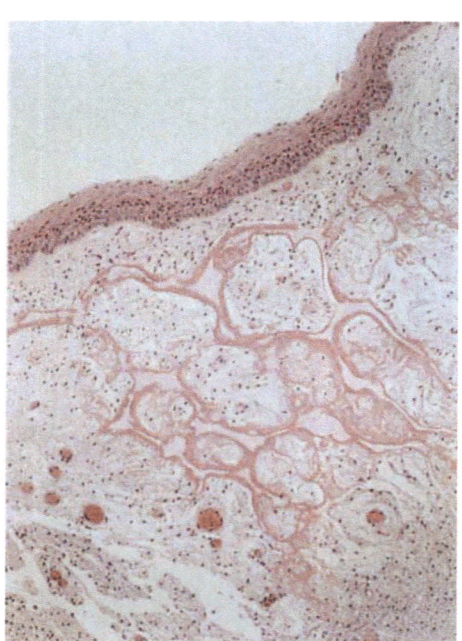

Figure 11.9 Higher power of fibrin exudate in Reinke's space from Figure 11.8. Note slight hyalinization of basement membrane. H & E (B)

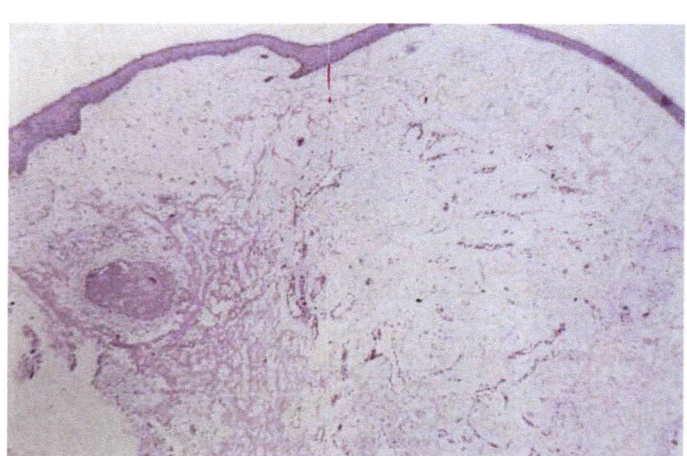

Figure 11.10 Thrombosed thin-walled blood vessel in vocal cord nodule. Note abundant fibrin and blood vessels in Reinke's space. H & E (A)

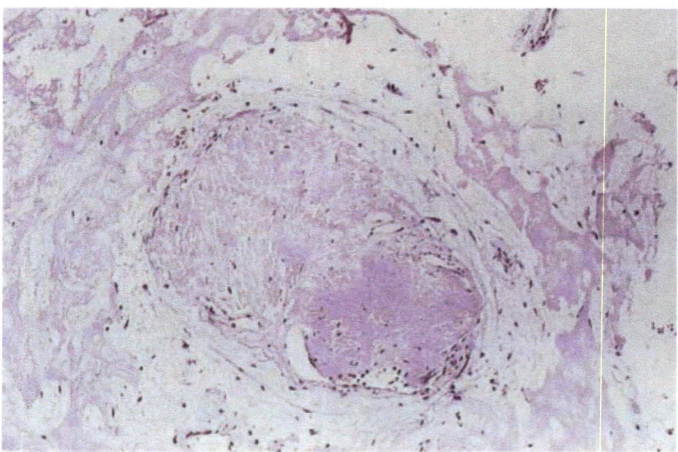

Figure 11.11 Higher power of thrombosed blood vessel in vocal cord nodule showing fibrin in blood vessel and surrounding it.   H & E (B)

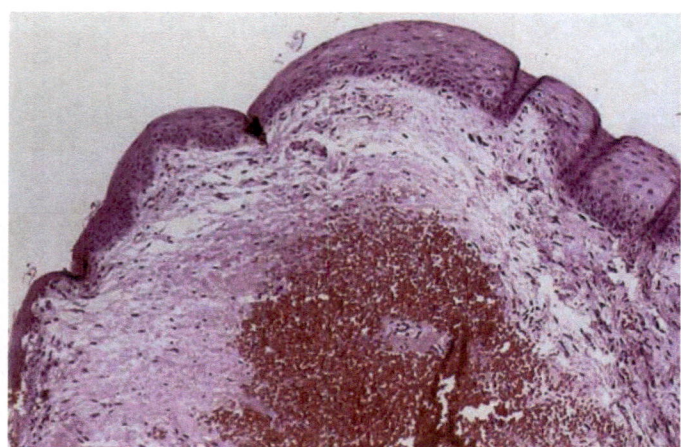

Figure 11.12 There is a large amount of fresh blood in this vocal cord polyp.   H & E (A)

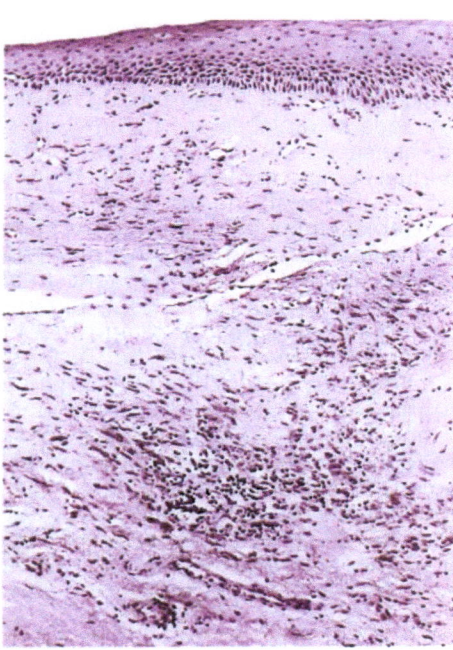

Figure 11.13 Fibrosis in vocal cord nodule. Note also haemosiderin (brown coloured) granules in histiocytes remote from surface epithelium. H & E (A)

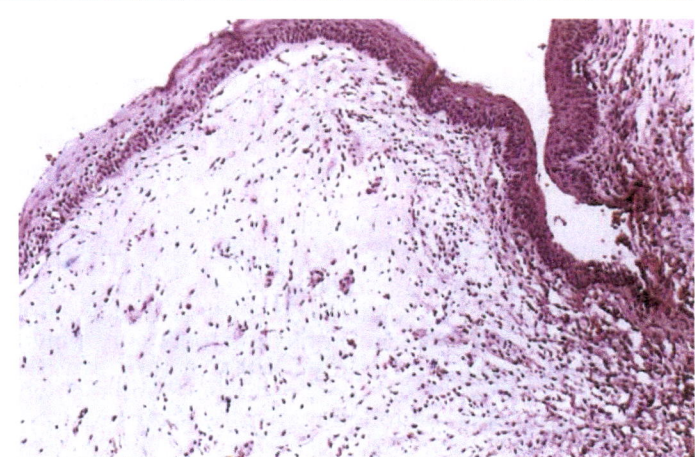

Figure 11.14 Myxoid appearance of connective tissue cells in laryngeal nodule. H & E (A)

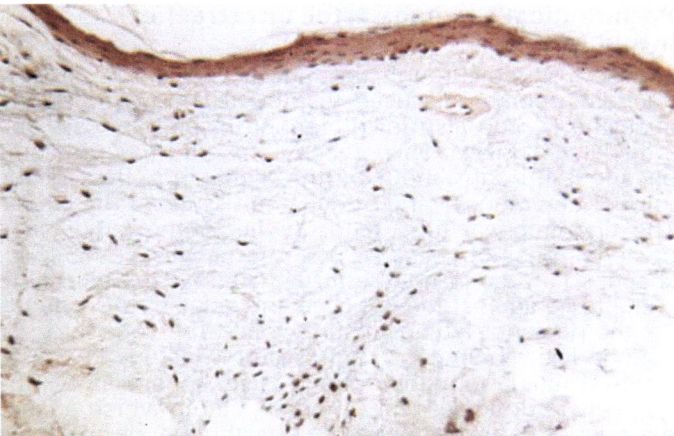

Figure 11.15 Reinke's oedema in a case of myxoedema. There is fibrin exudation and myxoid cells with a similar appearance to that of other types of vocal cord nodular change. H & E (B)

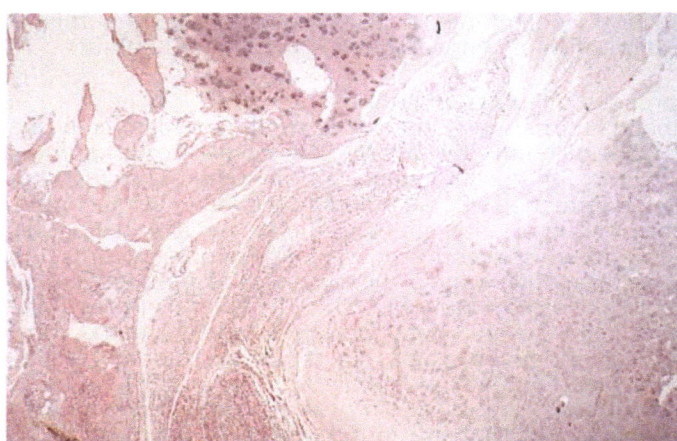

Figure 11.16 Cricoarytenoid joint in rheumatoid arthritis. The joint space is filled by fibrous tissue and there is erosion of the underlying cartilage. H & E (A)

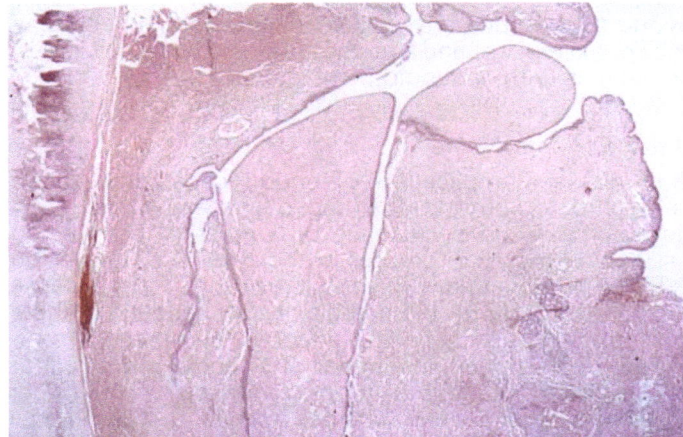

Figure 11.17 Amyloid deposit of false cord of larynx showing paucity of seromucinous glands. H & E (A)

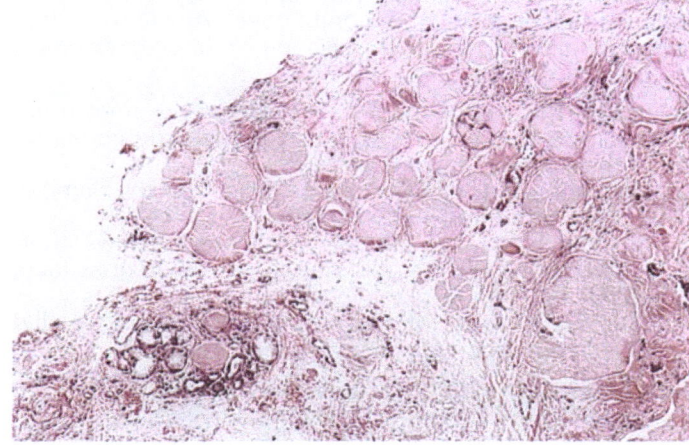

Figure 11.18 Amyloid deposit of false cord of larynx. Note numerous large round masses of amyloid and origin of two such 'balls' from seromucinous glands in lower right-hand corner. H & E (A)

Only a small number of Reinke's space exudative lesions show squamous epithelial changes. Within this category, one or more of the following may be present:

1. Hyaline thickening of the basement membrane (Figure 11.9);
2. Mild dysplasia of the epithelium;
3. Keratosis, rarely severe, of the epithelial surface.

Clearly, these changes are in reaction to the florid alterations taking place immediately below the epithelium and they rarely pose diagnostic problems. Vocal cord polyp and Reinke's oedema are so frequent that they may be found associated with vocal cord carcinoma, and the two conditions may even be found within the same biopsy.

Treatment
Exudative lesions of Reinke's space do not usually clear up by themselves and the treatment advised is endoscopic removal of the swollen mucosa with involved Reinke's space, following which the epithelium grows over and excellent healing usually takes place.

Arthritis of laryngeal joints
By far the commonest disease process producing inflammation of the laryngeal joints is rheumatoid arthritis.

Laryngeal rheumatoid arthritis
Rheumatoid arthritis may show itself in the larynx in one or both of two ways: by the development of an arthritis affecting the cricoarytenoid and cricothyroid joints; and by the formation of a granuloma – the rheumatoid nodule. Rheumatoid arthritis affecting the laryngeal joints passes through two successive phases of development: an acute phase of synovitis and a chronic phase of joint destruction and ankylosis (Figure 11.16). The latter is more dangerous, for the ankylosed laryngeal joints leave the vocal cords in adduction which may produce stridor and respiratory obstruction. Rheumatoid nodules may be found in the larynx in the subhyoid area (possibly in relation to the bursa occasionally found there) or the postcricoid region which is subject to recurrent trauma from deglutition[4] and may coexist with arthritis of the laryngeal joints.

Amyloid Deposits
Amyloidosis, whether primary or secondary, usually involves more than one internal organ. Solitary lesions of amyloid deposition giving rise to symptoms and signs also occur in, for example, the upper respiratory tract, urinary bladder, skin and conjunctiva. Amyloid of the upper respiratory tract shows the following characteristics[5]:

1. It may occur anywhere in the respiratory tract from the nose to the bronchi, but is particularly common in the false cord of the larynx.
2. Deposition of amyloid takes place in the lamina propria of the respiratory tract mucosa.
3. In most cases, the disease does not advance after initial diagnosis; in a few, slow progression does take place.
4. Surgical excision of the amyloid deposit is usually effective in treating the symptoms produced by it.

Localized amyloid of the upper respiratory tract has the same staining properties as systemic amyloid, appearing in haematoxylin and eosin-stained sections as pink, almost acellular, material, prominently infiltrating the lamina propria of the tissue, but always leaving intact the covering epithelium. In most biopsies, a striking feature is the disappearance of seromucinous glands in many areas – structures which normally constitute a large part of the tissues from which all the biopsies are derived – and their replacement by amyloid (Figure 11.17). The amyloid is deposited as thin flecks and also as large rounded masses of variable size. All stages of replacement by amyloid of seromucinous glands are seen in this process, from partial involvement of individual acini to the loss of entire glands, the final result being a number of uniform regular 'balls' of amyloid or a diffuse replacement of tissue (Figure 11.18 and 11.19). Perivascular deposit and foreign-body-type giant cell reaction to the amyloid are also frequent. In all cases, the amyloid stains positively with Congo red and gives a greenish birefringence (Figures 11.20 and 11.21). Laryngeal amyloid deposits tend to retain their Congo-red positivity after treatment by potassium permanganate solution, suggesting that they are composed of immunoglobulin amyloid. Trabeculae of woven bone are sometimes found in the amyloid material. A cartilage-like appearance is assumed by the amyloid in a few places (Figure 11.22). Irregular partly-ossified cartilaginous outgrowths derived from the tracheal rings are sometimes present, resembling tracheopathia osteoplastica[6]. (There is normally no evidence of amyloid in the latter condition – see Chapter 10.)

Pathological Changes after Intratracheal Intubation
A tube inserted through the mouth and larynx into the trachea is commonly used to provide an airway during anaesthesia, and also for prolonged respiratory care and artificial ventilation. This procedure is not free from complications brought about by the damaging effect of the tube on the mucosa and underlying tissues of the larynx. The endotracheal tube tends to lie in the larynx in a posterior position because the glottis has a triangular shape, so a tube inserted into the larynx is more likely to come to lie against the flat base and sides of the triangle, i.e. the posterior laryngeal surface and the vocal process region. The tendency of the posterior laryngeal wall to make contact with the tube is also enhanced by the normally lordotic cervical vertebral column which pushes the cricoid cartilage forward[7]. It is thus to be expected that pathological changes following prolonged intubation will be found principally in the posterolateral part of the larynx.

There are two groups of patients in whom intubation is especially frequently required, and so in whom the deleterious results of intubation represent a major problem: adults undergoing anaesthesia and resuscitation and neonates with respiratory distress. The pathological changes in the two groups are similar: inflammatory changes in the cricoid mucosa and over the arytenoid vocal processes, sometimes with arytenoid cartilage necrosis[8].

Intubation granuloma
An unusual complication of endotracheal anaesthesia is a chronic form of the above processes, the slow development and persistence of a mass of granulation tissue over the vocal process of the arytenoid. The lesion is found predominantly in adult females, perhaps because the smaller size of the female larynx renders it more susceptible to the damaging effect of the tube.

The gross appearance is that of a reddish spherical or oval swelling situated at the posterior end of the upper surface of a vocal cord. Microscopically, the granuloma has a round outline. The surface is usually covered by a layer of fibrin. The main component of the lesion is a network of capillary blood vessels, between which are plasma cells, lymphocytes, fibroblasts, neutrophils and eosinophils (Figures 11.23 and 11.24). At the base, the origin of this tissue from the underlying lamina propria can be identified.

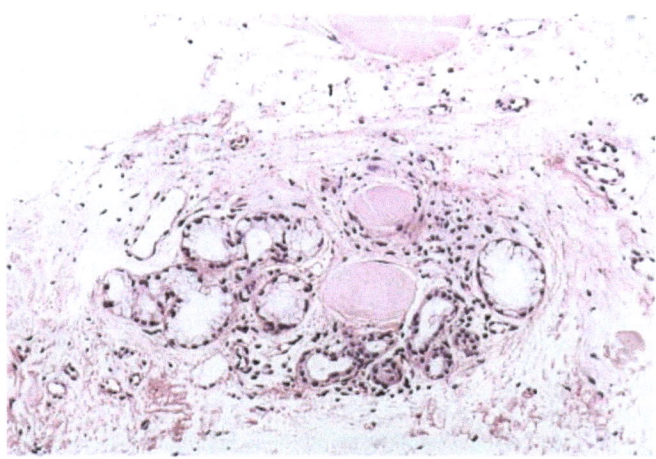

Figure 11.19 Higher power view of seromucinous glands from Figure 11.18 showing origin of amyloid. H & E (B)

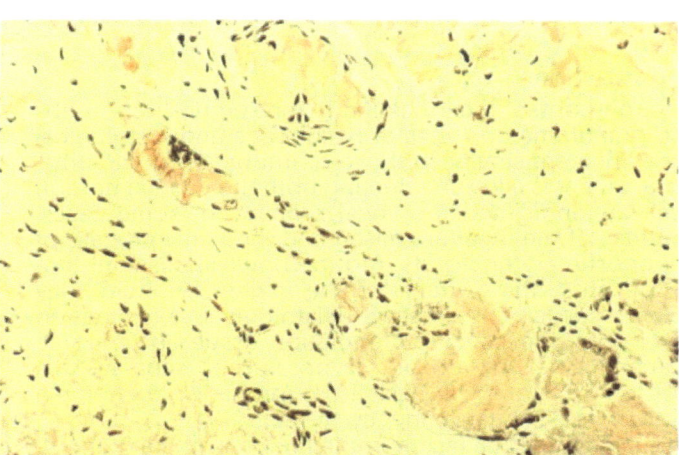

Figure 11.20 Amyloid deposit of false cord of larynx stained by Congo red. (B)

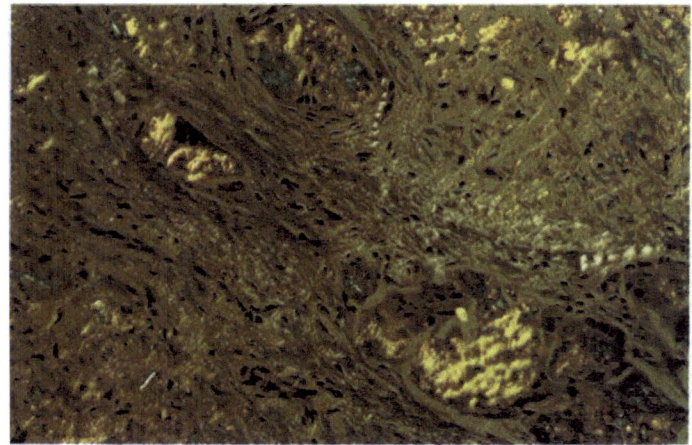

Figure 11.21 Same field of same Congo-red section as that depicted in Figure 11.20, viewed through crossed polaroids. The amyloid shows a greenish birefringence. (B)

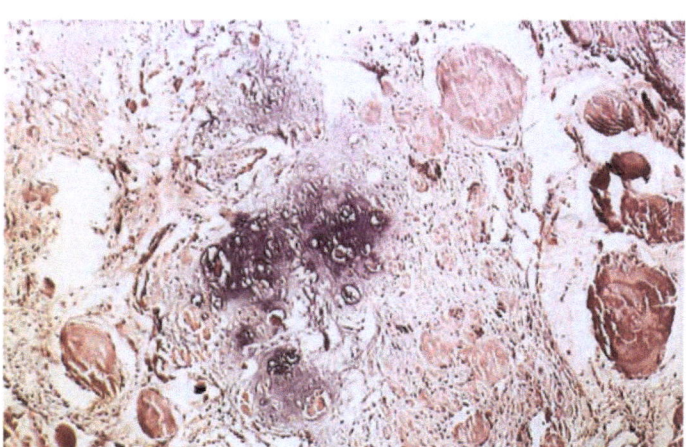

Figure 11.22 Metaplastic cartilage deposit in amyloid of trachea which is in the form of 'balls'. H & E (B)

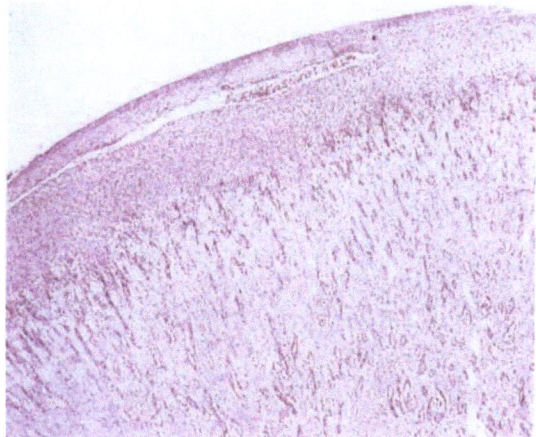

Figure 11.23 Intubation granuloma of arytenoid region of vocal cord. Note fibrin cap beneath which is inflammatory granulation tissue. There is surface ulceration. H & E (A)

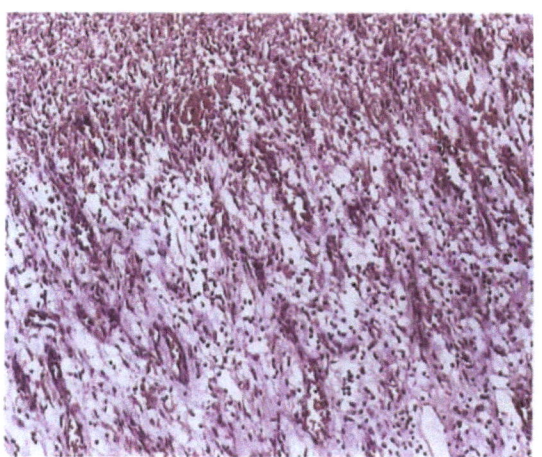

Figure 11.24 Higher power of intubation granuloma showing fibrin and inflammatory granulation tissue. H & E (C)

Contact Ulcer

Although contact ulcer has a different origin from intubation granuloma, the sites of occurrence and histological appearance are similar to those of intubation granuloma. Contact ulcer is a lesion affecting both the vertical portion of the arytenoid and the vocal process. In some cases, the edges of the ulcer are raised and the vocal process of the opposite arytenoid fits into the bowl-like lesion. In a few patients, the surface of the other arytenoid may become similarly ulcerated. Histological examination shows only non-specific granulation tissue and chronic inflammatory exudate. It is not possible to separate this lesion on a histological basis from intubation granuloma and there is a similar tendency to recur.

In a patient with a lesion in the region of the arytenoid, showing the histological features of pyogenic granuloma but without a history of intubation, possible causes of, or conditions related to, excess acidity and acid reflux, such as hiatus hernia, should be sought. It is possible that aspiration of excess acid onto the vocal cord surface during sleep may produce the lesion. Antacid treatment may lead to cure of the laryngeal condition[9].

References

1. Brenneman, J., Clifton, W. M., Frank, A. and Holinger, P. H. (1938). Acute laryngotracheobronchitis. *Am. J. Dis. Child.*, **55**, 667–695
2. Bull, T. R. (1966). Tuberculosis of the larynx. *Br. Med. J.*, **2**, 991–992
3. Kleinsasser, O. (1979). *Microlaryngoscopy and Endolaryngeal Microsurgery. Technique and Typical Findings*, 2nd Edn. (Baltimore: University Park Press)
4. Bridger, M. W. M., Jahn, A. F. and van Nostrand, A. W. P. (1980). Laryngeal rheumatoid arthritis. *Laryngoscope*, **90**, 296–303
5. Michaels, L. and Hyams, V. J. (1979). Amyloid in localised deposits and plasmacytomas of the respiratory tract. *J. Pathol.*, **128**, 29–38
6. Ashley, D. J. B. (1970). Bony metaplasia in trachea and bronchi. *J. Pathol.*, **102**, 186–188
7. Bergstrom, J., Moberg, A. and Drell, S. R. (1962). On the pathogenesis of laryngeal injuries following prolonged intubation. *Acta Otolaryngol. (Stockholm)*, **55**, 342–346
8. Michaels, L. (1987). *Ear, Nose and Throat Histopathology.* (London: Springer Verlag)
9. Miko, T. L. (1989). Peptic (contact ulcer) granuloma of the larynx. *J. Clin. Pathol.*, **42**, 800–804

Squamous Cell Neoplasms of the Larynx

12

Squamous Cell Papilloma

Squamous cell papillomas are frequent in the larynx of adults. They also present in children where, because of the much narrower diameter of the airway, the symptoms are more serious and treatment is more urgent and difficult. The pathological changes are, however, similar at all ages. By far the commonest site of occurrence of squamous papilloma of the larynx is the vocal cord and the anterior half of the cord is more frequently affected than the posterior.

Gross appearances

Squamous papillomas are delicate white, pink or red granular polypoid structures which vary from 1 to 10 mm in diameter, most being less than 5 mm. In florid cases which require laryngectomy, the papillomas form a solid field of mucosal thickening without invasion deep to mucosa (Figure 12.1). Under magnification, small individual papillae can be discerned as blunt finger-like processes with branches which never become long and filiform.

Microscopic appearances

The papillary processes arise from the epithelium of the larynx as cylindrical projections. Smaller cylindrical offshoots of squamous-cell-covered epithelium are usually present in the vicinity of the larger papillae and are cut in various planes. These represent second- or even third-order branching of the papillary structures (Figures 12.2 and 12.3). The numbers of layers of squamous epithelial cells lining the papilloma are related to the order of branching that the papilla represents. First-order papillae show up to 15 layers of squamous epithelium; third-order ones show only five or six.

In many papillomas, nuclei are retained up to the keratinized surface, but, in a minority of cases, there is keratosis in which several layers of completely keratinized anucleate cells are seen on the surface of the papillae (Figure 12.4). If keratosis is extensive in a papillary lesion, a careful histological study should be made to exclude squamous carcinoma, particularly that of the verrucous variety. In papillomas, the rete ridges of the squamous cell epithelium are always short and regular, unlike those in verrucous squamous carcinoma (see below).

The basal two or three layers of squamous papillomas are composed of small cells which are quite distinct from the more superficial 'prickle' cells. The basal cells lie loosely on a well-defined basement membrane which usually shows hyalinization (Figure 12.5). Sometimes cells of the squamous epithelial covering of the papillae show dysplastic changes, a situation which is usually related to the presence of koilocytosis (see below). The dysplastic changes are always slight or moderate in degree, and, in none of them, is there ever sufficient dysplasia to be considered as carcinoma in situ. Papillomas with dysplasia do not exhibit a tendency to recurrence or to develop malignant change (see below).

Koilocytosis is very frequently seen in the upper inter-mediate and superficial part of the squamous epithelium of squamous papillomas of the larynx (Figure 12.6). It consists of a spherical enlargement of the cells of the lesion, accompanied by perinuclear vacuolation, so that no stained cytoplasm is seen in the cell or, if it is, it is present as a thin rim around the cell periphery. The nucleus is central and often enlarged, angular or wrinkled. It may exhibit moderate degrees of dysplasia. Since infection of the cells of squamous papillomas of the larynx by human papillomavirus is very frequent, perhaps invariable (see below), it is not surprising that koilocytosis is so commonly seen in papillomas.

In a few cases of papillomatosis, some of the material shows a papillary process, not only of squamous cell epithelium, but also of respiratory epithelium. The latter comprises non-malignant respiratory epithelium featuring both ciliated cells and goblet cells. Areas of 'stratification' of this respiratory columnar epithelium are seen where cells are heaped up (Figure 12.7). Papillomas showing respiratory epithelial hyperplasia have a decided tendency to recur. The appearances of the columnar cell papillomas in papillomatosis of the larynx are similar to those of cylindric cell papilloma of the nose and paranasal sinuses (see Chapter 6).

Differential diagnosis

Difficulty may be experienced in distinguishing two other types of neoplastic lesion, which occur particularly often on the vocal cords, from squamous papilloma: keratotic plaque with dysplasia; and carcinoma of both verrucous squamous and usual types.

1. Keratotic plaque with dysplasia. Raised plaques composed of thickened squamous epithelium with keratinized surface are seen quite frequently in biopsy. They usually show a mild to severe degree of dysplasia of the deeper layers of their squamous cells. It is important to separate these lesions from squamous papillomas because they have a malignant potential which is not possessed by the latter. A careful examination of the whole biopsy for evidence of cylinders of papilloma formation and the branching that is associated with them will usually suffice to distinguish this lesion.

2. Carcinoma of both verrucous squamous and usual types. Squamous carcinoma may exhibit true papilloma formation and be mistaken for benign squamous papilloma (Figure 12.8). The pattern is not, however, as symmetrical as in papillomas and second- or third-degree branching is not seen. Verrucous squamous carcinoma often displays very long unbranched papillae composed largely of keratin (see below). The rete ridges are irregular and the basement membrane is not hyalinized in the same fashion. The latter is frequently seen in papillomas. Squamous cells of the intermediate layer in verrucous carcinomas are larger than those of the corresponding layer in squamous papillomas, showing a mean area of more than $300 \, \mu m^2$ (see below).

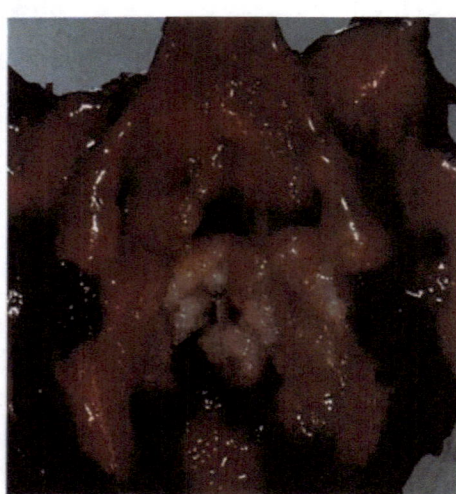

Figure 12.1 Squamous papillomas filling larynx of teen-age girl. A laryngectomy was required, since all other treatments had failed

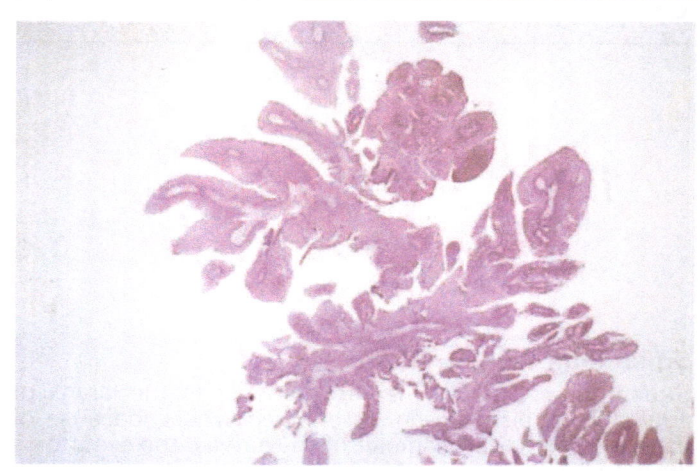

Figure 12.2 Squamous papilloma of larynx showing branching exophytic processes. H & E (A)

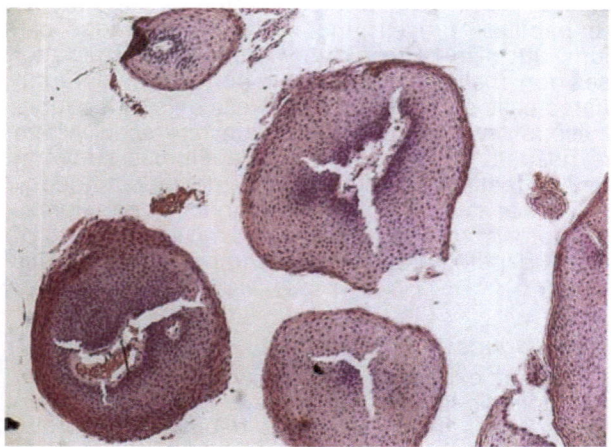

Figure 12.3 Juvenile papilloma of larynx showing thin cores of vascular connective tissue covered by stratified squamous epithelium. H & E (B)

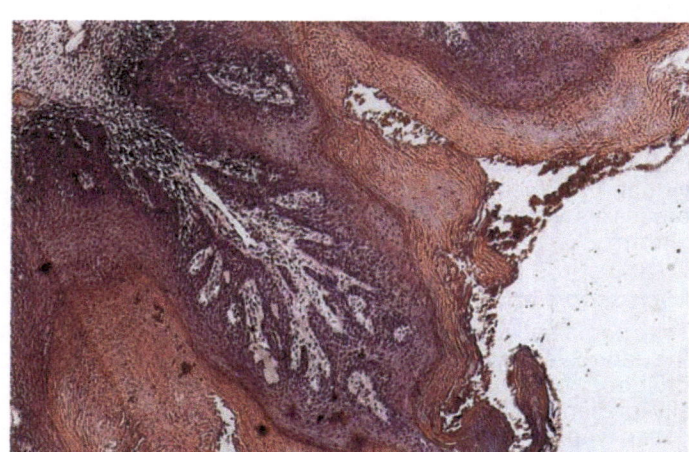

Figure 12.4 Keratotic squamous papilloma of voca cord showing papillary processes embedded in acellular keratin. H & E (B)

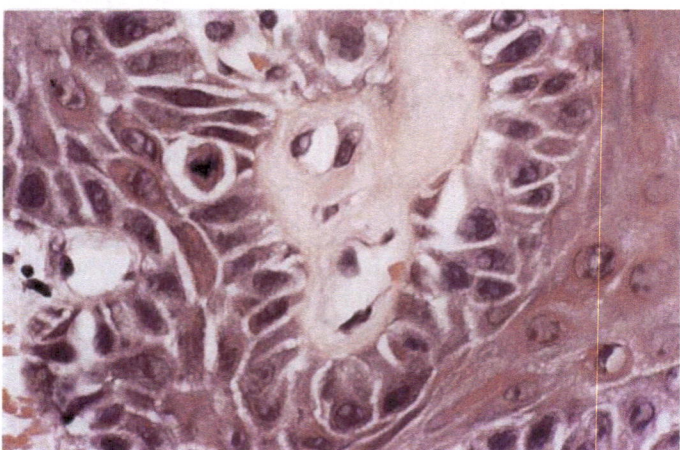

Figure 12.5 Basal cells and basement membranes of squamous papilloma of larynx showing hyalinization below epithelium. H & E (C)

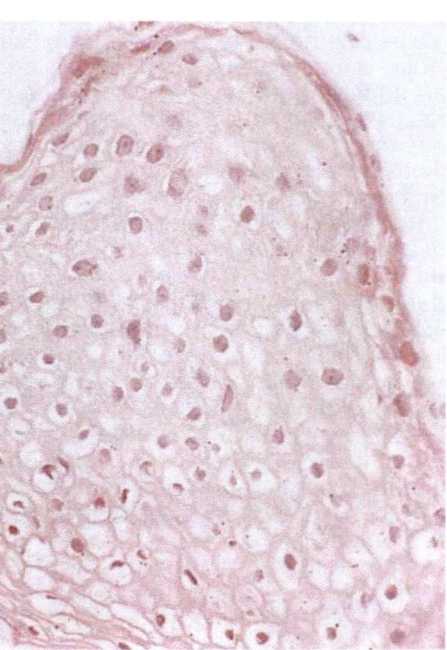

Figure 12.6 Koilocytosis of squamous epithelium on surface of squamous papilloma. H & E (C)

Natural history

Juvenile papilloma

Squamous papillomas arising in childhood have been regarded as distinct from the adult form because of their greater tendency to be multiple. Moreover, they affect both sexes equally, unlike those occurring in adults which have a male preponderance. They may arise at any age in childhood and have been described as early as 18 months.

Malignant alteration of juvenile papillomatosis has been described. Several cases are on record in which malignancy took place many years after treatment of juvenile papillomatosis by radiotherapy and there are even fewer on record who did not have irradiation therapy at any time[1].

Adult papilloma

In a large series of squamous papillomas in adults described from the Royal National Throat, Nose and Ear Hospital in London[2], 12 cases started as juvenile papillomas and continued into adult life. The maximum incidence of onset was in the fourth decade. Twice as many males as females were in the series. In none of the patients in this series did malignancy develop, although there were many recurrences, in some patients over a period of many years.

Relationship to human papillomavirus

Human papillomavirus (HPV) has been suspected as the causative agent of squamous papilloma of the larynx for many years. The localization of papillomavirus antigen using the immunoperoxidase method in paraffin sections of squamous papillomas has recently yielded encouraging results in support of this concept. The nuclei positive for this antigen are situated in the squamous cells of the papillomas, near the surface in each case. The technique of in situ DNA hybridization has also been used to detect the HPV genome in laryngeal papillomas with similar localization (Figure 12.9).

In both adults and children, HPV types 6 and 11 are usually present in squamous papillomas. The extent of virus deposition seems to be related to its tendency to recur[3].

Squamous Cell Carcinoma

Since the larynx is the commonest site for development of squamous cell carcinoma in the ear, nose and throat, this neoplasm will be discussed in detail here; the pathology of squamous carcinoma is similar in most other sites.

Surface origin

Squamous carcinomas in the larynx develop, not only from the epithelium of the vocal cord which is lined normally by squamous epithelium, but also from other areas of epithelium which are normally lined by respiratory epithelium (Figure 12.10). Even in large squamous carcinomas of the larynx, histological features are present by which the sites of surface origin of the growth may be detected. These features are: the presence of hyperplasia, carcinoma in situ or dysplasia of adjacent squamous epithelium (Figure 12.11); and the presence of a smooth covering of epithelium from the deep surface of which tongues of carcinoma are emanating. This epithelial surface is usually dysplastic itself (Figure 12.12); it may be keratinized or non-keratinized.

Although the growth of the cancer is at first in the form of a broad band emanating from the field of origin, at certain points, tongues of tumour appear to grow more rapidly and penetrate more deeply than the main tumour mass. This may occur anywhere in the field of tumour, and invasion will take place into anatomical structures – muscle, cartilage, ligaments, etc. – that are contiguous

with the tumour. Certain regions of the larynx, such as the connective tissue adjacent to the saccule or the anterior commissure, seem to be particularly favourable to the spread of squamous carcinoma, and tumour is often seen infiltrating these regions where it sends out malignant tongues away from the main field.

Precancerous states

A severe degree of dysplasia and carcinoma in situ are the precancerous states, which can be recognized by microscopic examination of the laryngeal epithelium.

Dysplasia (Figures 12.13 to 12.19)

Dysplasia of squamous epithelium is the presence of cells which have features of malignancy. A detailed analysis of such cells shows them to have many or all of the following characteristics: nuclear hyperchromatism, prominent nucleoli, increase in nuclear–cytoplasmic ratio, very large and very small nuclei, irregularity in nuclear membranes, increased numbers of mitoses, the presence of mitoses in the upper epidermal layers (i.e. away from the basal layer), and the presence of abnormal mitotic figures. Taking the squamous epithelium as a whole, dysplastic epithelium shows the following overall structural changes: hyperplasia of basal cells with disturbance of the normal maturational sequence; and, at a later stage, the presence of 'drop-shaped rete processes'. The rete processes normally taper progressively or else form structures with almost parallel sides and blunt ends. Rete processes which are wider at their deeper part than superficially are described as 'drop-shaped' and occur frequently in dysplastic epithelia.

It has become customary for dysplasia to be classified by degrees, as in the grades of uterine 'cervical intraepithelial *neoplasia*' (CIN). 'Neoplasia' is not a satisfactory designation for the lower grades of atypical change in the larynx, and 'laryngeal dysplasia' (LD) grades I, II and III would seem more appropriate to describe the severity of the precancerous change. Grade I shows a minor degree of atypical change confined to the basal third of the squamous epithelium. LD grade III embraces carcinoma in situ and is a rather better designation because not all cases go on to invasive carcinoma. It also embraces severe dysplasia, with and without surface keratosis, in which the atypical change involves at least two thirds of the epithelium. Grade II lies within the spectrum between grades I and III and shows involvement of one third to two thirds of the basal portion of the epithelium by the dysplastic change. Biopsies of laryngeal stratified squamous epithelium, taken after irradiation, frequently show severe degrees of dysplasia (Figure 12.20). The interpretation of such areas is less serious than is the case for unirradiated lesions. Extension of severe dysplasia along the ducts of seromucinous glands has no more significance than the presence of the dysplasia itself on the surface (Figure 12.21).

Invasive squamous cell carcinoma

Gross appearances

The commonest site for squamous carcinoma of the larynx is at the anterior part of the true cord but it may be seen anywhere in the larynx. It is least frequent in a posterior situation. Whatever its size and situation, by far the most usual gross appearance is that of a flat plaque with a well-defined somewhat-raised edge and a surface which ranges from occasional furrows to marked corrugation. Cut surface reveals this structure to consist of a pale-grey band of variable thickness. In a small proportion of cases, the tumours may show one or more papillary elements. These are most common in the glottic and subglottic regions, but are occasionally found in the supraglottic

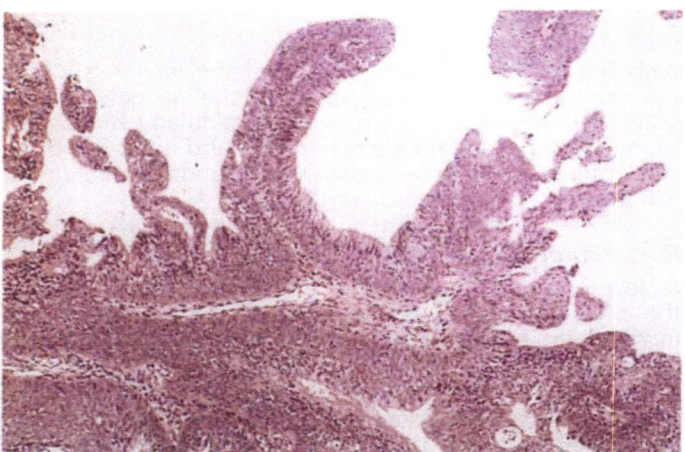

Figure 12.7 Papillomas of larynx lined by respiratory epithelium. H & E (B)

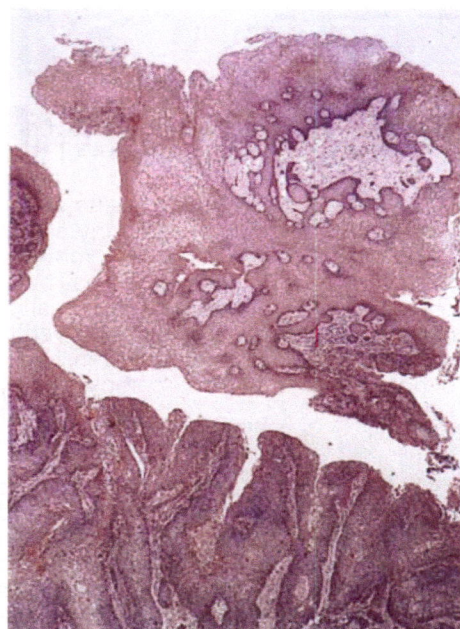

Figure 12.8 Benign appearing papillary outgrowth on surface of squamous carcinoma of larynx. H & E (B)

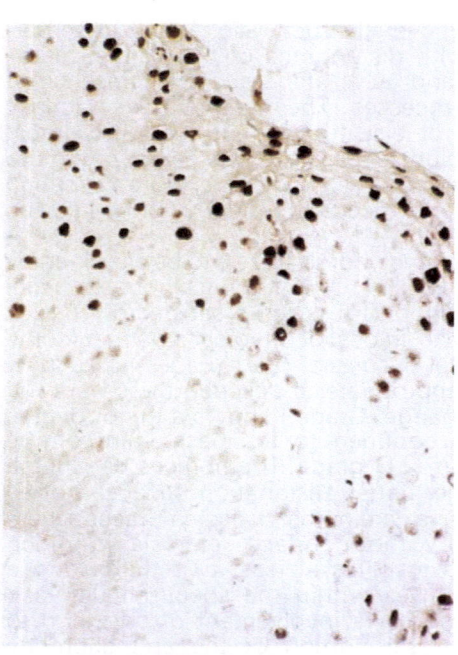

Figure 12.9 Localization of HPV type 6 in squamous papilloma of larynx. Virus is located in nuclei near surface of squamous epithelium. In situ hybridization (B)

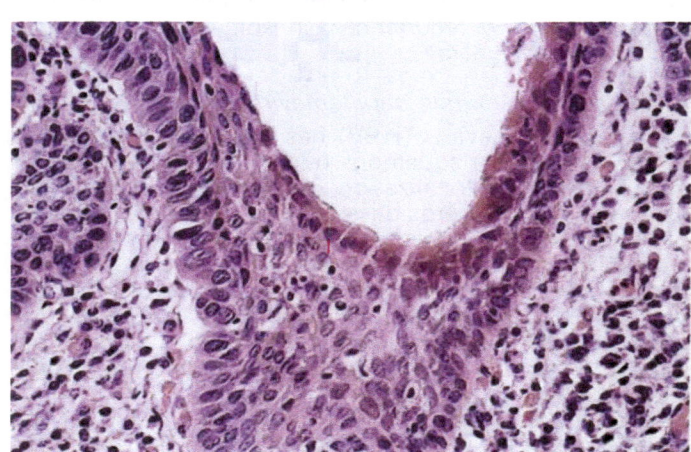

Figure 12.10 Origin of squamous carcinoma from respiratory epithelium. H & E (B)

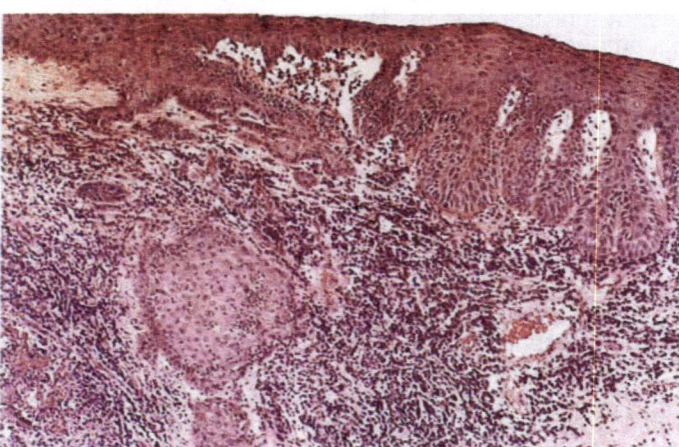

Figure 12.11 Dysplastic squamous epithelium at edge of invading squamous carcinoma. H & E (B)

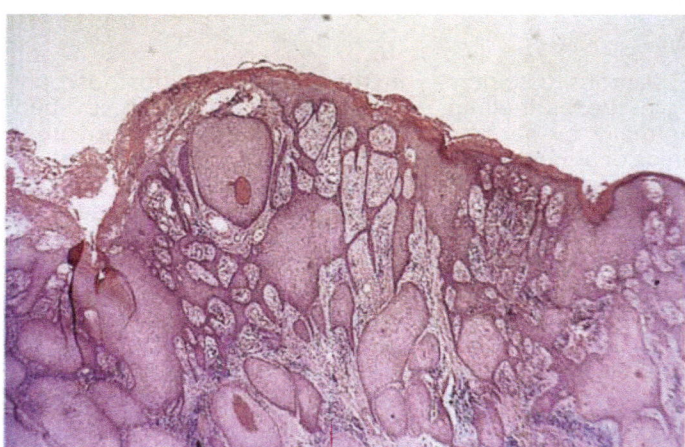

Figure 12.12 Origin of invading squamous carcinoma from surface epithelium. H & E (A)

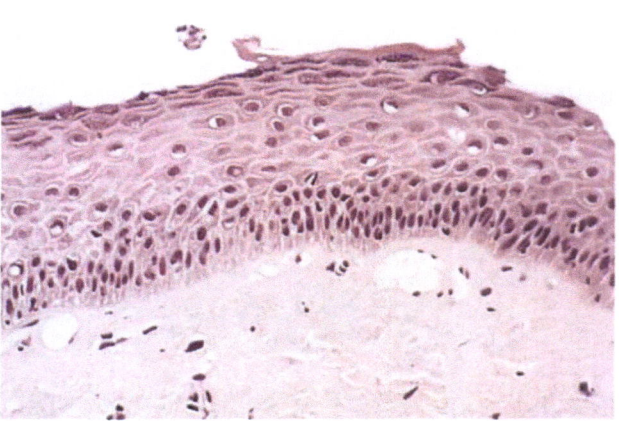

Figure 12.13 Laryngeal dysplasia grade II. H & E (B)

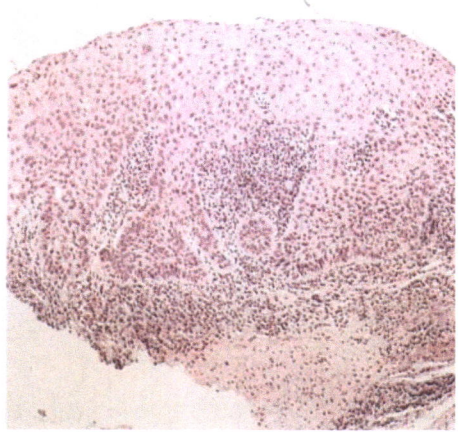

Figure 12.14 Laryngeal dysplasia grade III. H & E (B)

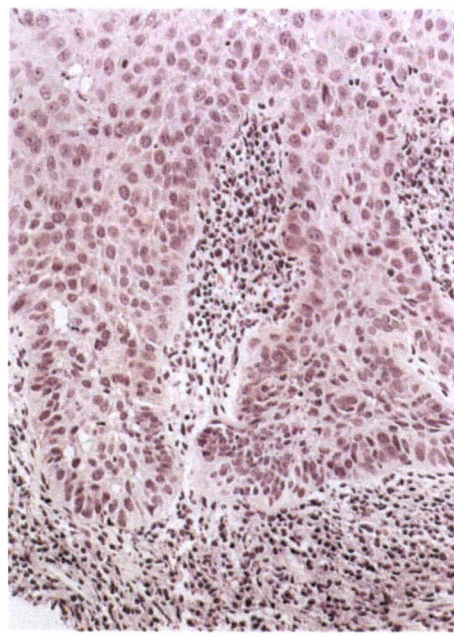

Figure 12.15 Laryngeal dysplasia grade III with 'drop-shaped' rete ridges and complete replacement of whole thickness of epithelium by dysplastic cells. H & E (B)

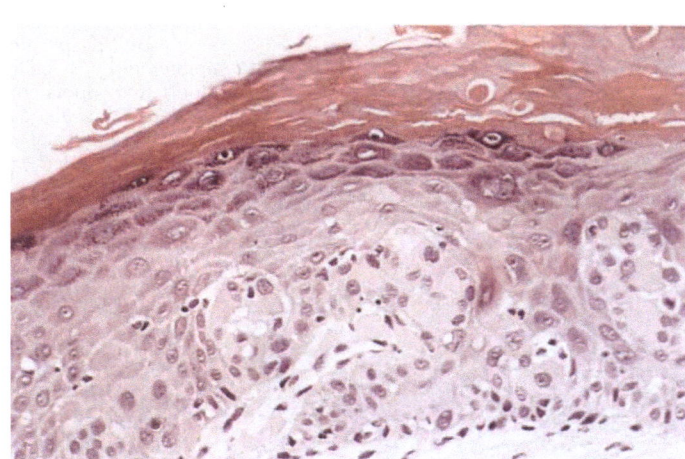

Figure 12.16 Laryngeal dysplasia grade III with prominent keratosis ('bowenoid' type). H & E (C)

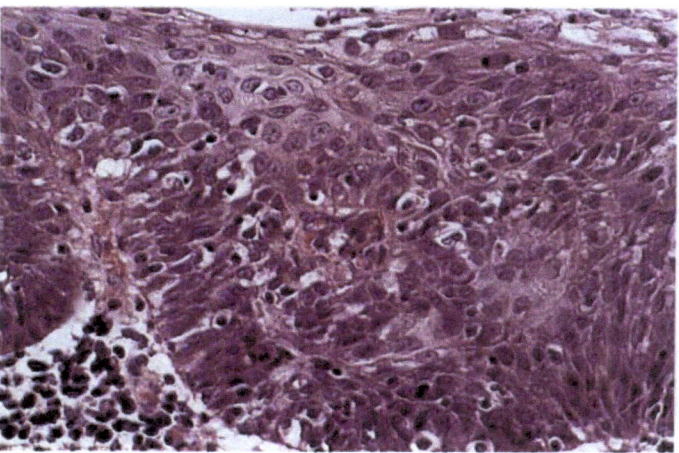

Figure 12.17 Laryngeal dysplasia grade III with replacement of whole thickness of epithelium by dysplastic cells ('pagetoid' type). H & E (C)

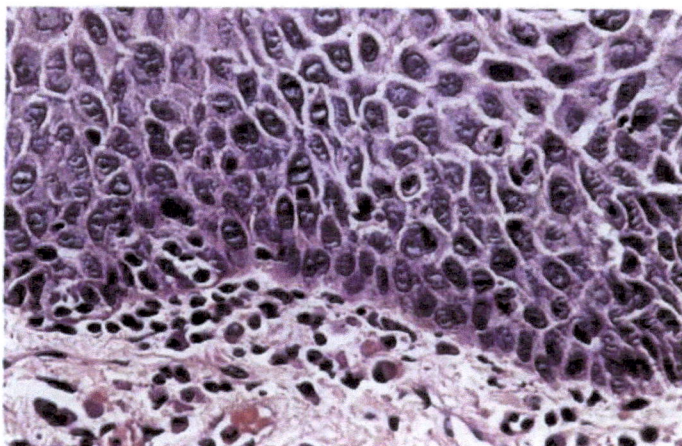

Figure 12.18 Laryngeal dysplasia grade III showing disturbance in polarity of basal layer. H & E (C)

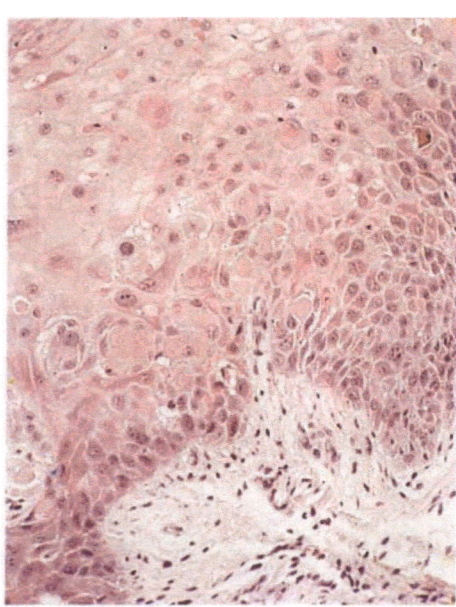

Figure 12.19 Laryngeal dysplasia grade III showing Civatte bodies. H & E (C)

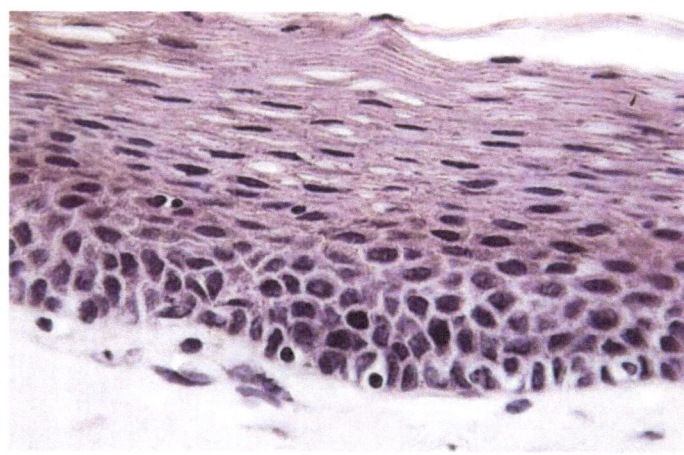

Figure 12.20 Squamous epithelium of vocal cord showing dysplasia after irradiation. H & E (C)

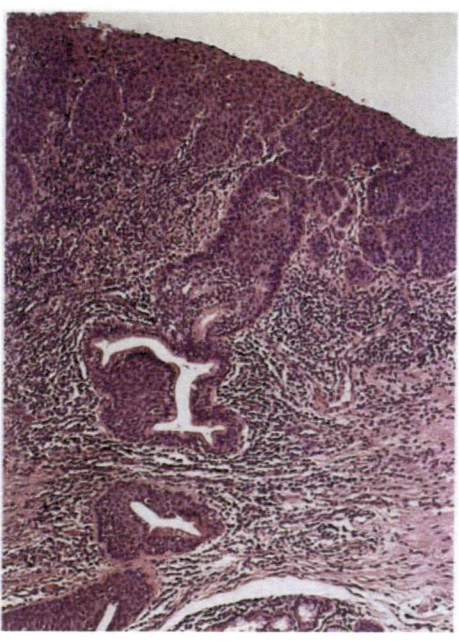

Figure 12.21 Extension of dysplastic epidermoid cells along the ducts of seromucinous glands in laryngeal dysplasia grade III. H & E (B)

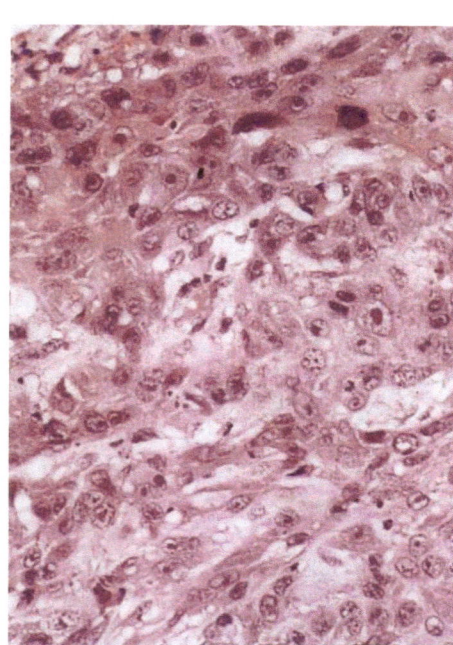

Figure 12.22 Squamous carcinoma of the larynx showing proliferated malpighian cells with no keratinization. H & E (B)

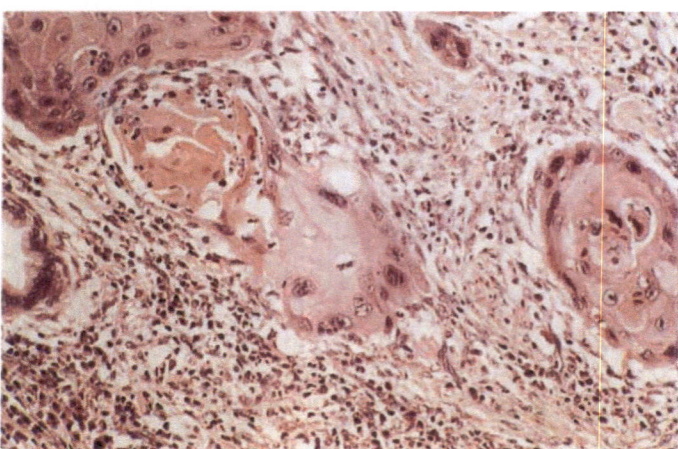

Figure 12.23 Keratinizing squamous cell carcinoma of the larynx. H & E (B)

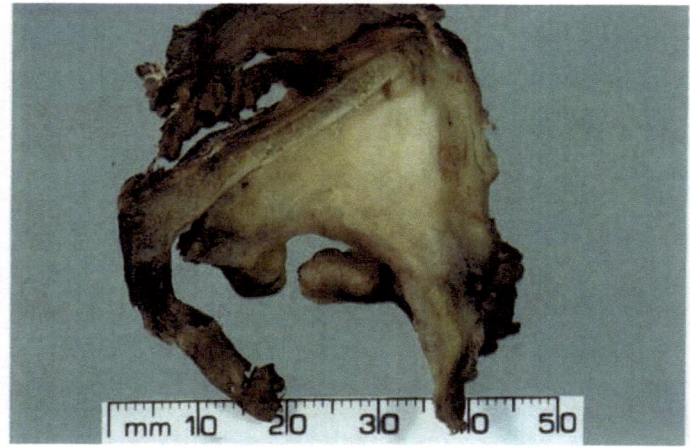

Figure 12.24 There is deep invasion of the pre-epiglottic space by carcinoma which has originated from the supraglottic epithelium. Note the pale-yellow bars of epiglottic cartilage

portion of a laryngeal neoplasm. When arising from the vocal cord, they may grow into the contralateral ventricle and, by occluding it, give rise to a mucocoele of the saccule on that side. Papillary areas of squamous cell carcinoma usually coexist with the flat type of neoplasm; they rarely exist as a single gross entity.

Microscopic appearances

The histological features of squamous carcinoma are extremely variable, and, in a particular neoplasm, result from the proportions of the different epidermoid components that are present. Like normal squamous cell epithelium, these include undifferentiated basal cells, intermediate 'prickle' cells, cells containing keratohyaline granules and acellular keratinous material. Glycogen is also found in varying amounts, sometimes large, within the epithelial cells of a squamous carcinoma. So squamous carcinoma of the larynx may display trabeculae formed largely of proliferated malignant basal cells, prominent groups of large pale cells with intercellular bridges ('prickles') (Figure 12.22), large areas of fully keratinized cells (Figure 12.23), often anucleate, or many cells vacuolated from the presence of cytoplasmic glycogen. Malignant basal type cells, sometimes including a few 'prickle' cells, in other instances composed of rows of single cell width, may give an irregular jagged margin to the tumour. Tumour edges composed of 'prickle' cells and keratinized cells tend to form large round masses, sometimes referred to as 'pushing' margins, suggesting that they invade by pressure rather than by cell infiltration. Some squamous carcinomas show a constant 'mix' of the squamous elements throughout the whole tumour. The majority, however, show considerable variation from one part of the neoplasm to another.

Assessment of the degree of differentiation is often carried out by pathologists to obtain an impression of the aggressiveness of the neoplasm. An overall impression of the degree of differentiation of the worst differentiated area is the method commonly used. This is of dubious validity because of its subjective nature and the variations in differentiation which may be frequently observed in different parts of the same neoplasm. The same considerations apply to the use of quantitative methods of assessing differentiation[4]. There is, however, some prognostic value in separating an extremely well-differentiated form – verrucous squamous carcinoma – although, even here, variations in structure across the tumour may lead to errors of diagnosis (see below).

Spread from laryngeal airway origin

The anatomical routes of invasion of squamous carcinoma arising from the epithelium of the laryngeal airway depend on the site of origin of the neoplasm within the larynx and can be studied in transverse slices of laryngectomy specimens. The tumour usually invades outwards at right angles to the surface of origin. In some places, the spread of the carcinoma is favoured in a different plane, e.g. adjacent to the saccule.

Supraglottic: In the supraglottis, tumours which arise from the laryngeal surface of the epiglottis invade towards and then through the epiglottic cartilage. The perforating seromucinous glands of that cartilage often provide pathways for its penetration, but penetration of the elastic cartilage itself by the tumour is sometimes seen. Anterior to the fixed portion of the epiglottis, lies a zone of adipose connective tissue – the pre-epiglottic space – and entry of carcinoma therein is frequent after its passage through the epiglottic cartilage (Figure 12.24). In some cases, the full thickness of the pre-epiglottic space is traversed by the neoplasm as far as the anterior boundary, which is the hyoid bone; sometimes, even that structure may be entered.

Thus, the hyoid bone should be examined for tumour grossly and microscopically, at least whenever the pre-epiglottic space has been found to be deeply invaded by neoplasm.

Lower down the supraglottis and more laterally, the aryepiglottic fold epithelium may be the source of tumour, which may invade that thin fold from medial to lateral side to attain, and even invade, the mucosa of the piriform fossa (Figure 12.25). Tumours originating on the false cords and glottis may also reach this surface since the piriform fossa extends downwards from a level behind the upper supraglottis to the upper subglottis. In its path of invasion, lower supraglottic tumour first encounters the thyroarytenoid muscle. The thyroid cartilage laterally and the arytenoid cartilage posteriorly may then be invaded by tumour arising at this level. Sometimes, squamous carcinoma arises from the posterior supraglottic epithelium. Invasion then is into the apical portion of the arytenoid cartilage.

Glottic: The field of carcinoma that includes the glottic area often shows origin of carcinoma in the region of the anterior commissure. Here the neoplasm is separated from the angle of the thyroid cartilage by only a very small band of connective tissue (Figure 12.26); as a result, invasion of the thyroid cartilage in this region is very common. More posteriorly, neoplasm arising on the vocal cord passes into the thyroarytenoid muscle and then on to the thyroid cartilage. Invading posterolaterally, it can reach the piriform fossa and posteriorly the arytenoid cartilage.

Subglottic: That portion of the neoplasm that arises in the subglottic region, if anterior, will come against the cricothyroid membrane. This sometimes, but not always, is penetrated by subglottic carcinoma. Frequently, penetrating tumour arises from above, where it is derived from neoplasm which has entered the thyroid cartilage in the supraglottic and/or glottic region, and then spreads within that cartilage as far as its inferior end. It then enters the cricothyroid ligament and may grow out of the larynx easily from that situation. In other parts of the subglottis, tumour will tend to invade the local muscles and cartilages in which it finds itself; the cricoarytenoid joint and cricoid lamina are sometimes invaded by posteriorly located neoplasm. On rare occasions, the tumour will penetrate the lamina of the cricoid and reach the posterior cricoarytenoid muscle. The lateral cricoarytenoid muscle, on the other hand, is frequently invaded by subglottic neoplasm, and the lower thyroid lamina above and the cricoid ring below are potential cartilage targets for invasion by such tumours.

Hypopharyngeal carcinoma: Carcinoma of the hypopharynx, that part of the food passage that extends from the level of the hyoid bone above to that of the lower border of the cricoid cartilage below, is closely related to the larynx. Indeed, when carcinoma extends forward from the hypopharynx into the larynx, it is sometimes mistaken for a primary tumour of the larynx. Although it is commonly stated that hypopharyngeal carcinoma has three main sites of origin: piriform sinus, postcricoid area and posterior pharyngeal wall, a study of specimens of surgically excised larynges shows that, in the majority, more than one of these sites are involved and usually all three (Figure 12.27). The laryngeal cartilages are resistant to invasion by hypopharyngeal carcinoma. Invasion of the laryngeal airway may take place, however, and the development of secondary infection with abscess formation, which occurs not uncommonly with this neoplasm, may exacerbate the airway obstruction (Figure 12.28). The thyroid gland is in close proximity and, when invaded by hypopharyngeal carcinoma (Figure 12.29), significantly reduces the patient's outlook[5].

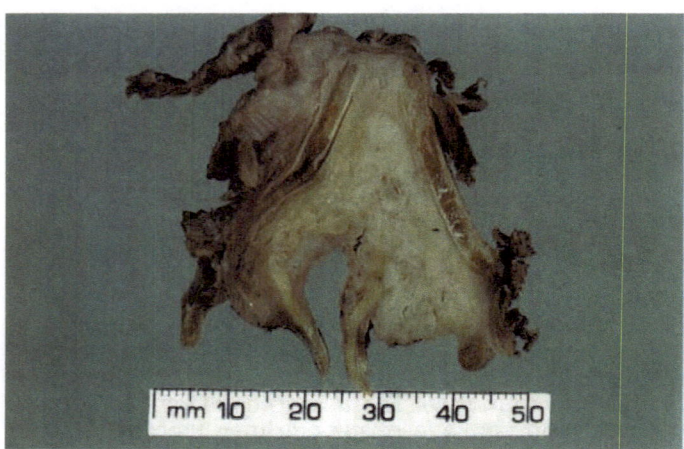

Figure 12.25 Supraglottic portion of origin of extensive carcinoma. There is penetration of the epiglottic cartilage by growth, and the tumour has reached the piriform fossa on the right side

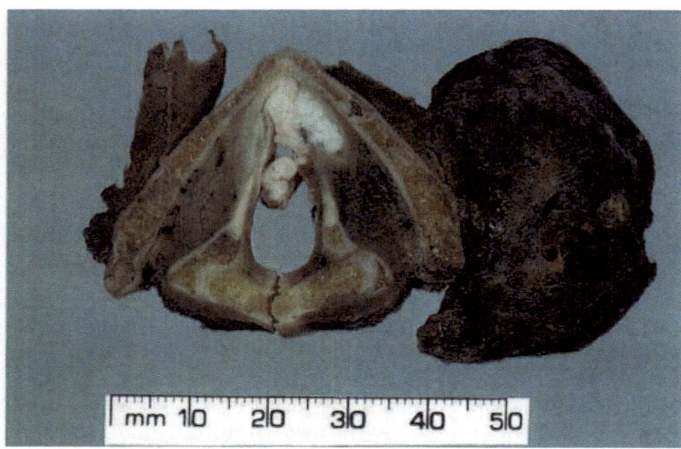

Figure 12.26 Carcinoma arising in the anterior glottic midline region and on the right just posterior to it. Note papillary protuberance of carcinoma

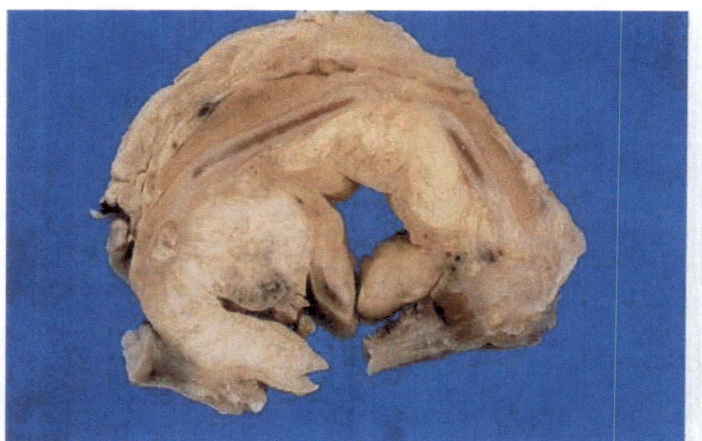

Figure 12.27 Carcinoma of hypopharynx affecting the left piriform fossa and the adjacent posterior wall

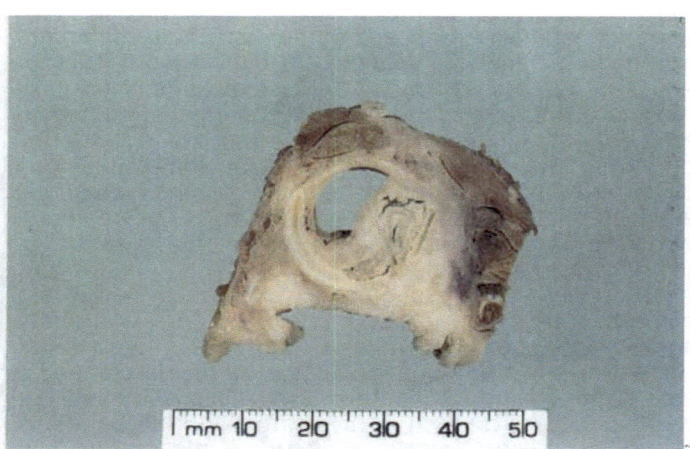

Figure 12.28 Carcinoma of hypopharynx in the postcricoid region. There is an abscess which had tracked into the right subglottic submucosa from the neoplasm and given rise to terminal asphyxia by compression of the airway

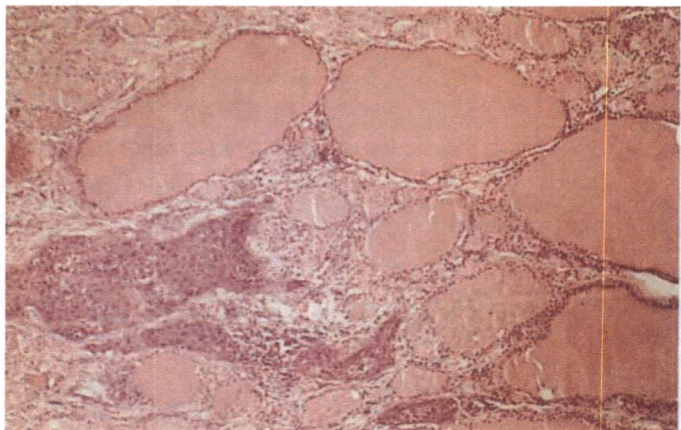

Figure 12.29 Squamous carcinoma originating in hypopharynx invading the thyroid gland. H & E (B)

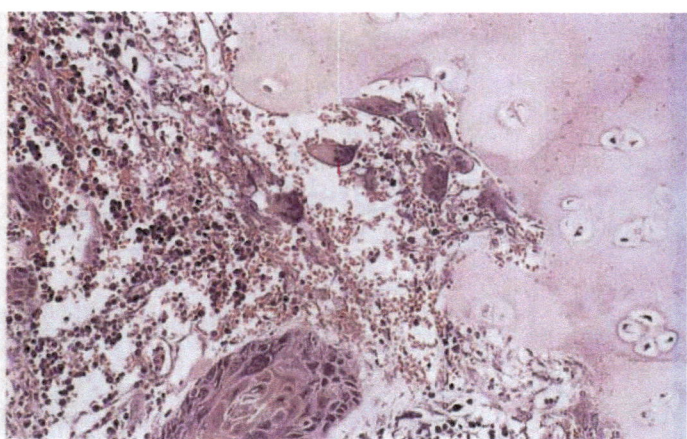

Figure 12.30 Invasion of non-ossified cricoid cartilage by squamous carcinoma. Note numerous giant cells between tumour and cartilage. H & E (B)

Invasion of the cartilaginous framework: Gross and microscopic study of laryngeal squamous carcinoma which is invading the cartilage frequently shows extensive invasion in non-ossified cricoid and thyroid cartilages[4]. The full thickness of cricoid or thyroid cartilage is often penetrated completely by tumour. Burrowing of squamous carcinoma into the depths of ossified cartilage is often seen, and the same is true of non-ossified tumour invasion to an equal extent. The interface of squamous carcinoma with cartilage shows multinucleated giant cells in most cases, and the giant cells are frequently lodged in lacunae, indicating that they are producing resorption of cartilage (Figure 12.30).

A striking mode of spread of squamous carcinoma through the thyroid cartilage – 'ballooning' – is seen in some cases. Tumour enters the thyroid cartilage, often in the anterior commissure region (see above), and then burrows through the cartilage and appears to blow out the outer shell of cartilage from within. Most of the ballooned thyroid cartilage is unossified. In this way, tumour frequently reaches the lower border of the thyroid cartilage, enters the cricothyroid membrane, and may leave the larynx.

Spread outside the larynx
Stomal recurrence: In some cases, the operation of laryngectomy for squamous carcinoma is followed by a carcinomatous deposit at the tracheostomy site which may arise within from a few months to more than 6 years. The deposits of carcinoma grow, not in the main skin scar, but in the mucocutaneous junction of the tracheostomy that is produced at the laryngectomy. There is a widespread feeling among surgeons (although it has not been statistically confirmed) that, if tracheostomy is required before laryngectomy, usually for severe stridor produced by the tumour, the incidence of stomal recurrence is higher. (It is also said to be higher with a predominantly subglottic component of malignancy.)

It has been suggested that the tracheostomal recurrence may result from deposition of cancer cells in the wound from the main specimen at the time of operation. Other suggestions that have been made are: extension from nearby lymph nodes involved by metastasis; development of an additional primary; and extension of neoplasm from the margin of resection. Recurrences nearly always take place in the presence of extensive inoperable neoplasm, although the latter is often occult. In two biopsy specimens of stomal recurrence that I have observed, the squamous carcinoma was clearly arising from the mucosal epithelial covering of the tracheostomy, suggesting that the presence of extensive local squamous carcinoma induces the epithelium of the tracheostomy to become malignant (Figure 12.31).

Lymph node metastasis: It was found by Tanner *et al.*[6] that, in 50 radical neck dissections that were examined from 50 patients with advanced irradiated squamous carcinoma of the head and neck, including 11 cases of laryngeal cancer, 36 specimens had metastatic carcinoma. The technique of isolating lymph nodes was so efficient that it resulted in a yield of up to 60 nodes per specimen. It consisted simply of fine slicing of the specimen systematically with a scalpel, using a new scalpel blade frequently, and embedding for section all areas that grossly suggested lymph node tissue. Involved nodes were mainly in the upper anterior neck, with sparing of the posterior triangle nodes. The proportion of nodes with metastatic carcinoma was low; the striking finding is that, in the great majority of necks with involved nodes, only one or two lymph nodes were so affected, the rest being free from tumour. Thus, 11 patients had only a single metastatic node, and ten patients had two involved nodes. Five

patients had three nodes involved, and smaller numbers of patients had more, up to a total of six positive nodes. Keratin granulomas were commonly found both with and without involved nodes. There was a high incidence of transcapsular spread. Large masses of keratin granuloma were found simulating lymph nodes in the radical neck specimens.

Bloodstream metastasis
In any postmortem study on patients who died of carcinoma of the larynx, it is found that the majority have bloodstream metastases[7,8]. It has been stated that supraglottic carcinomas show the greatest potential for distant metastases[9]. This is probably because they are usually larger than laryngeal cancers at other sites. Bloodstream metastases from squamous carcinoma of the larynx are most common in the lungs. They are also frequently seen in the liver and bones. In all cases showing bloodstream metastases, cervical lymph node metastases are present or have become manifest and have been treated.

Verrucous Squamous Carcinoma

Verrucous squamous carcinoma is a highly differentiated variant of squamous carcinoma which may develop in any mucosal surface of the ear, nose or throat, but, particularly, in the glottic region of the larynx. The gross appearance is usually that of a warty, grey-white lesion with filiform projections (Figure 12.32). Clefts are seen on the cut surface which extend from the surface into the substance of the growth[10]. Verrucous squamous carcinoma may arise from one, two or all three regions of the larynx.

Microscopically, the highly keratinizing surface of the neoplasm, the frequent presence of papillary areas, and the apparent absence of dysplastic change in the squamous epithelium make this lesion difficult to recognize when it first presents. A diagnosis of squamous papilloma is frequently rendered by the pathologist at this time and even after biopsy of one or more recurrences. Verrucous squamous carcinoma does, however, show a number of features in its histological picture which may suggest the correct diagnosis even at first presentation. Rete ridges are usually large, blunt-ended and irregular (Figure 12.33). Proliferating squamous masses often bulge outwards in a papillary fashion, but the symmetrical form of a benign squamous papilloma with branching is not seen (see above). Under the higher powers of the microscope, features of verrucous squamous carcinoma may be detected in each layer of the squamous epithelium. The basal cells show vesicular nuclei, usually containing a single eosinophilic nucleolus. These cells lie on a thin basement membrane, which, unlike squamous papilloma, does not appear wide and hyalinized even in the papillary areas of the tumour, and, in some areas, is not present at all. The basal cells appear to be crowded and even to be bulging the basement membrane outwards (Figure 12.34). More superficially, between the basal layers and the surface keratinizing cells, there are usually wide fields of squamous epithelium composed of cells which frequently have nuclei of 30–40 μm in diameter and a mean area of cytoplasm greater than 300 μm^2 and abundant pale cytoplasm. The large size of these cells, as compared with those from a similar region of squamous papilloma, is a useful diagnostic feature (Figures 12.35 and 12.36). Superficially, keratin is produced, often in great abundance. This is present in some fields with an externally pointed appearance – the 'church spire' effect (Figure 12.37). Parakeratosis is frequent. There is always a dense mononuclear cell exudate beneath the tumour processes; lymphocytes and plasma cells (the latter often in great abundance) are the component cells (Figure 12.34).

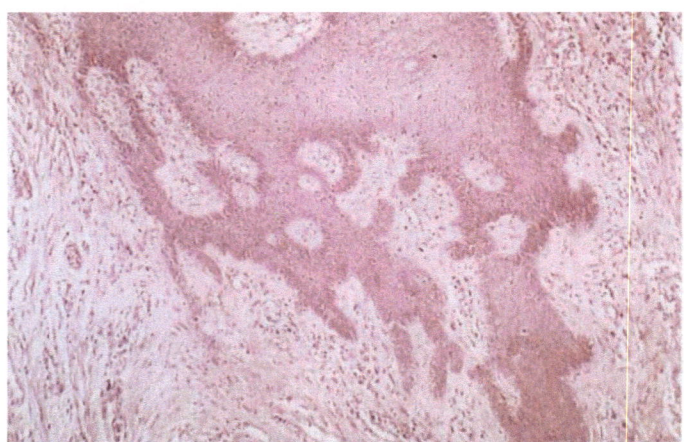

Figure 12.31 New primary squamous carcinoma in tracheostomy opening which had been made before resection of larynx. H & E (B)

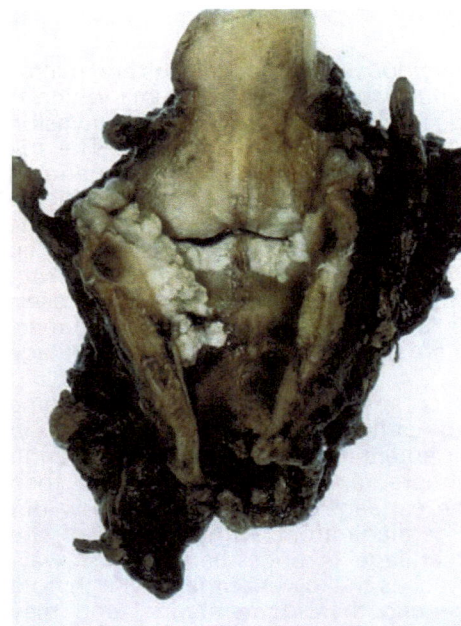

Figure 12.32 Larynx opened from behind to reveal verrucous carcinoma of supraglottis, glottis and subglottis. Note whitish (keratinized) outgrowths

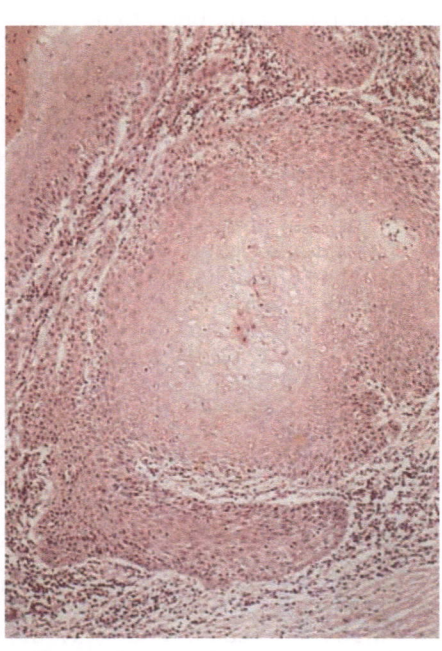

Figure 12.33 Verrucous squamous carcinoma showing atypical rete ridges. H & E (A)

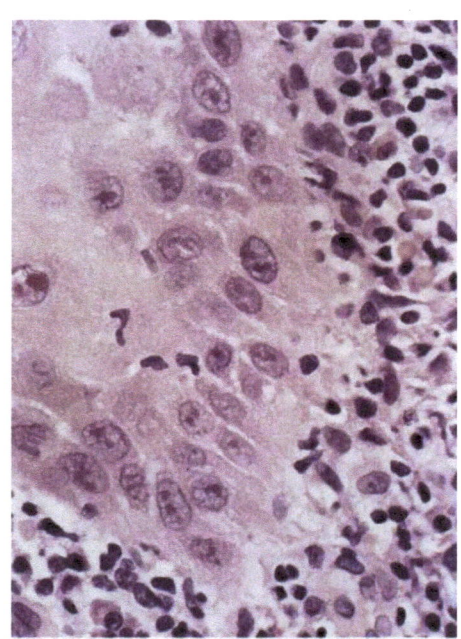

Figure 12.34 Basal layers of verrucous carcinoma. Note crowded appearance. There is a brisk lymphocyte and plasma cell infiltrate in the underlying lamina propria. H & E (C)

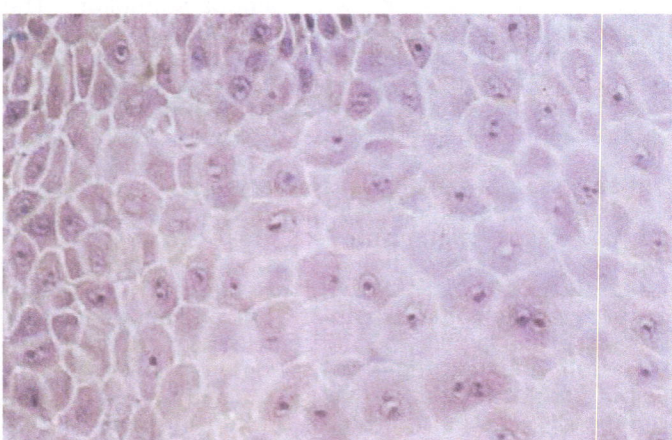

Figure 12.35 Squamous cells in malpighian layer of verrucous squamous carcinoma. Compare sizes of cells with those of squamous papilloma (Figure 12.36). H & E (C)

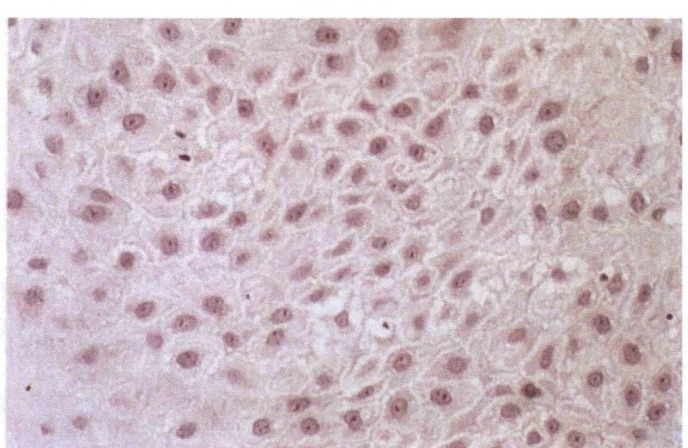

Figure 12.36 Malpighian squamous cells from squamous papilloma of larynx at same magnification as Figure 12.35. Note smaller size of papilloma cells. H & E (C)

Ventriculosaccular Carcinoma

Carcinoma of the saccule or ventricle has been considered to be a rare entity[11]. Michaels and Hassmann[12] described a series of patients with this tumour. After opening the larynx from behind in a laryngectomy specimen from a case of ventriculosaccular carcinoma, tumour is usually present in the ventricle, often filling it and covered by the stretched lips of the false cord and true cord, above and below respectively. Transverse slices of the larynx show a band of pale-grey tumour of mainly uniform thickness which surrounds the lumen of the ventricle and saccule (Figure 12.38). Microscopically, the carcinoma is a highly differentiated one of the squamous variety.

In none of the ten cases who were followed up after treatment for varying periods up to 27 years was there any recurrence of tumour locally or at a distance after laryngectomy; there were no cervical lymph node metastases at any stage of the disease, and there were no bloodstream metastases. In one case, symptoms were present for at least 6 years before the laryngectomy, but a positive biopsy could not be obtained during this time[12].

Spindle Cell Carcinoma

These lesions are carcinomas in which epithelial cells have taken on a mesenchymal appearance. The tumour has been encountered most frequently in the larynx, but it also occurs in the maxillary antrum, oral cavity, hypopharynx, oesophagus, skin and breast. The majority of laryngeal spindle cell carcinomas are polypoid. In the larynx, most of the lesions of spindle cell carcinoma are present on the vocal cord. The diagnosis of spindle cell carcinoma requires identification of squamous cell carcinoma in some part of the tumour. In many cases, however, a diligent search with multiple sections is required, since malignant epithelium is frequently scarce and may be absent from the surface in many areas. Sometimes, only carcinoma in situ without an invasive component is present and a diagnosis of spindle cell carcinoma can only be suspected. In the conventional squamous carcinomatous areas, a 'streaming' of malignant squamous cells into adjacent malignant stroma may be seen (Figures 12.39 to 12.41). The histological pattern of the spindle cell elements is extremely variable. At one end of the scale is a very cellular structure, composed of abundant parallel bipolar cells and containing a large round or oval nucleus with prominent single or multiple nucleoli and bipolar cytoplasmic processes. At the other end of the cellular spectrum are parts with a predominantly collagenous component and sparse spindle-shaped cells (Figure 12.42). Multinucleated giant cells may be found in variable numbers in addition to the spindle cell element. In the spindle cell component, a prominent collagen and reticulin fibre network is revealed by special stains. Histologically atypical cartilage (Figure 12.43) or osteoid tissue is sometimes present as a manifestation of the connective tissue component of the tumour. In the majority of cases that we have tested immunochemically, the spindle cells do not show cytokeratin. In some, they may stain for keratin markers, particularly those showing high molecular weight cytokeratins, such as LP34. Vimentin is usually positive. By the electron microscope, most cases show only cells of mesenchymal type.

In lymph node metastases from spindle cell carcinoma, there may be a squamous carcinomatous element only, both the squamous and the spindle cell element, or the spindle cell component alone. Similar variations of malignant cell types may be seen in more distant metastases. Such histological findings tend to confirm the concept that this lesion is a variant of squamous cell carcinoma.

It has been suggested that the prognosis of spindle cell carcinoma is better than that of squamous cell carcinoma,

but other studies present a somewhat less optimistic future[13,14], indicating that survival and reaction to treatment of spindle cell carcinoma are similar to those of conventional squamous cell carcinoma of the larynx, with particularly poor response to irradiation therapy alone.

Radiation Perichondritis

Clinical features suggestive of perichondritis of laryngeal cartilage are sometimes encountered at a later stage in patients who have been irradiated for malignant disease of the larynx. Gross examination of the larynx usually shows fibrous thickening of the mucosa with narrowing of the airway. Cartilaginous change is present at the perichondrial surface as a pale-yellow opaque area. Microscopically, the pale-yellow infiltrate of the cartilage and of the surrounding connective tissue represents a large acute abscess in each case. Neutrophils of the abscess encroach on and erode the cartilage in an irregular fashion. Small fragments of cartilage are sometimes seen loose within the abscess, but, even here, the chondrocytes, although often somewhat retracted from the wall of their lacunae in the cartilage, still show normally staining nucleus and cytoplasm (Figure 12.44). In the connective tissue around the abscess, in each case, there is an irregular deposition of fibrin, usually as a fine network. Collagen replacement of fibrin is frequent, and, within the collagen, fibroblasts are seen which are often the 'atypical' type frequently apparent after radiation damage and other changes characteristic of this state[15].

References

1. Bewtra, C., Krishnan, R. and Lee, S. S. (1982). Malignant change in non-irradiated juvenile laryngotracheal papillomatosis. *Arch. Otolaryngol.*, **108**, 114–116
2. Capper, J. W. R., Bailey, C. M. and Michaels, L. (1983). Squamous papillomas of the larynx in adults. A review of 63 cases. *Clin. Otolaryngol.*, **8**, 109–119
3. Quiney, R. E., Wells, M., Lewis, F. A., Terry, R. M., Michaels, L. and Croft, C. B. (1989). Laryngeal papillomatosis: correlation between severity of disease and presence of HPV 6 and 11 detected by in situ DNA hybridisation. *J. Clin. Pathol.*, **42**, 694–698
4. Michaels, L. (1984). *Pathology of the Larynx.* (Heidelberg, Berlin, New York: Springer)
5. Willatt, D. J., Jackson, S. R., McCormick, M. S., Lubsen, H., Michaels, L. and Stell, P. M. (1987). Vocal cord paralysis and tumour length in staging postcricoid carcinoma. *Eur. J. Surg. Oncol.*, **13**, 131–137
6. Tanner, N. S. B., Carter, R. L., Dalley, V. M., Clifford, P. and Shaw, H. J. (1980). The irradiated radical neck dissection in squamous carcinoma: a clinico pathological study. *Clin. Otolaryngol.*, **5**, 259–271
7. Harrer, W. V. and Lewis, P. L. (1970). Carcinoma of the larynx with cardiac metastases. *Arch. Otolaryngol.*, **91**, 382–384
8. O'Brien, P. H., Carlson, R., Stuebner, E. A. *et al.* (1971) Distant metastases in epidermoid cell carcinoma of the head and neck. *Cancer*, **27**, 304–307
9. Alonso, J. M. (1967). Metastasis of laryngeal and hypopharyngeal carcinoma. *Acta Otolaryngol. (Stockholm)*, **64**, 353–360
10. Dockerty, M. B., Parkhill, E. M., Dahlin, D. C. *et al.* (1968). *Tumours of the Oral Cavity and Pharynx. Atlas of Tumor Pathology.* (Washington DC: Armed Forces Institute of Pathology, section IV, fascicle 10b)
11. Olofsson, J. and van Nostrand, A. W. P. (1973). Growth and spread of laryngeal and hypopharyngeal carcinoma with reflections on the effect of preoperative irradiation. 139 cases studied by whole organ sectioning. *Acta Otolaryngol. (Stockholm)*, (Suppl.), **308**, 1–84
12. Michaels, L. and Hassmann, E. (1982). Ventriculosaccular carcinoma of the larynx. *Clin. Otolaryngol.*, **7**, 165–173
13. Appelman, H. D. and Overman, H. A. (1965). Squamous cell carcinoma of the larynx with sarcoma-like stroma. A clinico-pathologic assessment of spindle cell carcinoma and 'pseudosarcoma'. *Am. J. Clin. Pathol.*, **44**, 135–145
14. Hyams, V. J. (1975). Spindle cell carcinoma of the larynx. *Can. J. Otolaryngol.*, **4**, 307–313
15. Fajardo, L. F. and Berthrong, M. (1978). Radiation injury in surgical pathology. Part I. *Am. J. Surg. Pathol.*, **2**, 159–199

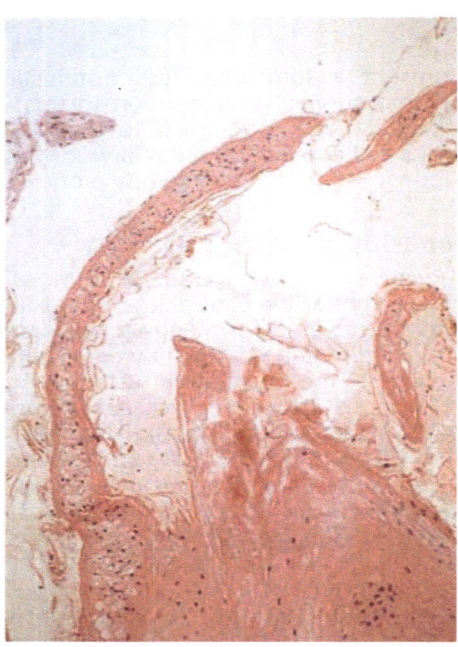

Figure 12.37 Long thin keratinous 'spires' on surface of verrucous carcinoma. H & E (A)

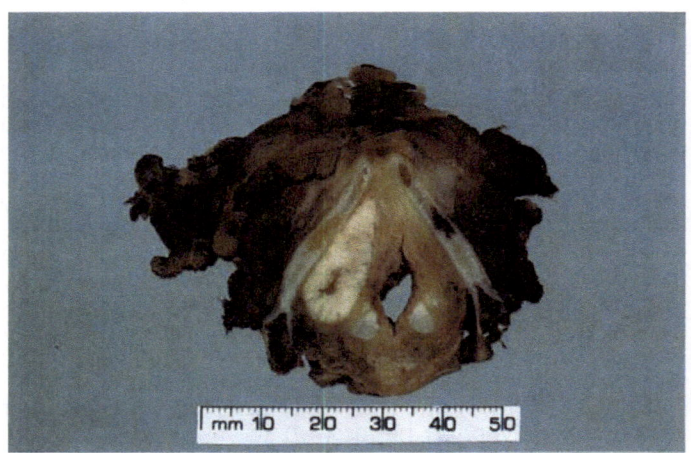

Figure 12.38 Saccular component of ventriculosaccular carcinoma of larynx in transverse slice. The lateral edge of the neoplasm lies against the thyroid cartilage but does not invade it

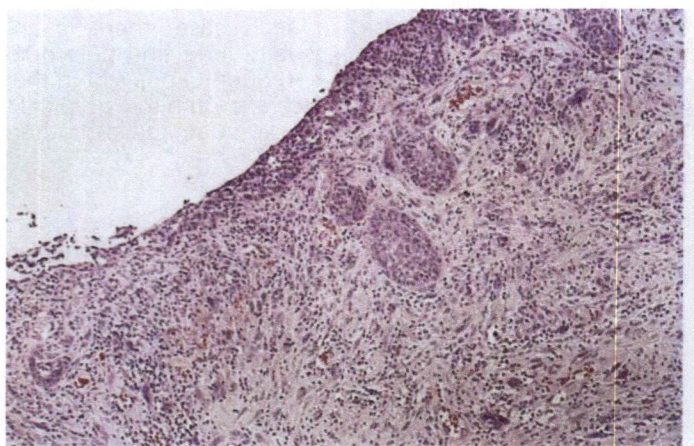

Figure 12.39 Origin of spindle cell carcinoma of vocal cord from squamous carcinoma. H & E (B)

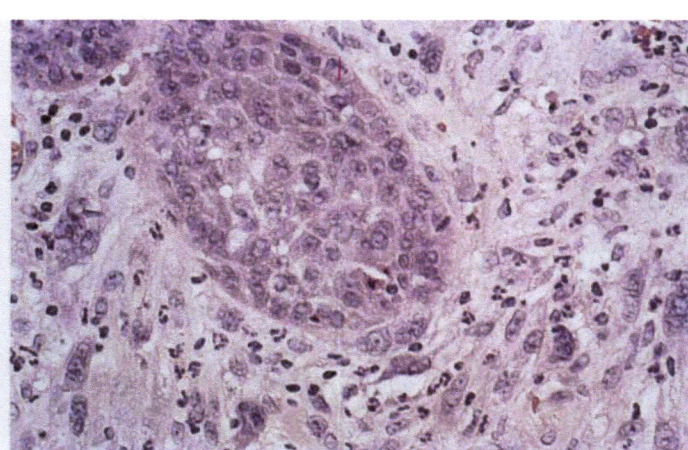

Figure 12.40 Higher power of spindle cell carcinoma cells and true squamous carcinoma. H & E (C)

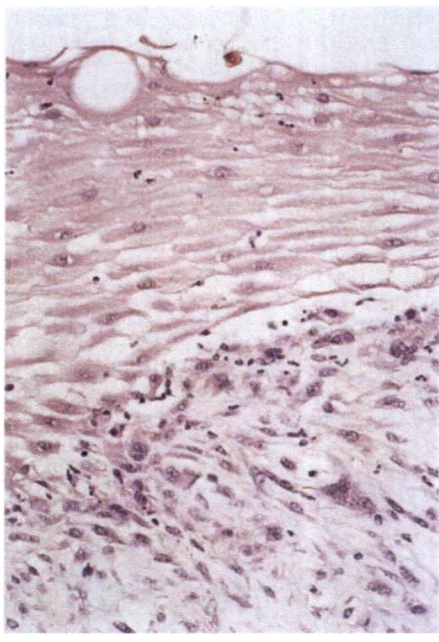

Figure 12.41 Dysplastic surface and spindle cell carcinoma cells 'raining' down from it. H & E (C)

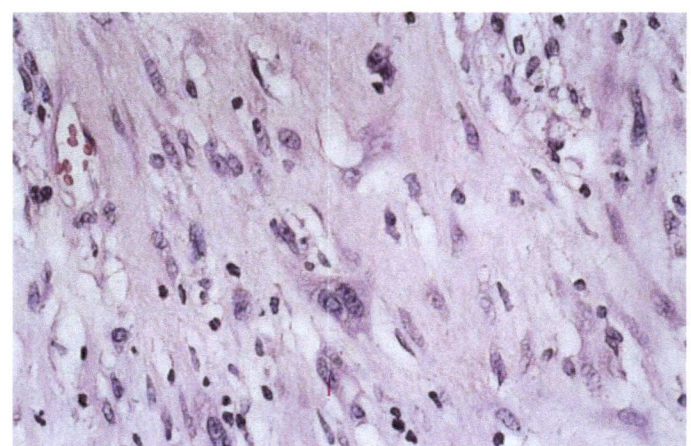

Figure 12.42 Spindle cell carcinoma showing bizarre elongated mesenchymal-appearing cells. H & E (C)

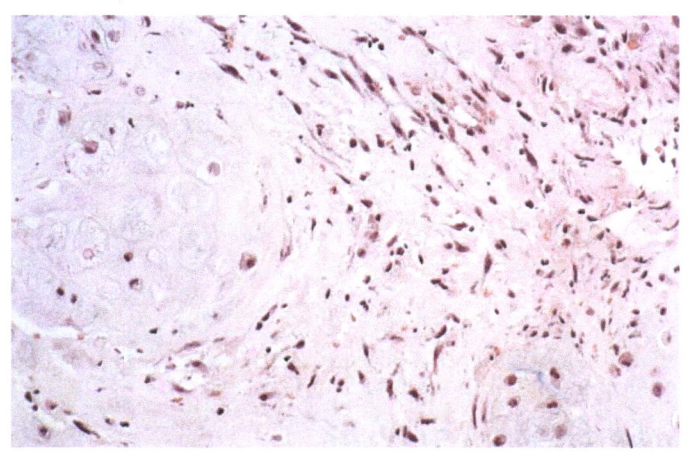

Figure 12.43 Spindle cell carcinoma showing chondroid change. H & E (B)

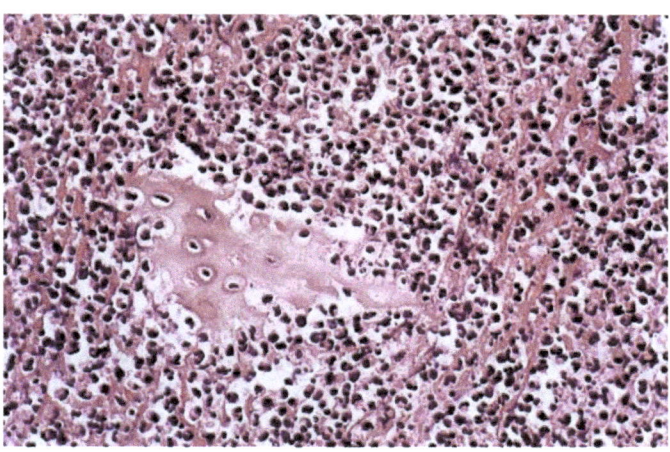

Figure 12.44 Radionecrosis of larynx showing eroded fragment of cartilage in pus. H & E (C)

Adenocarcinoma and Adenoid Cystic Carcinoma

Most of the benign and malignant epithelial neoplasms of the larynx are epidermoid but a small proportion are not. The latter may occasionally arise from the respiratory epithelium which covers most of the larynx, but more usually emanate from the cells lining the seromucinous glands, which are abundant in the larynx, particularly in the false cord and adjacent to the saccule. Benign neoplasms arising from seromucinous glands of the larynx are very rare. Malignant tumours originating from seromucinous glands are in the form of adenocarcinomas and of adenoid cystic carcinomas. Although more frequent than benign seromucinous gland neoplasms, they are usually thought to constitute less than 1% of all laryngeal neoplasms. A third group of non-epidermoid carcinomas, possibly of the same source, and thought to be the largest group – the neuroendocrine carcinomas – is considered below.

Malignant non-epidermoid epithelial tumours usually produce large non-ulcerated masses with either a smooth or a granular surface. There may be a polypoid configuration. On slicing, the tumours are seen always to invade the underlying intrinsic muscles, and invasion of the thyroid and cricoid cartilages, and epiglottic cartilage in the case of supraglottic tumours, is frequent. One or other lobes of the thyroid gland may be ultimately involved by deeply invading tumours.

Approximately two thirds of the cases of non-epidermoid carcinomas are adenocarcinomas. The great majority of the other cases show an adenoid cystic histological appearance[1]. Their constituent neoplastic cells are usually arranged in a glandular configuration with varying degrees of pleomorphism. Solid trabeculae of tumours of this type sometimes occur. Adenoid cystic carcinomas are usually considered as a myoepithelial cell-derived variant of adenocarcinoma with a very specific histological pattern (Figure 13.1) (see Chapter 6). As in major and minor salivary glands, invasion of tumour along perineural spaces is frequently seen in histological sections of larynges bearing adenoid cystic carcinoma.

A small number of cases of glandular carcinomas with histological features other than those of simple adenocarcinoma or adenoid cystic carcinoma have been described. They have been mostly classified under the designation of mucoepidermoid carcinoma (Figures 13.2 and 13.3), although other histological patterns are also possible[1]. In every adenocarcinoma of the larynx, particularly one with a papillary pattern, the possibility of extension from an adenocarcinoma of the thyroid should be considered (Figure 13.4).

Adenocarcinoma of the larynx has a bad prognosis. Lymph node and bloodstream metastases are common and most patients die with metastases within 2 years of the onset in spite of radiotherapy and surgical treatment. Lymph node metastases are rare in adenoid cystic carcinoma. Recurrence usually follows local excision within 2 years, but, in some cases, a delay in recurrence of 5 years or more is seen (as in adenoid cystic carcinoma of minor salivary glands) and a similar delay may occur in the development of bloodstream metastases.

Neuroectodermal Tumours

Granular cell tumour

Granular cell tumour, a benign lesion, which is commonly seen in surgical histology practice in such sites as the subcutaneous tissue, the tongue and other mucosal surfaces, also presents sometimes in the larynx. The most common site for this lesion is on the vocal cord. It is usually a small sessile raised swelling with a smooth mucosal surface arising from the vocal cord. The histological characteristic of the lesion is the presence of rows of cells with granular eosinophilic cytoplasm. The nuclei are usually small and inconspicuous ((Figure 13.5). Interstitial fibrous tissue is commonly found and the base of the lesion may thus give an impression of deep invasion which belies the benign course of the disease. The cytoplasmic granules are eosinophilic by ordinary staining and positive by the periodic acid–Schiff method. In the larynx, as in other mucosal surfaces, pseudoepitheliomatous hyperplasia of the overlying squamous epithelium commonly, but not always, takes place. The squamous cells do not have significant dysplastic features (Figures 13.6 and 13.7).

Neurogenic tumours

Neurogenic tumours appear, in most cases, as a supraglottic bulge covered by mucosa. The neurilemmomas are invariably firm spherical swellings with well-defined outlines. Neurofibromas may be more diffuse and less well defined. A major nerve trunk is sometimes identified in relation to the neoplasm in laryngeal tumours.

Histologically, in a typical neurilemmoma, Antoni A areas of palisaded Schwann cells are prominent; they are often whorled into Verocay bodies. Antoni B areas are almost invariably present in the same tumours and represent looser reticular, often mucoid, areas between the Antoni A regions (Figure 13.8) (see Chapter 3). Neurofibromas are typically fibrous lesions with frequent nerve fibres traversing the tumour (Figure 13.9). Ash et al.[2] stated that laryngeal neurogenic tumours are mostly of the neurofibromatous variety; more proximally, in the mouth and pharynx, neurilemmomas will predominate.

Neuroendocrine carcinoma

A concept of 'endocrine' or 'neuroendocrine' carcinoma has arisen in recent years and includes carcinoid tumours of intestine and lung and a wide variety of other tumours of endodermal or neuroectodermal origin, including oat cell carcinoma. These tumours have an epithelial, often glandular, structure and are usually argentaffin or argyrophil. Immunostaining reveals the presence of neurone-specific enolase and inappropriate hormone secretion within the tumour cells, such as adrenocorticotrophic hormone or calcitonin. In the larynx, two forms of neuroendocrine carcinoma have been described in recent years: large-cell neuroendocrine carcinoma, which is a

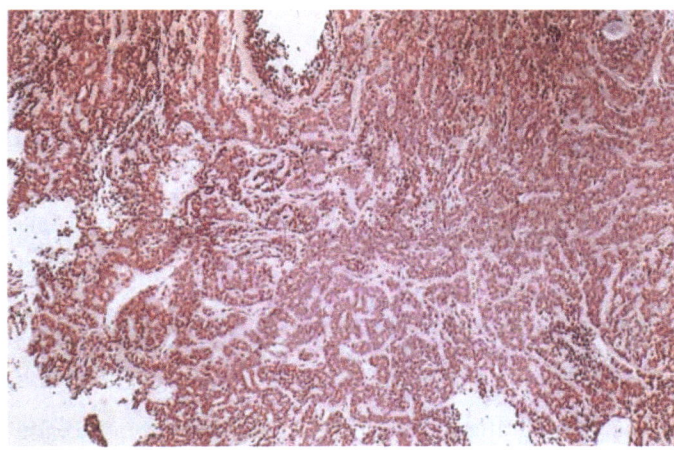

Figure 13.1 Adenocystic carcinoma of the larynx. H & E (A)

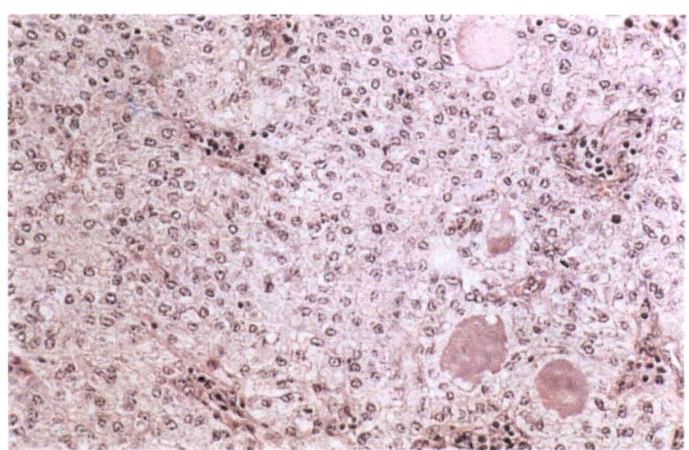

Figure 13.2 Mucoepidermoid carcinoma of the larynx. Uniform epidermoid cells in association with small mucus-containing glands. H & E (B)

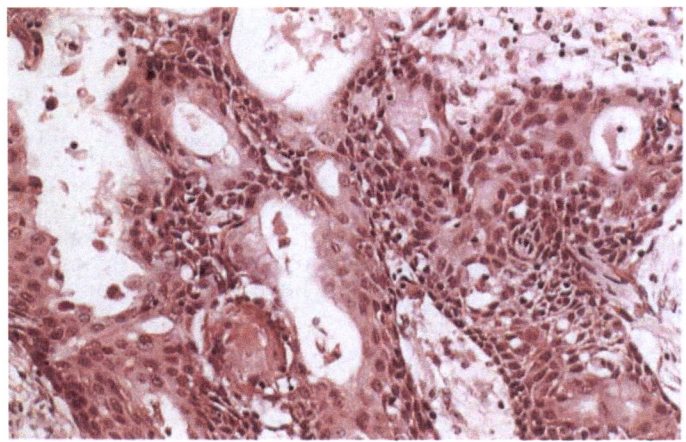

Figure 13.3 Mucoepidermoid carcinoma of the larynx. Large mucus-containing glands with malignant epidermoid foci. H & E (B)

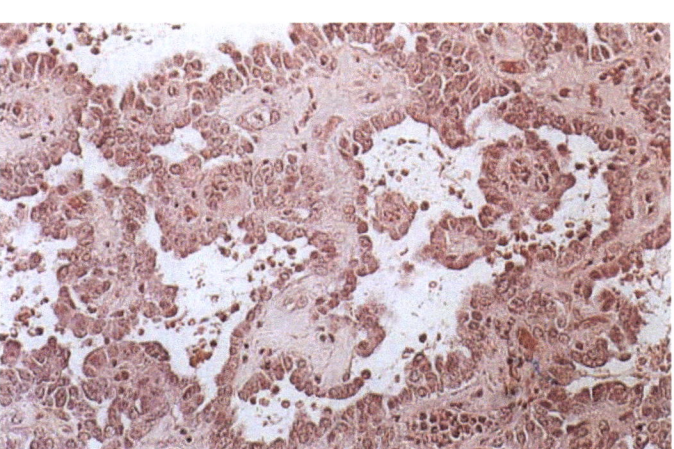

Figure 13.4 Papillary adenocarcinoma of the thyroid presenting as a laryngeal tumour. H & E (B)

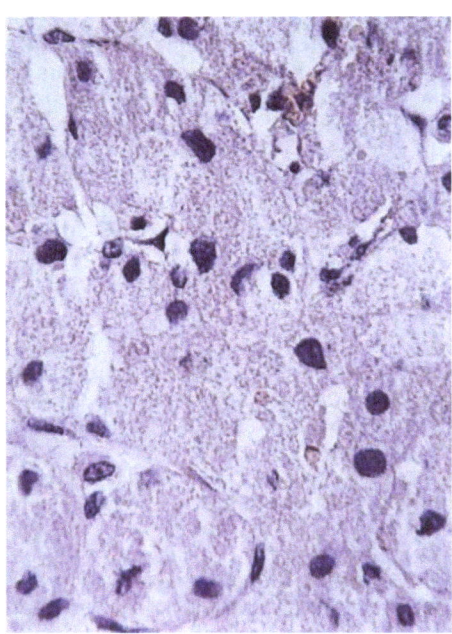

Figure 13.5 Granular cell tumour of the vocal cord. The tumour is composed of large cells with eosinophilic granular cytoplasm and small inconspicuous nuclei. (C)

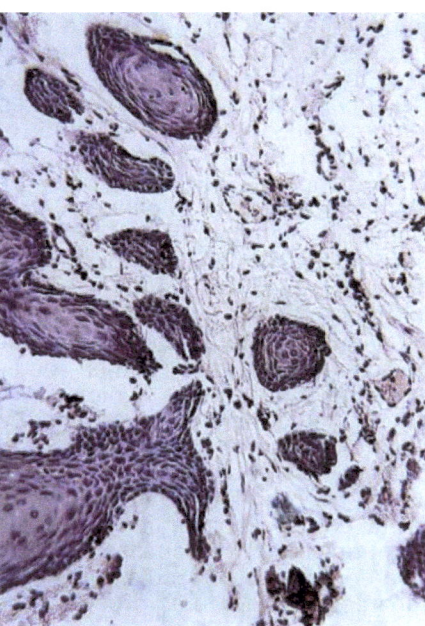

Figure 13.6 Hyperplasia of squamous epithelium associated with granular cell tumour of vocal cord. H & E (B)

less differentiated form of the carcinoid type of tumour; and small-cell neuroendocrine carcinoma, which is histologically similar to oat cell carcinoma. A third type of tumour, paraganglioma, which is said to be derived from laryngeal paranganglia, has some features in common with large-cell neuroendocrine carcinoma. Woodruff et al.[3] suggest that neuroendocrine carcinomas are the largest group of non-epidermoid carcinomas of the larynx, having found 13 out of 22 tumours of the latter type to be neuroendocrine carcinoma, and Wenig et al.[4] came to a similar conclusion.

Large-cell neuroendocrine carcinoma
The slowly growing well-differentiated carcinoid type 'adenoma' found in the bronchus has not been observed in the larynx. A tumour which is less differentiated histologically and more aggressive in its behaviour would seem to be the laryngeal variant of this neoplasm. Most of the tumours arise in the supraglottis. The neoplasm is composed of epithelial cells forming nests, cords and acini (Figure 13.10). The tumour cells contain eosinophilic cytoplasm, are often argyrophilic and, on electron microscopy, always contain dense-core neurosecretory granules which range from 90 to 250 nm in diameter. Neurone-specific enolase is present on immunostaining in all large-cell neuroendocrine carcinomas (Figure 13.11) and calcitonin in the majority of those examined by Woodruff et al., who found the detection of calcitonin to be a valuable feature in the differential diagnosis of these tumours from laryngeal paraganglioma. A total of 60% of the reported patients had died of the tumour at the time of reporting, with a mean survival time of 2 years and 6 months after diagnosis.

Small-cell neuroendocrine carcinoma
This tumour resembles oat cell carcinoma of the larynx, with small tumour cells showing little cytoplasm and containing darkly staining nuclei. Tubule formation may be present (Figures 13.12 and 13.13). Argyrophilia is not present in the majority of these tumours. Ultrastructural examination shows neurosecretory granules between 100 and 380 nm in diameter. Immunohistochemical staining is positive for neurone-specific enolase, and other antigens, such as carcinoembryonic antigen and serotonin, may also be positive. Small-cell neuroendocrine carcinomas are very aggressive neoplasms with a mean survival time from diagnosis of only 13 months[3].

Paraganglioma
The rarity of paraganglioma of the larynx, the difficulty of its histological diagnosis and its malignant behaviour in contrast to all other paragangliomas, make this a difficult tumour to describe. It should be emphasized that the histological impression gained in the study of paragangliomas of the carotid body, vagus nerve and jugular and tympanic paraganglioma is usually one of a bland uniform neoplasm composed of 'Zellballen' and blood vessels (see Chapter 3). Paragangliomas are positive for neurone-specific enolase. Material has been studied at our hospital from three patients with laryngeal neoplasms thought originally to be paraganglioma; in each of these patients, multiple painful skin metastases developed. Such behaviour is unlike other paragangliomas, such as carotid body tumour, which rarely manifest metastatic activity. Paragangliomas arising in the larynx thus seem to be unique among paragangliomas in general in their malignant behaviour. It is possible that, in many cases, a large-cell neuroendocrine carcinoma of the larynx has been mistaken for paraganglioma. Such a histological misinterpretation would be quite easily made if the carcinoma showed considerable vascularity. Only a single case showing characteristic features of a benign-appearing laryngeal paraganglioma has been identified at our centre in recent years. Cells of sustentacular appearance, staining positively for S100 protein, were observed around the periphery of the Zellballen (Figures 13.14 and 13.15). Neuroendocrine granules and neurone-specific enolase are found, on electron microscopy and immunostaining respectively, in both neuroendocrine carcinoma and paraganglioma tumour types. Woodruff et al.[3] recommend the use of calcitonin as an immunochemical marker to distinguish between large-cell neuroendocrine carcinoma and paraganglioma of the larynx. This substance was stated by them to be present in the majority of cases of the former but is usually not found in the latter.

Touch preparations, dried over phosphorus pentoxide and exposed to paraformaldehyde vapour have been found useful in the diagnosis of neuroendocrine carcinoma (Figure 13.16).

Vascular Neoplasms
Haemangioma
Haemangiomas in the adult larynx are unusual and clinically not distinctive lesions. In infants, on the other hand, laryngeal haemangiomas represent a distinctive and dangerous entity.

Adult form
In the larynx of the older child and adult, pyogenic granuloma and a vascular vocal cord polyp may be confused with haemangioma of the vocal cord and it is likely that, in some of the reports of vocal cord haemangioma in adults, this has given rise to misinterpretation. Supraglottic capillary haemangiomas do grow occasionally in adults and cavernous haemangioma has been described[5].

Infantile form
The infant larynx may be the site of a similar haemangioma to that commonly seen in the skin of infants. The lesion is almost always subglottic. The growth of infantile haemangioma in this position is dangerous because, since the subglottis is very narrow in the infant, airway obstruction soon takes place. Frequently, the tumour is not visible, even on direct laryngoscopy, and the infant may die of respiratory obstruction without the diagnosis having been suspected[6]. Even at necropsy, the haemangioma may not be seen grossly or may appear too small to be a cause of respiratory obstruction as the blood drains from the vessels after death and the lesion shrinks.

Microscopically, the infantile haemangioma appears as small sinusoidal or capillary blood channels. Usually arranged in lobules, it is situated in the submucosa or on the luminal side of the cricoid cartilage perichondrium in contact with the the the latter (Figures 13.17 and 13.18). If, as is usually the case, the lesion is composed of capillaries, the endothelial cells may be swollen and the lumina difficult to identify.

Haemangiosarcoma
This rare lesion has a haemorrhagic and cystic gross appearance and appears in the supraglottis where it is widely invasive[7]. Microscopically, a spectrum of appearances can be recognized in haemangiosarcomas, from a well-differentiated angiomatous pattern to a poorly differentiated solid pattern (Figures 13.19 and 13.20). It is important to identify that the actual lining blood vessels have malignant features. Stains for factor VIII or the Ulex marker may help in this determination. In laryngeal haemangiosarcoma, the neoplasm metastasizes early and the patients usually die of the metastases within one year.

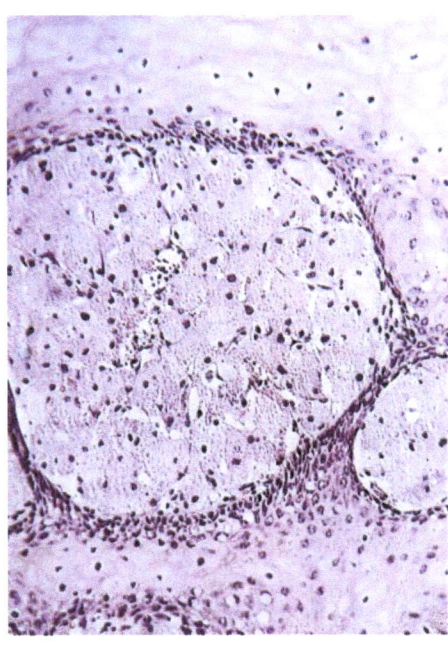

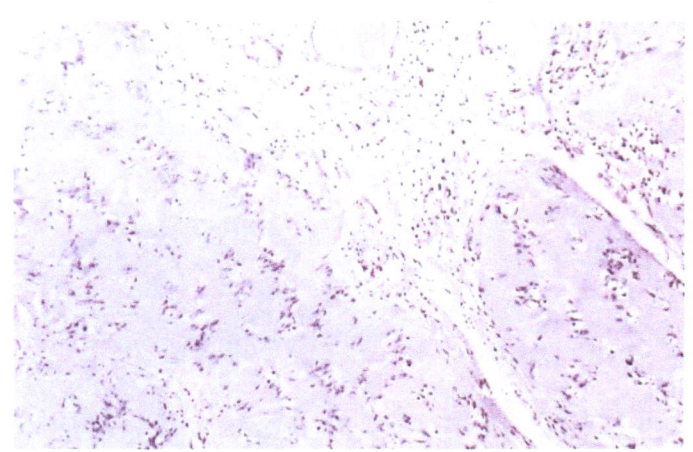

Figure 13.7 Hyperplastic squamous epithelium of vocal cord in association with granular cell tumour. Note that there is no dysplasia of the epithelium. H & E (C)

Figure 13.8 Neurilemmoma (schwannoma) of larynx showing Antoni A and B areas. H & E (A)

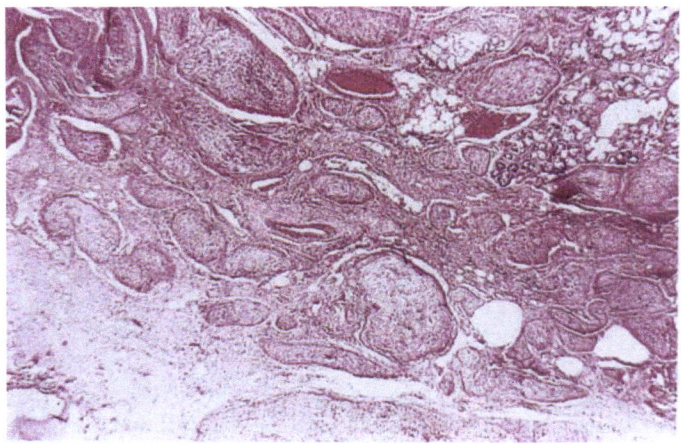

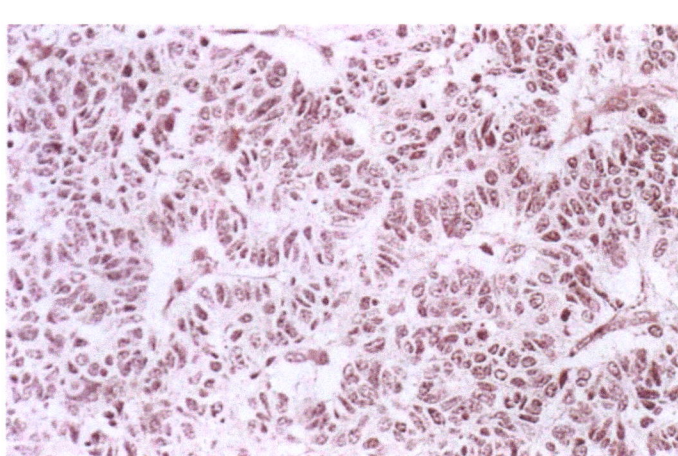

Figure 13.9 Plexiform neurofibroma from region of superior laryngeal nerve. Groups of proliferated nerve fibres are set in a fibrous background. H & E (A)

Figure 13.10 Large-cell neuroendocrine carcinoma of larynx. Nests and acini of tumour cells. H & E (C)

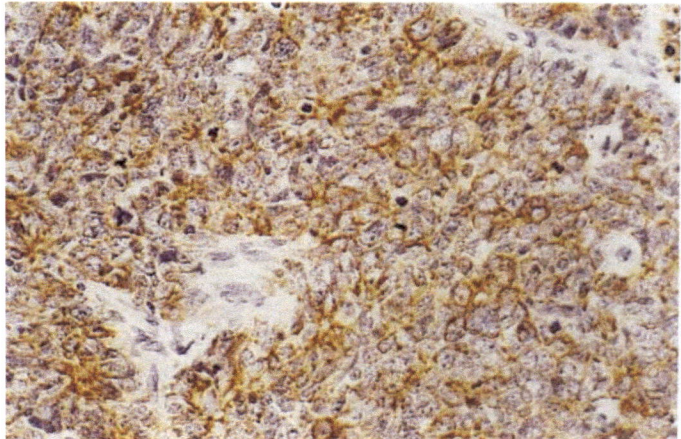

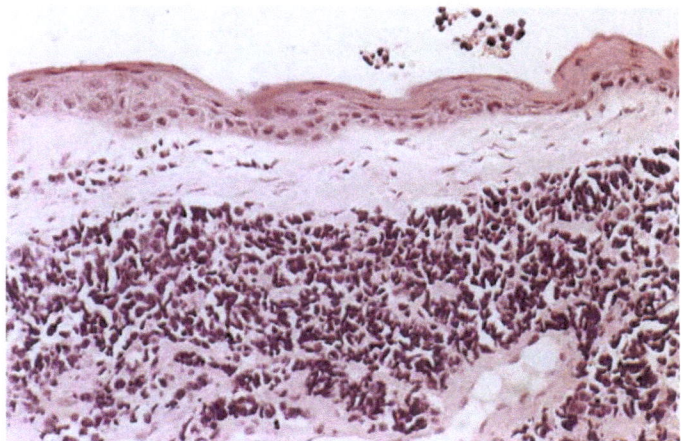

Figure 13.11 Large-cell neuroendocrine carcinoma of larynx. Immunochemical staining for neurone-specific enolase showing positive reaction of the tumour cells. (C)

Figure 13.12 Small-cell neuroendocrine carcinoma of the larynx beneath the epithelium of the mucosa. H & E (B)

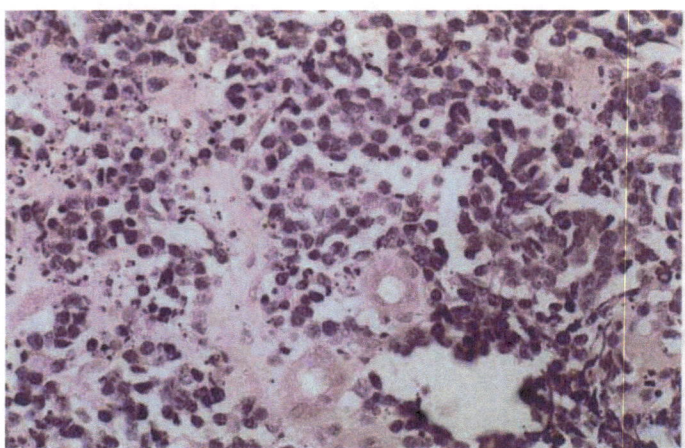

Figure 13.13 Small-cell neuroendocrine carcinoma of the larynx showing some attempts at tubule formation.   H & E (C)

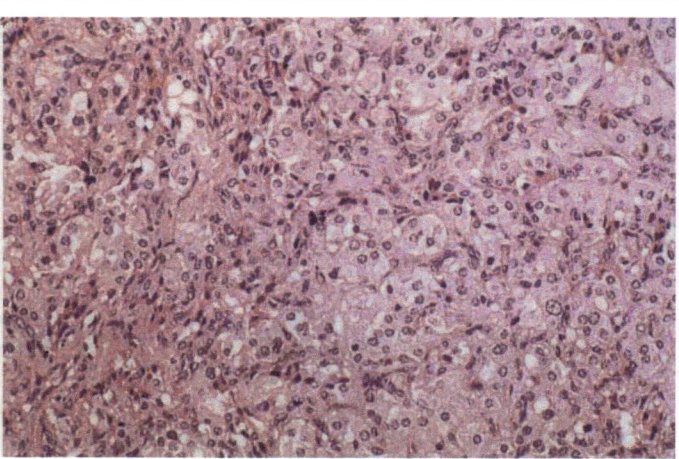

Figure 13.14 Paraganglioma of the larynx. Note arrangement of cells into small packets – 'Zellballen'.   H & E (B)

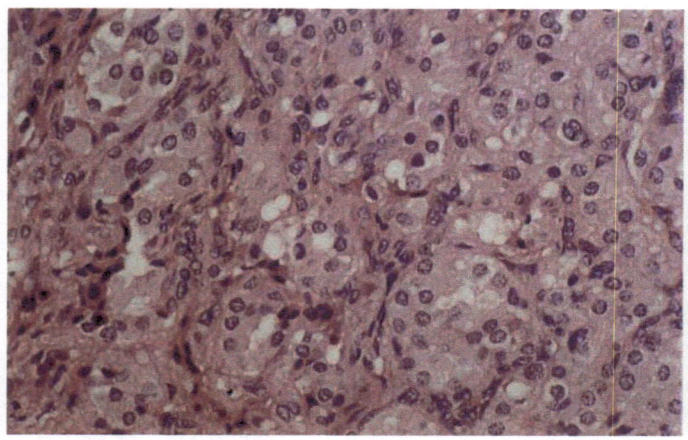

Figure 13.15 Higher power of paraganglioma of larynx shown in Figure 13.14. Note regular cells and peripheral flattened sustentacular cells.   H & E (C)

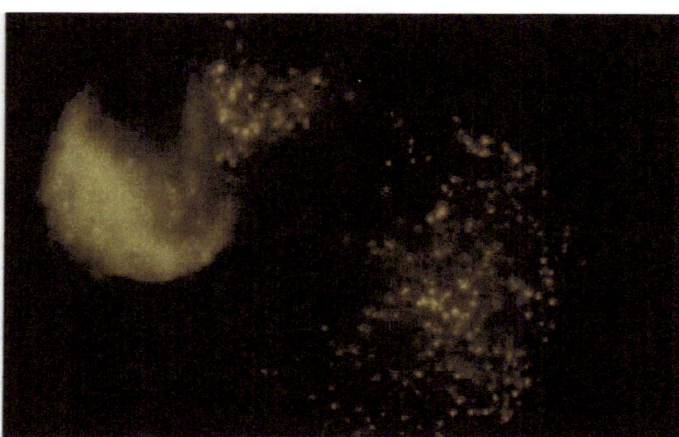

Figure 13.16 Touch preparation of large-cell neuroendocrine carcinoma of larynx which had been exposed to paraformaldehyde vapour. Two tumour cells are seen, both showing granular fluorescence of catecholamines. Photographed in ultraviolet light (D)

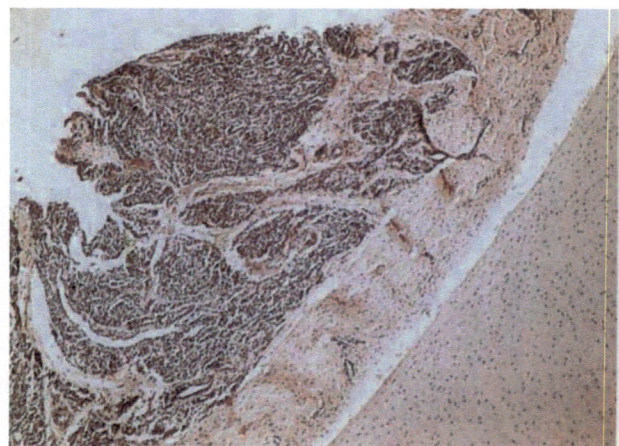

Figure 13.17 Subglottic haemangioma from an infant aged 18 months. It shows closely packed capillaries extending to the cricoid cartilage.   H & E (A)

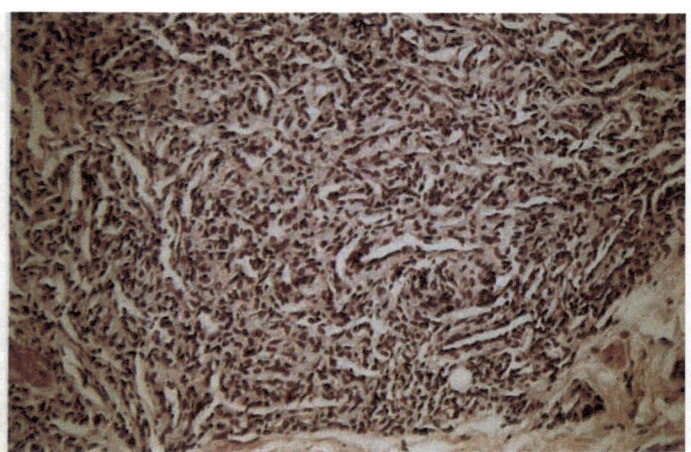

Figure 13.18 Higher power of Figure 13.17 showing closely packed capillary blood vessels.   H & E (B)

Neoplastic Collagenous Lesions

It is doubtful whether benign neoplasms in this category exist. The great majority of collections of fibrocytic cells with collagen are reactive in nature or fibromatoses. Malignant tumours in this category – 'fibrosarcoma' of high-grade fibrosarcomas have been described in the larynx in small numbers[8]. Microscopically, they are composed of elongated spindle cells in bundles, often with a 'herringbone' pattern. The rate of growth is related to the degree of differentiation. It should be stressed, however, that, in the larynx, a pedunculated lesion with a malignant fibroblastic histological appearance growing in the region of the anterior vocal cord is most likely to be a spindle cell carcinoma (see Chapter 12).

Myogenic Neoplasms

Smooth muscle neoplasms of the larynx are very rare.

Neoplasms of striated muscle

Benign rhabdomyoma
The larynx is an occasional site of presentation for benign rhabdomyoma. Two forms of rhabdomyoma are recognized: adult and fetal. The site of origin of rhabdomyomas may be anywhere in the larynx[9].

Adult rhabdomyoma: This benign lesion is well circumscribed or encapsulated and usually presents in the supraglottis. Histologically, adult rhabdomyomas are composed of large uniform round-to-polygonal cells with abundant acidophil, fibrillary cytoplasm and large vesicles, often peripheral nuclei and prominent acidophil nucleoli. Cross-striations are difficult to find. Glycogen is plentiful in the cytoplasm of the cells and may be demonstrated by the periodic acid–Schiff stain with and without diastase. A feature of this tumour is the so-called 'spider cells' in which there is a large peripheral cytoplasmic clear zone transversed by thin cytoplasmic strands extending from the central acidophilic cytoplasm to the periphery, the result of the loss of glycogen in the periphery of the cells by solution during fixation and processing (Figures 13.21 and 13.22). Desmin is strongly expressed on immunochemical staining in the cytoplasm of these tumours (Figure 13.23).

Fetal rhabdomyoma: Fetal rhabdomyomas are rare neoplasms which have been described mainly in the postauricular subcutaneous tissue of young children and in the vulvovaginal region of middle-aged women[10]. They may also occur as polypoid lesions in the upper respiratory tract, including the larynx, of adults in the second and third decades[11] (Figure 13.24). Histological appearances range from a 'cellular' (Figure 13.25) to a 'myxoid' arrangement of spindle cells, which may form a cambial layer similar to that of embryonal rhabdomyosarcoma. Occasional spindle cells may contain multiple nuclei which are situated in tandem (Figure 13.26). All tumours display occasional groups of adult skeletal muscle cells (Figure 13.27). Desmin and myoglobin are uncommonly expressed by the undifferentiated spindle cells but are always shown by the differentiated cells. Local recurrence may occur but not invasion or metastasis.

Alveolar Soft Part Sarcoma

Also known as malignant granular cell myoblastoma, alveolar soft part sarcoma is a malignant tumour which usually occurs in the muscles of the extremities, but which occasionally presents in the head and neck, including the larynx. The tumour is characterized by the arrangement of the cells in compact groups composed of 5–50 cells. The component cells are large, polyhedral and eosinophilic, with finely granular cytoplasm. The nuclei are eccentrically situated, vesicular and contain one or more distinct nucleoli (Figures 13.28 and 13.29). Large crystals may be found by light and electron microscopy in the cytoplasm of many alveolar soft part sarcomas. Metastasis often occurs; in some cases, local lymph node metastasis is reported, but, more frequently, this stage is bypassed and bloodstream metastases are the first sign of spread[12].

Neoplasms of Hyaline Cartilage

Neoplasms of the laryngeal cartilage are surprisingly rare in spite of the considerable bulk of that tissue. All are derived from and are composed of hyaline cartilage. Benign and malignant neoplasms of hyaline cartilage are found in the larynx. Although extreme degrees of malignancy are easy to recognize, the distinction between benign chondromas and low-grade chondrosarcomas is often not easy, and the two types of tumour will be considered as one entity. By far the most usual site of origin of cartilaginous neoplasms in the larynx is the posterior lamina of the cricoid cartilage; a smaller number arise from the thyroid cartilage. The arytenoid cartilage is rarely a site of cartilaginous tumour origin[13,14]. Diagnosis is usually made following biopsy of a mass protruding into the laryngeal airway. In some cases, the presence of highly atypical cartilage cells in the biopsy fragment may enable a diagnosis of chondrosarcoma to be made easily. In other cases, cartilage showing only slightly atypical changes may be obtained in the biopsy material, and the pathologist may be under the impression that this is normal cartilage removed at a rather deep bite by the biopsy forceps. In bronchial biopsies, normal cartilage is frequently removed and its presence is of no significance in the pathological assessment. In endoscopic biopsies of the larynx, however, cartilage is rarely removed unless it is pathological, usually as a result of either perichondritis (see Chapter 12) or a cartilaginous neoplasm.

The majority of neoplasms of hyaline cartilage in the larynx are smooth protrusions of the cricoid lamina projecting from the posterior subglottic wall into the lumen. On opening the larynx, the tumour is seen to be arising from the central portion of the cartilage, usually on one side but sometimes involving both sides of the cricoid lamina. The lesion has a faint bluish or grey hyaline appearance with a gently lobulated surface (Figure 13.30). Thyroid and arytenoid cartilage neoplasms present focal bulges from these cartilages with similar cut-surface appearances. The cells may be grouped in small clusters like normal cartilage but are always surrounded by large amounts of metachromatic hyaline ground substance containing fine collagen fibres. In a chondroma, there is a resemblance of all cartilage cells to normal cells. In chondrosarcoma, the differences from normal may be quite subtle. These differences were summarized by Lichenstein and Jaffe[15] and their severity provides an indication of the propensity for aggressive growth of laryngeal cartilage neoplasms. These criteria are as follows:

1. There are too many cells;
2. The cells and nuclei are too irregular, i.e. pleomorphism is present;
3. Nuclei stain too darkly;
4. Large or giant cells with single, double or multiple nuclei are present.

Huizenga and Balogh[13] found that more malignant tumours had numbers of 'plump' nuclei in many of the high-power fields, and increase of nuclear size seemed important as a criterion of malignancy up to a maximum nuclear size in the malignant lesions of 18–26 μm compared with the benign lesions which showed maximum nuclear diameters of only 10–12 μm. Another feature of early malignant change was an irregularity of cell clustering. Areas of calcification may be seen in this neoplasm

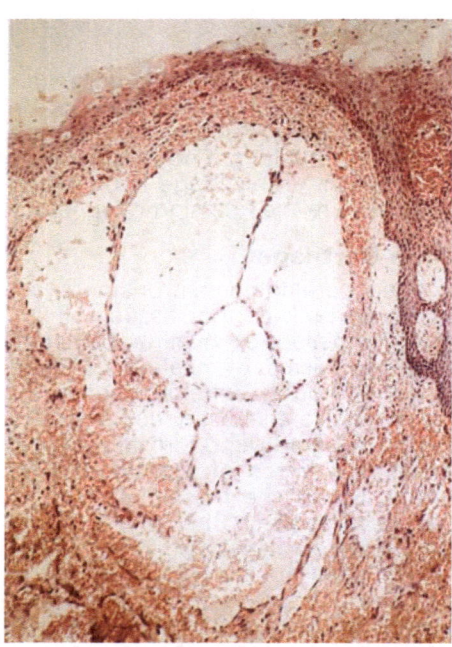

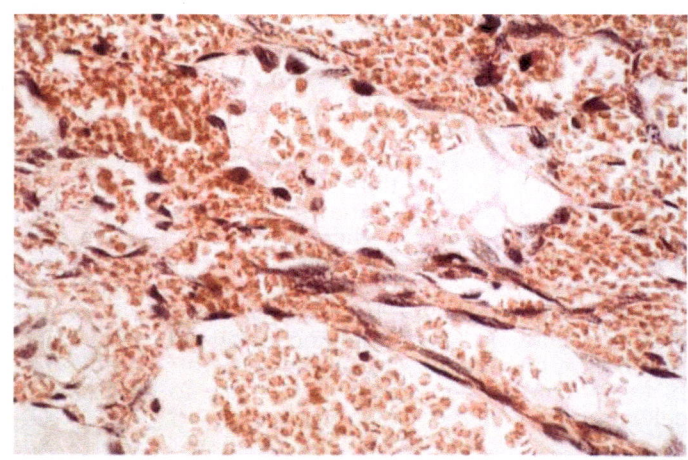

Figure 13.19 Angio-sarcoma of the larynx showing large irregular thin-walled blood vessels beneath squamous epithelium of larynx.   H & E (A)

Figure 13.20   Higher power of tumour shown in Figure 13.19 showing highly atypical endothelial cells lining the vessels.   H & E (C)

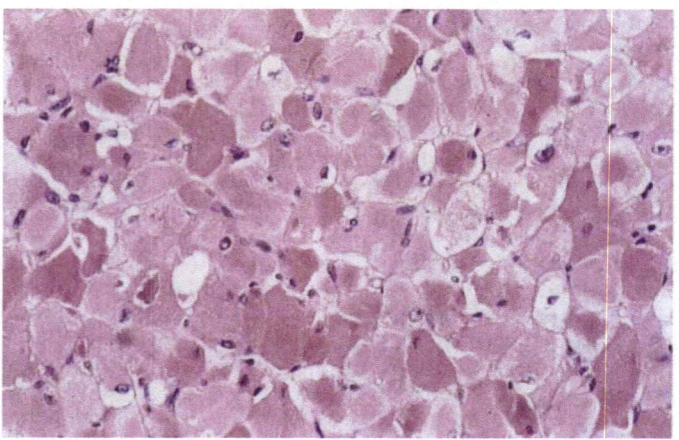

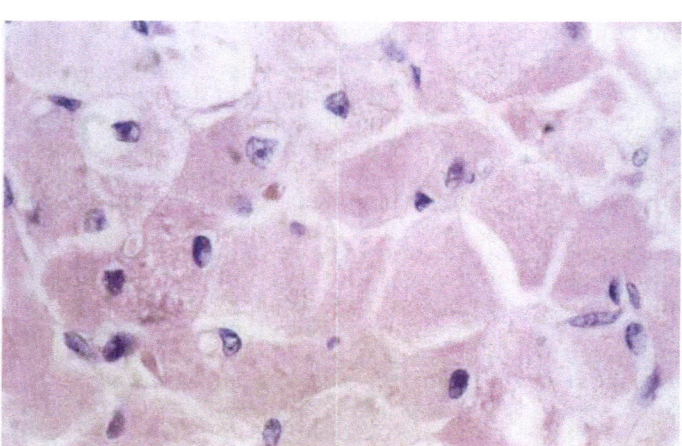

Figure 13.21   Adult rhabdomyoma of larynx showing cells with abundant acidophil cytoplasm. There are occasional 'spider cells', with thin cytoplasmic strands around the periphery.   H & E (B)

Figure 13.22   Adult rhabdomyoma of larynx at higher power. The cells do not contain cross-striations which are usually difficult to find in this tumour.   H & E (C)

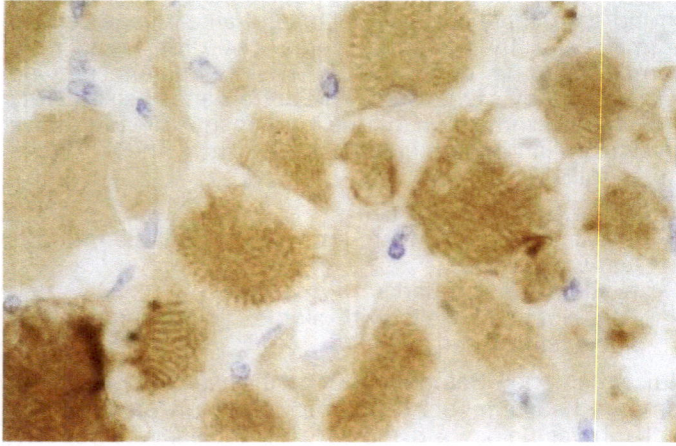

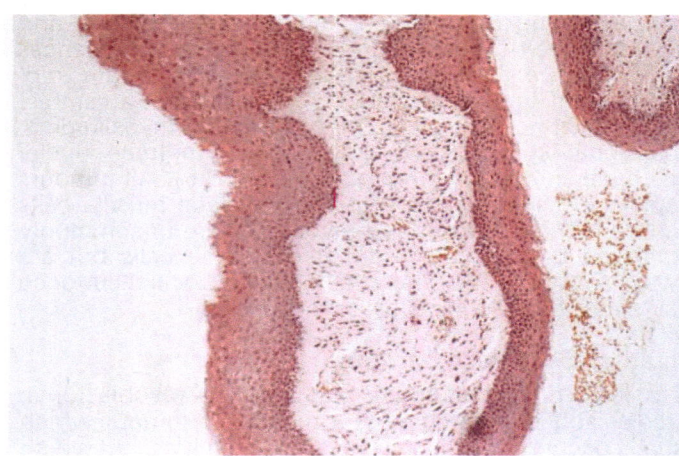

Figure 13.23   Immunochemical staining for desmin in the rhabdomyoma reveals numerous cross-striations.   (C)

Figure 13.24   Fetal rhabdomyoma of myxoid variety presenting as a polyp of the vocal cord. Note myxoid appearance of cells in lamina propria.   H & E (B)

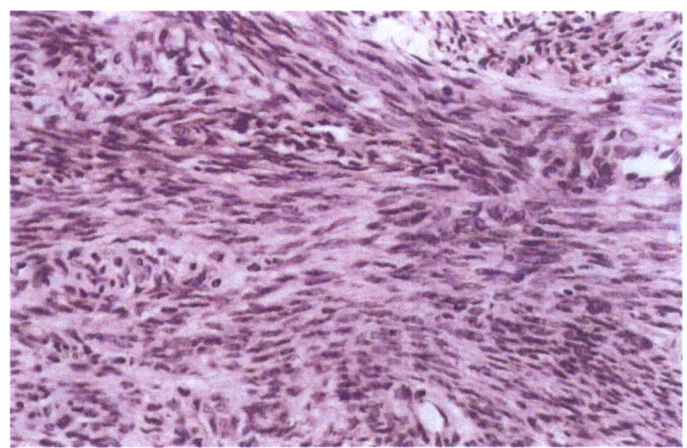

Figure 13.25 Tumour with appearances suggestive of the cellular type of fetal rhabdomyoma. This tumour was found in the nasopharynx. Note abundant closely packed undifferentiated spindle cells.　H & E (B)

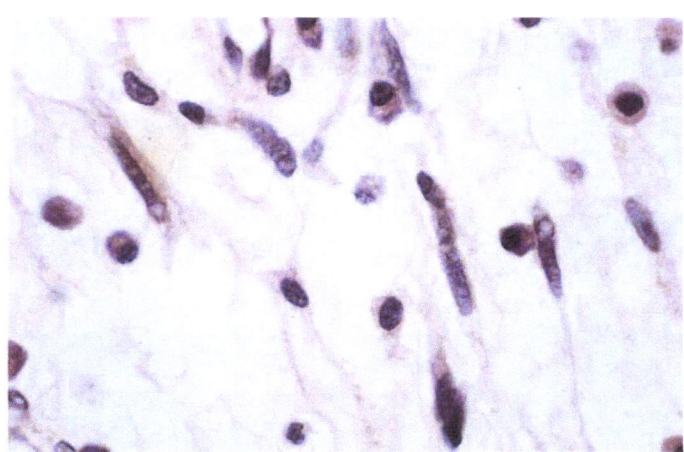

Figure 13.26 End-to-end arrangement of nuclei in tandem in fetal rhabdomyoma.　H & E (C)

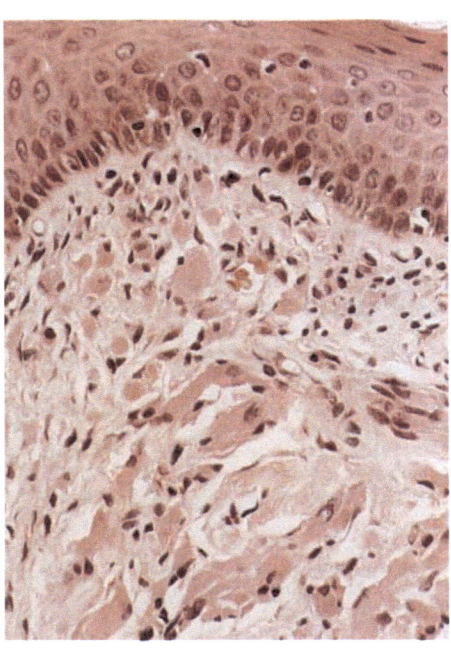

Figure 13.27 Fetal rhabdomyoma of larynx showing an area of differentiated striated muscle cells. H & E (B)

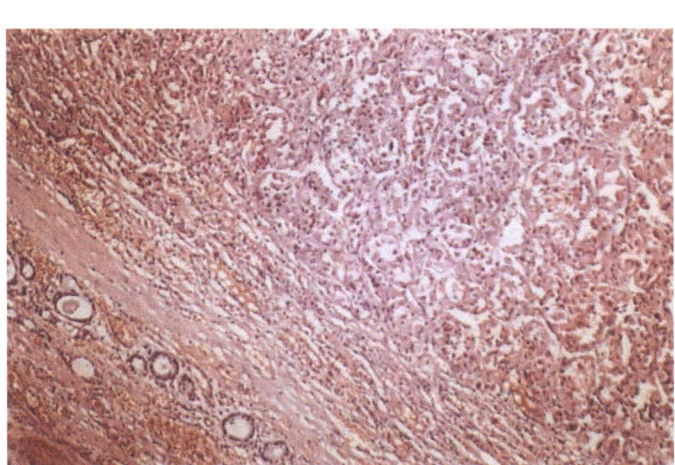

Figure 13.28 Alveolar soft part sarcoma of larynx showing round clumps of eosinophilic cells near laryngeal glands.　H & E (B)

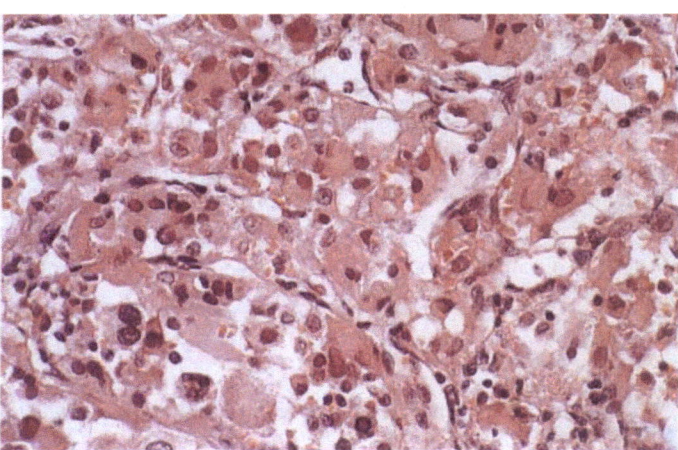

Figure 13.29 Alveolar soft part sarcoma showing large, eosinophilic polyhedral cells with finely granular cytoplasm.　H & E (C)

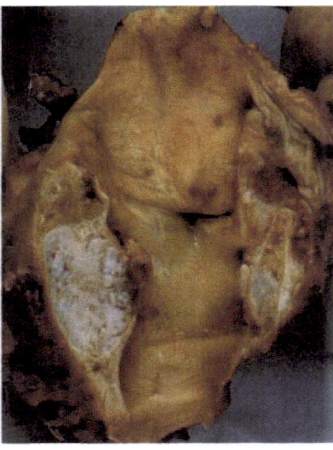

Figure 13.30 Chondrosarcoma of cricoid lamina. Larynx opened through the cricoid lamina which is expanded by a pale-grey tumour of hyaline appearance

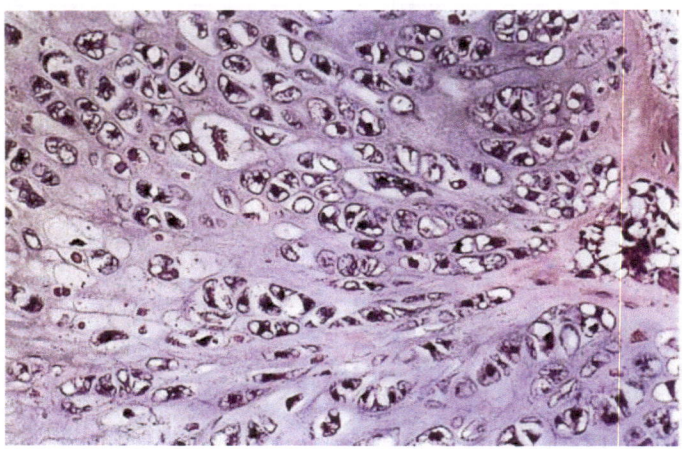

Figure 13.31 Chondrosarcoma of cricoid cartilage. The tumour cells are larger, more darkly staining, more numerous and more variable in size than normal cartilage cells.   H & E (B)

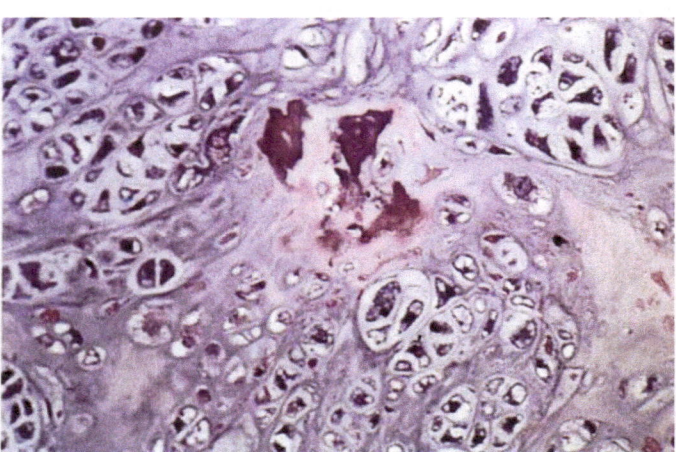

Figure 13.32 Chondrosarcoma of cricoid cartilage. There is calcification among the tumour cells.   H & E (B)

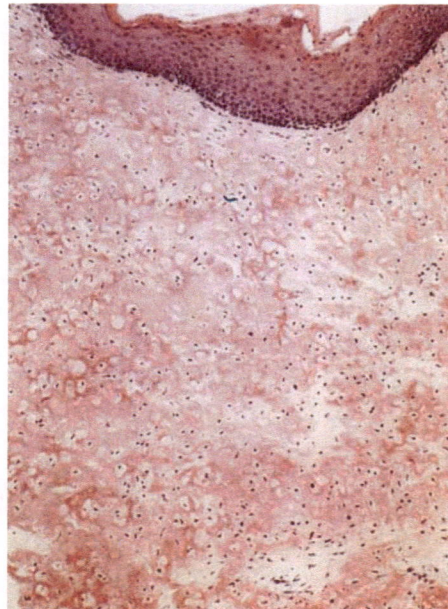

Figure 13.33 Elastic cartilage metaplasia in connective tissue of false cord which normally consists of glands, connective and adipose tissue.   H & E (B)

as in chondrosarcomas at other sites (Figures 13.31 and 13.32).

Elastic Cartilage Metaplasia

Nodules of elastic cartilage are quite commonly found in the false cord or true cord. In the true cord, their presence rarely causes a clinical problem. In the false cord, such nodules may produce symptoms and may be detected radiologically or observed as smooth bulges protruding into the laryngeal lumen at direct laryngoscopy. Histologically, these lesions are seen as adult elastic cartilage (Figure 13.33). Fibroblasts at the periphery of the lesions show a transition to chondrocytes in the main part of the lesion[16].

References

1. Fechner, R. E. (1975). Adenocarcinoma of the larynx. *Can. J. Otolaryngol.*, **4**, 284–289
2. Ash, J. E., Beck, M. R. and Wilkes, J. D. (1964). *Tumours of the Upper Respiratory Tract and Ear. Atlas of Tumor Pathology.* (Washington DC: Armed Forces Institute of Pathology, section 4, fascicles 12 and 13)
3. Woodruff, J. M., Huvos, A. G., Erlandson, R. A., Shah, J. P. and Gerold, F. P. (1985). Neuroendocrine carcinomas of the larynx. A study of two types, one of which mimics thyroid medullary carcinoma. *Am. J. Surg. Pathol.*, **9**, 771–790
4. Wenig, B. M. and Heffner, D. K. (1988). Moderately differentiated neuroendocrine carcinoma of the larynx. A clinicopathologic study of 54 cases. *Cancer*, **62**, 2658–2676
5. Bridger, G. P., Nassar, V. H. and Skinner, H. G. (1970). Haemangioma in the adult larynx. *Arch. Otolaryngol.*, **92**, 493–498
6. Ferguson, C. F. and Flake, C. G. (1961). Subglottic haemangioma as a cause of respiratory obstruction in infants. *Trans. Am. Bronchoesoph. Assoc.*, **41**, 27–47
7. Pratt, L. W. and Goodof, I. I. (1968). Hemangioendotheliosarcoma of the larynx. *Arch. Otolaryngol.*, **87**, 484–489
8. Batsakis, J. G. and Fox, J. E. (1970). Supporting tissue neoplasms of the larynx. *Surg. Gynecol. Obstet.*, **131**, 989–997
9. Ferlito, A. and Frugoni, P. (1975). Rhabdomyoma purum of the larynx. *J. Laryngol. Otol.*, **89**, 1131–1141
10. Di Sant'Agnese, P. A. and Knowles, D. M. (1980). Extracardiac rhabdomyoma: a clinicopathologic study and review of the literature. *Cancer*, **46**, 780–789
11. Helliwell, T. R., Sissons, M. C. J., Stoney, P. J. and Ashworth, M. T. (1988). Immunochemistry and electron microscopy of head and neck rhabdomyoma. *J. Clin. Pathol.*, **41**, 1058–1063
12. Hajdu, S. I. (1979). *Pathology of Soft Tissue Tumors.* (Philadelphia: Lea and Febiger)
13. Huizenga, C. and Balogh, K. (1970). Cartilaginous tumors of the larynx. A clinicopathologic study of 10 new cases and a review of the literature. *Cancer*, **26**, 201–210
14. Hyams, V. J. and Rabuzzi, D. D. (1970). Cartilaginous tumours of the larynx. *Laryngoscope*, **80**, 755–767
15. Lichenstein, L. and Jaffe, H. L. (1943). Chondrosarcoma of bone. *Am. J. Pathol.*, **19**, 553–589
16. Hill, B. J., Taylor, C. L. and Scott, G. B. D. (1980). Chondromatous metaplasia in the human larynx. *Histopathology*, **4**, 205–212

Index

Italic references are to figures